Basic Pathology

Fourth edition

Basic Pathology

An introduction to the mechanisms of disease

Sunil R Lakhani BSc MBBS MD FRCPath FRCPA
Professor and Head, Molecular and Cellular Pathology,
School of Medicine, University of Queensland,
Mayne Medical School, Brisbane,
Australia

Susan A Dilly BSc MBBS FRCPath
Professor and Institute Director,
Institute of Health Sciences Education,
Barts and The London,
Queen Mary's School of Medicine and Dentistry,
London, UK

Caroline J Finlayson MBBS FRCPath
Honorary Senior Lecturer and Consultant in Histopathology,
St George's Hospital Medical School,
London, UK

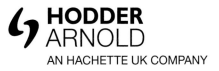

**HODDER
ARNOLD**
AN HACHETTE UK COMPANY

First published in Great Britain in 1993
Second edition 1998
Third edition 2003
This fourth edition published in 2009 by
Hodder Arnold, an imprint of Hodder Education, an Hachette UK Company,
338 Euston Road, London NW1 3BH

http://www.hoddereducation.com

British Library Cataloguing in Publication Data
A catalogue record for this book is available from the British Library

Library of Congress Cataloging-in-Publication Data
A catalog record for this book is available from the Library of Congress

ISBN   978 0 340 95003 6

2 3 4 5 6 7 8 9 10

Commissioning Editor: Sara Purdy
Production Editor: Jane Tod
Production Controller: Karen Dyer
Cover Designer: Helen Townson
Indexer: John Sampson

Typeset in 10.5 Perpetua by Macmillan Publishing Solutions
Printed and bound in Italy

What do you think about this book? Or any other Hodder Arnold title?
Please visit our website: www.hoddereducation.com

Preface   vii
Acknowledgements   ix

PART 1   Introduction: what is a disease?   1

Prologue: What is a disease?   3

              Chapter 1:   Causes and mechanisms – general principles   7
              Chapter 2:   What causes disease?   29

PART 2   Defence against disease   75

              Introduction: The role of epidemiology in disease   77
              Chapter 3:   The body's response to infection   79
              Chapter 4:   The acute inflammatory response   89
              Chapter 5:   Chronic and granulomatous inflammation,
                            healing and repair   115
              Chapter 6:   The immune defence against infection   139

PART 3   Circulatory disorders   163

              Introduction: Features of circulatory disorders   165
              Chapter 7:   Vascular occlusion and thrombosis   169
              Chapter 8:   Atherosclerosis and hypertension   189
              Chapter 9:   Circulatory failure   211

PART 4   Cell growth and its disorders   239

              Introduction: A brief history of cancer   241
              Chapter 10:   Benign grown disorders   243
              Chapter 11:   Malignant neoplasms   251
              Chapter 12:   What causes cancer?   263
              Chapter 13:   Molecular genetics of cancer   273
              Chapter 14:   The behaviour of tumours   291
              Chapter 15:   The clinical effects of tumours   297

Epilogue   307
Index   309

What is the use of a book', thought Alice, 'without pictures or conversations'.

Lewis Carroll

Any artist will tell you that in drawing objects, you cannot ignore the spaces in between. The picture ceases to exist when only one aspect is viewed in isolation. Musical pieces composed entirely of notes and without pauses would be nothing more than a noise and an irritation. Yet when it comes to teaching, we may ignore this fact and fail to put our own specialty into the context of the whole curriculum.

Over the last decade, there has been a trend towards a more integrated approach to medical education. We are delighted that such an approach, which we have always used in our teaching, is now widely adopted in the UK and abroad.

Our aim in this book has been to create a tutorial on the mechanisms of disease over a background of history, science and clinical relevance. The goal is to give the student a sense of belonging to a movement, the movement from past to present and from laboratory to patient.

This book has been written in the hope that the student will read the text fully and at leisure. This not only contains detail about the disease processes but also historical anecdotes and clinical scenarios. The cartoons are intended to amuse as well as illustrate the importance of certain topics, and we sincerely hope that students reading the book will be able to shed the dull, dreary image of histopathology that they all seem to be born with. Pathology is one of the most fascinating and fun subjects students are likely to encounter during their undergraduate training. If you understand the basic principles then the interpretation of clinical symptoms and signs, the rationale behind investigation and treatment and the unravelling of complex cases becomes more logical. Time spent building a framework of mechanisms will assist your clinical practice.

To help you with this, we have produced a companion volume called *Pathology in Clinical Practice: 50 Case Studies*. These are designed to help you to use your pathology knowledge in clinical settings by taking a clinical presentation, such as you might come across on the wards or in a case-based learning tutorial, and to pose you a number of questions, then guide you with the answers. This is divided into sections based on symptoms, signs, investigation, patient management and complex cases. It helps you to add clinical information on to the basic science and to recognize some of the processes of clinical reasoning that you must master. We hope that you will also find it stimulating and fun.

This pair of books is primarily intended for undergraduate medical students, but should also be useful to students of dentistry, human biology and other health professions. Postgraduate students studying for pathology or surgical exams may also wish to consult these books.

To access the image library on the website
www.hodderplus.co.uk/basicpathology
please register using the serial number **student09**.
Once you have registered you will not need the serial number but can log in using the username and password you will create during registration.

ACKNOWLEDGEMENTS

When we set out 15 years ago to write a textbook in which we would take the students on a journey, from past to present and from patient to the cell and back again, the phrase 'integrated curriculum' was not in common usage. Today, most medical schools have switched to the new style curriculum in which pathology is supposedly taught as an integrated subject with other disciplines. We have always believed that pathology should be taught in the context of the clinical situation and hope that this has been reflected by the content of this and the previous editions. It is a shame, however, that in many schools, pathology rather than being integrated with clinical work has been dis-integrated and lost as it is not deemed as important as clinical training for the new generation of doctors, nurses and disciplines allied to medicine.

Pathology is the study of the mechanism of disease. It has therefore been, and hopefully will remain, at the heart of anybody's desire to understand and manage disease. It is the core discipline of medical education and the very fabric that underpins clinical medical practice. That is not intended to imply that the non-biomedical aspects—ethics, communication, developing empathy and understanding—are not important. These aspects have to be taught side by side, not instead of, the mechanisms of disease.

Our endeavours to produce this fourth edition have been considerably aided by help, comments and constructive criticism from a number of people and we would like to acknowledge their time and effort. They include Professor Philip Butcher, Professor Mike Davies and Dr Grant Robinson at St George's Hospital who helped us with the second edition and whose efforts are still included in the current work. Dr Ahmet Dogan, one of our co-authors from the third edition, had to withdraw due to other work commitments but has kindly agreed to let us use his previous contributions. We are grateful for his generosity and continued support. We would like to acknowledge the work that Drs Pria Pakkiri, Leonard Da Silva and Professor Frederique Penault-Llorca have put in to read and review the changes and the images kindly provided by Dr Mitesh Gandhi.

Finally and most importantly, we would like to thank our families for their encouragement and support. But for their understanding, it would be difficult to get away with the disproportionate amount of time that such projects consume.

SRL
SAD
CJF
2009

PART I

INTRODUCTION: WHAT IS A DISEASE?

Prologue: What is a disease? 3

Chapter 1: Causes and mechanisms –
general principles 7

What are the most common
mechanisms? 7
Clinical case: myocardial
infarction 8
Biochemical changes in the
cells 9
Clinical relevance of cell
changes 12
Sub-lethal cell injury 13
Necrosis 15
Apoptosis and autophagy 19
Treating diseases by interfering
with cell death 24
Ageing 27

Chapter 2: What causes disease? 29

Clinical case: frostbite 31
Biological agents as causes of
diseases 33
Hypersensitivity and autoimmune
disease 44
Nutritional diseases 49
Coeliac disease: genetic
predisposition and hypersensitivity 50
Genetic causes of disease 51
Clinical case: Turner's syndrome 57
What are the commonest
genetic diseases? 57
How can genetic disorders be
diagnosed? 63
Methods of genetic analysis 65
Who should have their genes
examined? 69

Medicine, to produce health, has to examine disease.

Plutarch (c.46–120)
Greek biographer and essayist

You have just opened a book entitled *Basic Pathology – An introduction to the principles and mechanisms of disease*. Is it fair to face you with an enormous challenge in the opening paragraph by asking, 'What is a disease'? Although you might expect the authors to offer you a definition, we would prefer you to think it through with friends and colleagues because there is no simple answer.

This book will adopt a strongly biomedical concept of disease. This is a mechanistic model that regards the body as a machine with repairable or replaceable parts. It looks for specific underlying biological causes and places a high emphasis on the scientific evidence-base for untangling cause and effect in both the disease and its treatment, because this is important for patient care and prognosis. However, it is important that you appreciate that defining diseases is fraught with problems. Disease definitions change with time and across cultures and social classes. Naming a condition can create a spurious impression of understanding and inhibit further patient investigation or research. Measuring biochemical changes in the blood can provide an early warning of the onset of disease but does a person have the disease before the symptoms appear? Do you, in fact, need to suffer from a disease as part of the definition? If you do not, then where do you draw the line for deciding who has a disease when the 'marker' follows a normal pattern of distribution within the population? For example, is hypertension a disease defined by a particular level of blood pressure? Alternatively, should we talk of cardiovascular disease and define that through the symptoms of strokes and heart attacks. Then the 'marker' of raised blood pressure is but one consideration in a complex multi-factorial process. In psychiatric practice, doctors have no problems is dissecting the symptoms from the 'disease' or 'illness'. A person presenting with a phobia today almost certainly started their mental 'illness/disease' many years previously.

Although it is sometimes said that 'health' should not be defined as merely the absence of disease, as pathologists, we might argue that disease is best defined as a reduction in health; then it embraces almost everything. This also reflects the origin of the word 'disease' which is from the French: des = from, aise = ease.

With all those caveats, we shall offer a biomedical definition of disease. 'Disease is a consequence of a failure of homeostasis', where homeostasis is the concept of equilibrium within the body despite changes in the internal or external environment. If you accept this definition then understanding the mechanisms of disease will involve understanding the processes for maintaining homeostasis, identifying the agents and events that disrupt homeostasis, trying to determine why homeostatic mechanisms fail and whether any intervention can prevent or correct this sequence that results in a disease. Rather arbitrarily, we shall decide that a disease should have the potential to produce some impairment of function, but may be detected and defined whilst asymptomatic. It may also be treated or heal through the body's normal processes so that no permanent damage is produced.

Diseases have causes (aetiology) and mechanisms (pathogenesis). They may result in symptoms (experienced by the patient) and signs (elicited by the physician). There may be structural changes that are visible to the naked eye (gross or macroscopical appearances), or only detectable down a microscope (microscopical appearances). Functional changes may be detectable by an ever increasing range of clinical and laboratory techniques. All of this is pathology, and pathology is the study (logos) of suffering (pathos).

Although we are adopting a mechanistic model, it is a complex model with multiple parts that interconnect (Fig. 2). A change in one area is likely to affect another. Thus maintaining homeostasis is not a simple single feedback loop and it is perfectly acceptable that a new equilibrium is achieved under a new set of circumstances, a new baseline; you do not have to return to the original state. Let us take the example of lobar pneumonia (see chapter 4) and introduce a diagram that helps to illustrate the various components of the disease process (Fig. 3).

In its simplest form, an intrinsic or external factor (the cause) acts on a cell, tissue, organ or whole person

Figure 1 Defining disease is not as easy as it sounds. This diagram will help with the terminology

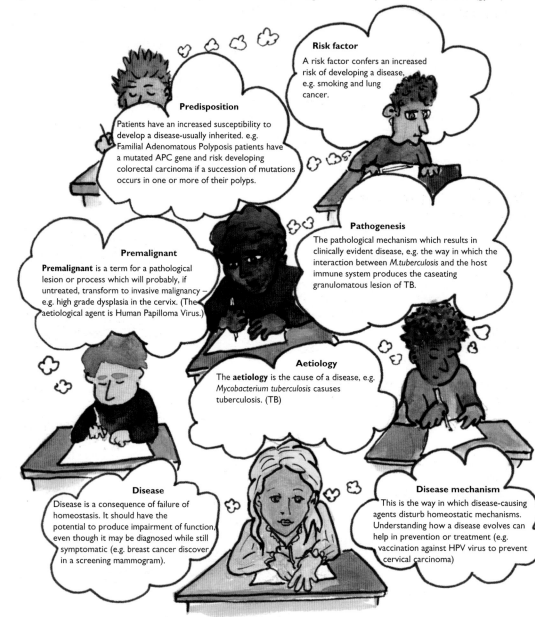

Risk factor

A risk factor confers an increased risk of developing a disease, e.g. smoking and lung cancer.

Predisposition

Patients have an increased susceptibility to develop a disease-usually inherited. e.g. Familial Adenomatous Polyposis patients have a mutated APC gene and risk developing colorectal carcinoma if a succession of mutations occurs in one or more of their polyps.

Pathogenesis

The pathological mechanism which results in clinically evident disease, e.g. the way in which the interaction between *M.tuberculosis* and the host immune system produces the caseating granulomatous lesion of TB.

Premalignant

Premalignant is a term for a pathological lesion or process which will probably, if untreated, transform to invasive malignancy – e.g. high grade dysplasia in the cervix. (The aetiological agent is Human Papilloma Virus.)

Aetiology

The **aetiology** is the cause of a disease, e.g. *Mycobacterium tuberculosis* casuses tuberculosis. (TB)

Disease

Disease is a consequence of failure of homeostasis. It should have the potential to produce impairment of function, even though it may be diagnosed while still symptomatic (e.g. breast cancer discover in a screening mammogram).

Disease mechanism

This is the way in which disease-causing agents disturb homeostatic mechanisms. Understanding how a disease evolves can help in prevention or treatment (e.g. vaccination against HPV virus to prevent cervical carcinoma)

to produce structural or functional changes and a response. If an adaptive response is 100% successful, then homeostasis is maintained and no symptoms or signs result. If unsuccessful, then the disease manifests and the structural and functional changes may have an impact on another cell, tissue or organ to produce another set of reactions. Thus in lobar pneumonia, the extrinsic cause is the bacterium, *Streptococcus pneumoniae*, which affects the lung. This stimulates an acute inflammatory response that can produce the structural changes of consolidation and functional changes of reduced gas transfer in alveoli.

Figure 2 Aspects of the disease process

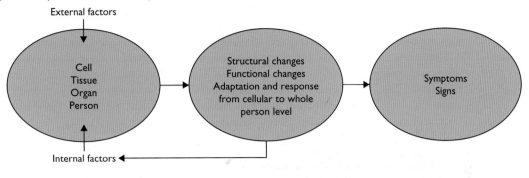

External factors

Cell
Tissue
Organ
Person

Internal factors

Structural changes
Functional changes
Adaptation and response
from cellular to whole
person level

Symptoms
Signs

Figure 3 Lobar pneumonia: primary mechanism

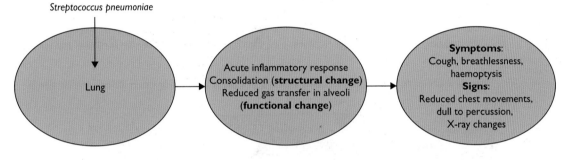

Streptococcus pneumoniae

Lung

Acute inflammatory response
Consolidation (**structural change**)
Reduced gas transfer in alveoli
(**functional change**)

Symptoms:
Cough, breathlessness,
haemoptysis
Signs:
Reduced chest movements,
dull to percussion,
X-ray changes

Figure 4 Lobar pneumonia: additional secondary mechanism

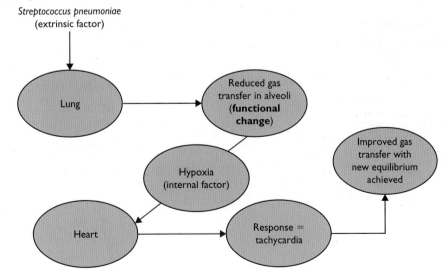

Streptococcus pneumoniae
(extrinsic factor)

Lung

Reduced gas
transfer in alveoli
(**functional
change**)

Hypoxia
(internal factor)

Improved gas
transfer with
new equilibrium
achieved

Heart

Response =
tachycardia

Dictionary

Consolidation: The process by which the
tissue becomes solid; process of
solidification

The patient suffers from cough, breathlessness and,
even, haemoptysis (coughing up blood). The physician
may detect the signs of reduced chest movements, an area
that is dull to percussion and X-ray opacity reflecting lung
solidification. However, that is not the end of the story.

We can produce another 'disease sequence' where the reduced gas transfer results in hypoxia (reduced oxygen saturation in the blood), which acts as an internal factor that leads to the heart responding with an increased heart rate (tachycardia). More blood is pumped through the part of the lung which is not consolidated, so increasing gas transfer, and this may successfully compensate so that the hypoxia is corrected, i.e. a new equilibrium is achieved (Fig. 4). But before you relax, look at page 109 where we explain about pyrogens that may accompany the inflammatory response to bacteria and the effect that they may have on the heart. Yes, that is another route for producing a tachycardia and so our diagram could become almost infinitely complex as we add the different pathways. This complexity is not unique to pathology or the human body but is true of almost everything as our knowledge and understanding increases. In order to avoid being confused, you need to appreciate and accept the 'interconnectedness'. It is important not to divide the phenomenon into different pieces, as in a jigsaw, but to think of them as interlacing connections. In any one situation, it is the unique combination of these connections that produces the final picture. The idea that it is connections rather than individual objects that are important is well recognized in atomic physics. As Heisenberg (of Heisenberg's uncertainty principle) said:

> (In modern physics), one has now divided the world not into different groups of objects but into different groups of connections. What can be distinguished is the kind of connection which is primarily important in a certain phenomenon... The world thus appears as a complicated tissue of events, in which connections of different kinds alternate or overlap or combine and thereby determine the texture of the whole.

Figure 5 The disease process can be viewed as being made up of many interlacing connections, rather like a road map

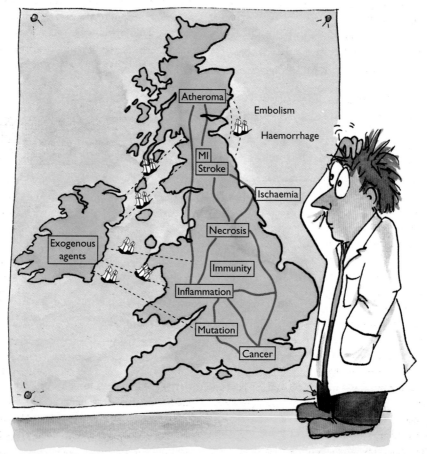

CHAPTER 1

CAUSES AND MECHANISMS – GENERAL PRINCIPLES

Those who are enamoured of practice without science are like a pilot who goes into a ship without rudder or compass and never has any certainty where he is going. Practice should always be based upon a sound knowledge of theory.

Leonardo da Vinci (1452–1519); Italian artist, sculptor, architect and engineer

Almost anything can cause 'disease' if the conditions are right. For example, water is essential for life but if taken in extreme excess or given intravenously, particularly in a patient with kidney failure, it can cause problems. In this situation, the body is unable to respond adequately so homeostasis is not maintained and a 'disease state' occurs. What may be harmless to one person may cause disease in another. A sudden drop in oxygen during a flight may not affect most of the passengers but could be potentially serious to a person with sickle cell disease (page 69). Thus there is interplay between the potential causes of disease and the potential victim. Factors that predispose an individual to disease may occur at many levels. They may be genetic and inherited from parents, such as a predisposition to cancer or Huntington's chorea (a neurological disorder), congenital, i.e. present from birth but not necessarily genetic and could be acquired during fetal life because of conditions in the uterus, or may be acquired during life. Such factors often combine with others to produce disease.

Life is fairly simple when a single cause produces a clearly defined and easily recognized disease, especially if that disease is uncommon (e.g. abnormal short limbs due to the drug thalidomide). It is much more difficult to disentangle 'cause and effect' from 'associated with' for most health problems and it is important to appreciate how new causes of disease may be identified. Often the starting point is information gathered by epidemiologists. On page 77, we describe how John Snow postulated that cholera was spread by water before bacteria had been identified. He tested his hypothesis by mapping the positions of the cholera cases and the water pumps. Thus, he established an association and some ideas about a mechanism. From this first clue that a disease state and a potential causative agent are 'associated', it is important to try to establish a mechanism whereby an agent could produce the necessary changes. The precise approach will depend on the agent and the disease but this is a crucial step, not only for establishing causation but also for identifying possible methods of treatment. This is why a basic understanding of the principles of the mechanisms of disease (i.e. the subject of this book) is so important. Learning details of specific diseases and treatments can follow or be looked up when required, but understanding the mechanisms will allow you to identify new diseases or develop new treatments. Think big – someone has to win the Nobel prizes!

WHAT ARE THE MOST COMMON MECHANISMS?

We are viewing diseases from a biomedical standpoint that regards the body as a machine and disease as some impairment of function. That impairment of function or homeostasis can affect the whole person, a particular tissue or a cell and this will influence the symptoms. The common building blocks for most parts of the body are cells and these have a common genetic code and a broadly similar set of metabolic pathways, though each will express different pathways dependent on its specialized function. Almost always, something goes wrong at a cellular level leading to dysfunction within the tissue or organ. The ramifications may be quite complex and impact on many other areas of the body.

Thus we will work through the common mechanisms by considering the cell as the key building block. Let us take the most extreme example first of complete failure of cell function, either due to cell damage or cell death: what are the biochemical changes that occur in an injured cell and what distinguishes reversible from irreversible damage? Rather than discuss this exclusively as a cellular problem, let us consider its clinical importance by using the example of heart muscle cells suddenly being deprived of oxygen and nutrients (also known as ischaemia) because a coronary artery is blocked with thrombus, i.e. a heart attack.

CLINICAL CASE: MYOCARDIAL INFARCTION

A 60-year-old man complained of sudden onset of chest pain which had started 2 hours previously. It radiated down his left arm. He was found to be in shock with a blood pressure of 90/50 mmHg and his electrocardiogram (ECG) showed evidence of an anterior myocardial infarction. He also had bilateral pulmonary oedema. The serum cardiac markers were elevated, including the creatinine kinase MB isoenzyme. Before he could be transferred to the coronary care unit, he developed ventricular fibrillation and, despite resuscitation attempts, died.

The following day, an autopsy was carried out and part of the report is illustrated below.

Let us use this example to consider the changes that take place in myocardial cells following an ischaemic insult. We know that the final outcome is dependent on a number of variables. These include the severity and duration of the ischaemia and the volume of heart muscle affected. It will also be influenced by any collateral circulation and the metabolic demands of the myocardial cells at the time of the insult. Hence, the extent of cell damage and death and whether the injury is reversible or irreversible depends on a number of factors and may be altered by medical intervention. The changes in the heart following ischaemia also vary with time.

MACROSCOPIC APPEARANCE

Although biochemical changes may take place very quickly, the gross appearance of the myocardium is generally entirely normal for the first 6 to 12 hours. The NBTZ test can be used to highlight the area of infarction in this early period (page 216) and this is what was done in the patient described above. After about 18 hours, the myocardium generally appears slightly pale but may look red–blue due to the entrapped red blood cells within the area of infarction. Each day that follows makes the area of infarction a little more defined, paler and softer. By the end of the first week, there is usually a rim of hyperaemia surrounding the pale yellow–brown area of infarction. This is due to the ingrowth of richly vascularized connective tissue that will be involved in the healing and repair process. As time goes by, the dead myocardial cell debris is removed and a pale firm fibrous scar laid down; a process which is complete by 6 weeks.

Autopsy report

Name: I B EDE
Age: 60 years
Date of admission: 24.7.08
Date of death: 24.7.08
Date of autopsy: 25.7.08

External findings
The body was that of a Caucasian male. A central venous line in the right jugular vein and peripheral cannula in the left arm were present. There was bruising on the chest related to the resuscitation. No other abnormalities seen.

Internal examination
Cardiovascular system
There was marked atheroma within the aorta and large vessels. The left coronary artery and the left anterior descending (LAD) artery both showed atheroma with 90 per cent occlusion. In addition, there was an acute thrombus at the origin of the LAD. The right coronary artery showed 50 per cent occlusion. There was no macroscopic evidence of an infarction, however, staining with NBTZ confirmed a full thickness anterior infarct.

Respiratory system
Both lungs showed evidence of pulmonary oedema.

Renal system
The kidneys showed evidence of ischaemic scarring.

Central nervous system
There was marked atheroma in the carotids and cerebral vessels but no evidence of a cerebral infarction.

Cause of death
 1a: Myocardial infarction
due to 1b: Coronary artery thrombosis
due to 1c: Coronary artery atheroma

MICROSCOPIC APPEARANCE

As with the gross appearance, the changes seen by light microscopy lag behind the biochemical changes. The earliest change (4–12 hours) is mild oedema and separation of the muscle fibres. The cells adjacent to the area of infarction may also show small droplets within the cytoplasm and this phenomenon is called vacuolar degeneration. By 24 hours, neutrophil polymorphs infiltrate the area of necrosis and the necrotic myocytes undergo cytoplasmic and nuclear changes typical of necrosis. The cytoplasm appears more pink (eosinophilic) and the nuclei become pyknotic. Later the nuclei are lost and the cross-striations disappear. By day 3, the infiltrate of neutrophils is heavy and, by the end of the week, the cellular debris from dead cells is being removed by macrophages. The fibrovascular connective tissue, which gives the hyperaemia seen macroscopically, is also evident. Examination at later stages shows the varying amounts of fibrous scar tissue seen on gross inspection.

Figure 1.1 summarizes the main findings on gross and microscopic examination of the myocardium at different times following the ischaemic episode.

BIOCHEMICAL CHANGES IN THE CELLS

There are two important questions to consider:

- What are the biochemical changes that occur in an injured cell?
- What distinguishes reversible from irreversible injury?

There are four sites within the cell which are of paramount importance in cell damage and death. These are the:

- mitochondria
- plasma membrane
- ionic channels in cell membranes
- cytoskeleton.

The first effect of ischaemia is to reduce the production of adenosine triphosphate (ATP) by the mitochondrial oxidative phosphorylation system (Fig. 1.2). If the production of energy slows down or stops, then the cells cannot function; in the case of heart muscle, the cell cannot contract: it is as simple as that! Obviously, if the ischaemic cells cannot partake in aerobic metabolism, then they will switch over to anaerobic metabolism to derive energy from the stored glycogen. The enzyme creatinine kinase, which is present in the myocardial cells, is also utilized to produce energy from the anaerobic metabolism of creatinine phosphate. The net effect of these mechanisms is to deplete the cells of glycogen and to produce acidosis within the cells by the production of lactic acid and inorganic phosphates. This further inhibits the normal function of the myocardial cells. The acidosis within the cells is thought to be responsible for one of the observed histological hallmarks of cell damage – the clumping of the nuclear chromatin and pyknosis of the nuclei. Ischaemia also has profound effects on the plasma membranes and on the ionic channels situated within the membranes. You will recall that these are vital in maintaining the normal ionic gradients across the cell membranes, with sodium and calcium at low concentrations inside the cells and potassium lower in the extracellular space. These concentrations are maintained by pumps that are energy dependent; hence it is not difficult to see that the loss of oxidative phosphorylation and any direct damage to the membranes will disrupt the function of these pumps. So what is the effect?

First, the failure of the pumps will result in the leakage of sodium into the cells and potassium out of the cells. Sodium has a larger hydration shell than potassium so more water moves in association with sodium ions than exits with the potassium. Additional water enters because the acidosis and raised intracellular concentrations of high molecular weight phosphates will increase the osmotic pressure inside the cell. The result is acute swelling of the cell due to cellular oedema. The endoplasmic reticulum also swells, the ribosomes detach from the endoplasmic reticulum, the mitochondria become swollen and blebs begin to appear on the cell surface. This last phenomenon is intriguing as the changes in cell shape and surface blebbing implies alterations in the cytoskeleton of the cell. The changes in the microfilaments of the cytoskeleton are believed to be due to the increased concentration of calcium which also results from the failure of the membrane pumps. Calcium is a very important ion in cell death and we shall see why in a minute.

You might find it difficult to believe but all the changes described so far are reversible! If the oxygen supply is restored, the cells still have the capacity to return to the normal state and the ability of the myocardial cells to contract is restored. So what are the changes that finally tip the cell beyond the point of no return?

The morphological hallmarks are a severe disruption of the mitochondrial membranes with deposition of matrix lipoproteins, disruption of the plasma membranes and rupture of lysosomes with release of enzymes. Calcium is thought to play a central role in this final progression to irreversible cell death.

Figure 1.1 Myocardial infarction: changes with time

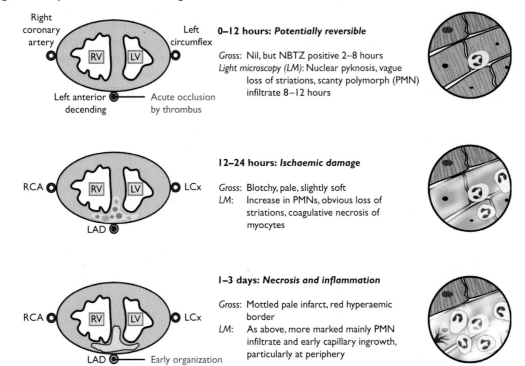

0–12 hours: *Potentially reversible*

Gross: Nil, but NBTZ positive 2–8 hours
Light microscopy (LM): Nuclear pyknosis, vague loss of striations, scanty polymorph (PMN) infiltrate 8–12 hours

12–24 hours: *Ischaemic damage*

Gross: Blotchy, pale, slightly soft
LM: Increase in PMNs, obvious loss of striations, coagulative necrosis of myocytes

1–3 days: *Necrosis and inflammation*

Gross: Mottled pale infarct, red hyperaemic border
LM: As above, more marked mainly PMN infiltrate and early capillary ingrowth, particularly at periphery

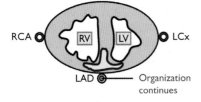
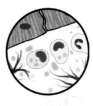

4–7 days: *Removal of debris, early organization*

Gross: Depressed, soft, yellow infarct, prominent hyperaemic edge
LM: As before, with increased macrophages phagocytosing debris from dead myocytes, peripheral granulation tissue formation

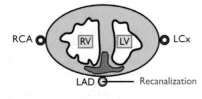
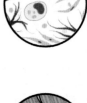

7–14 days: *Organization*

Gross: 'Bruised' look: red/purple colour, increasingly firm as granulation tissue forms
LM: Decreased inflammation as dead tissue is cleared, granulation tissue replaces damaged area

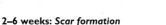

2–6 weeks: *Scar formation*

Gross: Infarct becomes firm and white and eventually contracts, the LV wall is thinned
LM: Capillaries and fibroblasts are replaced by acellular fibrous scar tissue

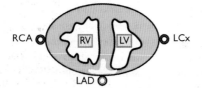

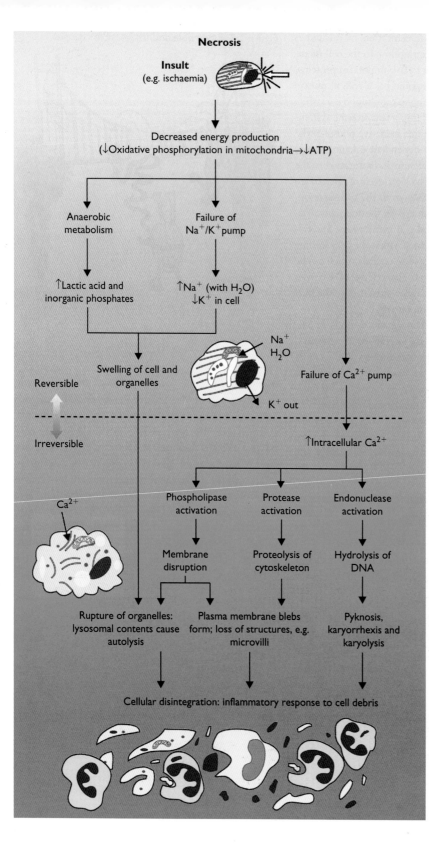

Necrosis

Insult
(e.g. ischaemia)

Decreased energy production
($\downarrow$Oxidative phosphorylation in mitochondria$\rightarrow\downarrow$ATP)

Anaerobic
metabolism

Failure of
Na^+/K^+ pump

$\uparrow$Lactic acid and
inorganic phosphates

$\uparrow Na^+$ (with H_2O)
$\downarrow K^+$ in cell

Swelling of cell and
organelles

Na^+
H_2O

K^+ out

Failure of Ca^{2+} pump

Reversible

- -

Irreversible

$\uparrow$Intracellular Ca^{2+}

Ca^{2+}

Phospholipase
activation

Protease
activation

Endonuclease
activation

Membrane
disruption

Proteolysis of
cytoskeleton

Hydrolysis of
DNA

Rupture of organelles:
lysosomal contents cause
autolysis

Plasma membrane blebs
form; loss of structures, e.g.
microvilli

Pyknosis,
karyorrhexis and
karyolysis

Cellular disintegration: inflammatory response to cell debris

Figure 1.2 Necrosis is the culmination of a series of events, the first phases of which are reversible. The failure of the calcium pump marks the onset of irreversible change. In necrosis, a response to extreme adversity such as ischaemia, the cell breaks down and its contents are exposed to the extracellular space, with leakage of lysosomal membranes and other cellular constituents. The cells appear swollen and degenerate under the microscope

In the normal cell, the concentration of calcium is tightly controlled by the calcium pump in the cell membrane. Inside the cell, it binds to two important proteins, troponin and calmodulin. Troponin has a role in muscle contraction and calcium binding to calmodulin is a switch to turn on phosphorylation of important enzyme systems inside the cell. Ischaemia disrupts oxidative phosphorylation, so affecting the energy dependent calcium pump, leading to a rapid influx of calcium and saturation of the calcium regulating proteins. The high levels of calcium are toxic to the cell leading to changes in the cytoskeleton, cell surface blebbing, and damage to the mitochondria, the lysosomal membranes and cell membranes. The calcium also binds to the phosphates within the cells leading to a precipitation of hydroxyapatite crystals which can be observed in the mitochondria. The release of enzymes from the ruptured lysosomes also contributes to the final destruction of the cellular components.

The biochemistry of cell damage and death is a complex process, with many systems interacting. In summary, ischaemia decreases the energy production by the oxidative phosphorylation system in mitochondria, which leads to loss of integrity of the plasma membrane, loss of function of the Na^+/K^+ and Ca^{2+} pumps and severe injury to the mitochondria, nucleus, cytoskeleton and lysosomes. Experimental evidence suggests that calcium has a pivotal role in pushing the cell into irreversible cell damage and death (Fig. 1.3).

CLINICAL RELEVANCE OF CELL CHANGES

So much for science. Do these biochemical and microscopical changes help us to understand any of the clinical

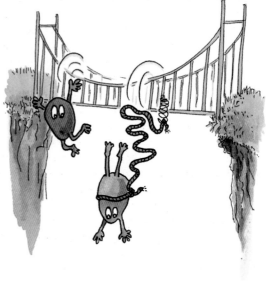

Figure 1.3 Reversible and irreversible changes

manifestations of our patient with myocardial infarction, chest pain and cardiac failure? We know that ischaemia leads to a decrease in mitochondrial function and, hence, a decrease in ATP formation so that the cells stop contracting. What is absolutely staggering is that an ischaemic episode lasting only 1 minute can produce this change!

The cellular damage may be reversible but the changes still profoundly affect the function of the organ. If the area of ischaemia is large, enough cells stop contracting to reduce the pumping power of the heart and cause cardiac failure. Any arrhythmia will exacerbate the cardiac failure. You will know that the rhythmic contraction of the heart is due to the passage of electrical impulses down

Key facts

Features of reversible and irreversible cell damage

Reversible	Irreversible
Cell swelling	Release of lysosomal enzymes
Mitochondrial swelling	Protein digestion
Endoplasmic reticulum swelling	Loss of basophilia
Detachment of ribosomes	Membrane disruption
'Myelin' figures	Leakage of cell enzymes and proteins
Loss of microvilli	Nuclear changes: pyknosis, karyorrhexis, karyolysis
Surface blebs	
Clumping of nuclear chromatin	
Lipid deposition (fatty change)	

the specialized conduction pathways and within the myocardium. Abnormal conduction can occur if there is damage to the sinoatrial or atrioventricular nodes, the conduction bundles or the myocardium. Conduction of electrical impulses requires an intact cell membrane and functioning ionic channels within the membrane. Ischaemia interferes with membrane and ionic channel function and produces abnormal conduction.

The right coronary artery supplies the A–V node in 85 per cent of people; hence, right coronary artery occlusion can produce complete heart block as well as inferior infarction. If the area of ischaemia involves the specialized bundles, the bundles may be selectively affected resulting in either a right bundle branch block or a left bundle branch block. Occlusion of the left anterior descending artery produces an anterior infarction which may be complicated by blockage of both conduction bundles. This is frequently fatal, not purely because of the conduction problem, but because it is associated with a large area of infarction. Finally, the myocardium itself may affect the passage of impulses. An infarcted area of myocardium may not only slow down or stop the passage of electrical current, but may also generate an arrhythmia.

An ECG is a standard investigation for these patients and will detect disorders of cardiac rhythm, and the approximate position and size of the infarction. The 12-lead ECG essentially produces a three-dimensional electrical picture of the heart. When part of the myocardium is damaged by ischaemia, the normal path of the electrical wave is impeded and the impulse has to travel via an alternative route. Consequently, the ECG pattern is altered and the type of change on the tracing helps to identify the area and the approximate size of the infarction.

Our patient had elevated levels of cardiac enzymes in the blood. Many enzymes are common to a variety of cells but other enzymes are associated with the cell's specialist functions and will be restricted to only a few cell types. The cardiac muscle cell contains creatinine kinase (CK), aspartate aminotransferase (AST) and lactate dehydrogenase (LDH). Ischaemic damage to the myocardial cells disrupts the cell membranes, allowing leakage of these enzymes. If it is suspected that a patient has suffered a myocardial infarction, then serial measurements of these 'cardiac enzymes' can be helpful to confirm the diagnosis and give a rough indication of the size of the damage. The same is true of other cell markers and, in recent years, troponins have largely replaced enzymes as markers of myocardial infarction.

You can see how knowledge of the cellular events helps us to understand the gross and histological appearances as well as the clinical measurements that are useful in diagnosis and management of the patient. Since mild reversible injury to cells is probably more common than irreversible injury we will examine the histological patterns of reversible sub-lethal injury before going on to look at types of necrosis.

SUB-LETHAL CELL INJURY

The changes of reversible, sub-lethal injury are often difficult to demonstrate in human tissues. There are two patterns that can be identified in tissues using light microscopy: cloudy swelling and fatty change.

CLOUDY SWELLING

This has already been mentioned when considering myocardial ischaemia. The insult affects membrane ion exchange mechanisms to alter the ionic gradients leading to increased intracellular sodium and water. This produces acute cellular oedema or 'cloudy swelling'. At the light-microscopy level, this appears as expansion of the cell and a pale granular look to the cytoplasm. Vesicles may also appear due to the distension of the endoplasmic reticulum. This picture of cellular oedema is also referred to as hydropic or vacuolar degeneration. Remember that a whole range of insults may precipitate cellular oedema and that it is not specific to ischaemia. Chemical toxins, infections and radiation can all induce similar changes. Remember also that cellular oedema is reversible.

FATTY CHANGE

This refers to an excess of intracellular lipid which appears as vacuoles of varying size within the cytoplasm. Like cellular oedema, it is entirely reversible and is a non-specific reaction to a variety of insults. Sometimes it is present adjacent to tissues that are more severely damaged or show frank evidence of necrosis. Fatty change can occur in any organ but is most frequent in the liver, which is not surprising since the liver is the major site of lipid metabolism. For this reason, we will use the liver as an example to discuss the pathogenesis of fatty change (Figs 1.5 and 1.6).

Figure 1.6 illustrates the main causes and effects of fatty change in the liver. Very simply, adipose tissue releases fat as free fatty acids which enter the hepatocytes, where they are converted to triglycerides and, to a

Figure 1.4 Normal and fatty liver (pale)

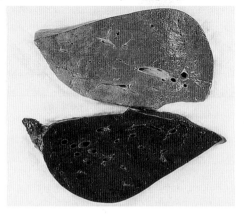

Figure 1.5 Photomicrograph of liver showing fatty change (vacuoles arrowed)

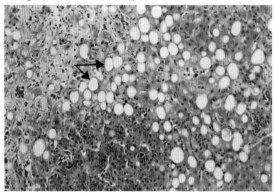

Figure 1.6 Fatty liver: main causes of fat accumulation and their deleterious effects

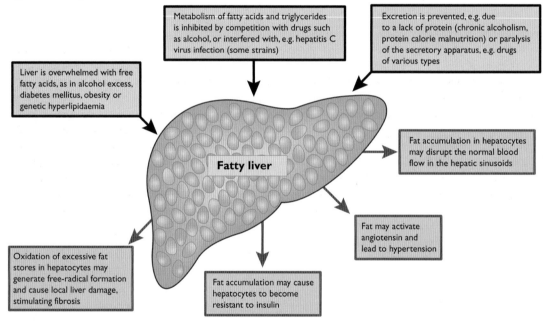

Metabolism of fatty acids and triglycerides is inhibited by competition with drugs such as alcohol, or interfered with, e.g. hepatitis C virus infection (some strains)

Excretion is prevented, e.g. due to a lack of protein (chronic alcoholism, protein calorie malnutrition) or paralysis of the secretory apparatus, e.g. drugs of various types

Liver is overwhelmed with free fatty acids, as in alcohol excess, diabetes mellitus, obesity or genetic hyperlipidaemia

Fat accumulation in hepatocytes may disrupt the normal blood flow in the hepatic sinusoids

Fatty liver

Fat may activate angiotensin and lead to hypertension

Oxidation of excessive fat stores in hepatocytes may generate free-radical formation and cause local liver damage, stimulating fibrosis

Fat accumulation may cause hepatocytes to become resistant to insulin

smaller extent, cholesterol. Triglycerides are complexed with apoproteins to form lipoproteins which are then secreted into the blood. Changes will lead to lipid accumulation within the hepatocytes. The liver appears enlarged and pale (Fig. 1.4) and fat globules are seen microscopically (Fig. 1.5).

This is not just a hypothetical model derived from experimental systems but a common problem in people who abuse alcohol. Alcohol is a hepatotoxin that has wide ranging effects on fatty acid metabolism. It increases peripheral tissue release of fatty acids so that more are delivered to the liver and, within the liver, it is implicated in increasing fatty acid synthesis, in decreasing the utilization of triglycerides, decreasing fatty acid oxidation and blocking lipoprotein excretion. Thus, it is common for the causative agent to interfere with a variety of biochemical pathways. Malnutrition particularly affects two steps. It increases the release of fatty acids from peripheral tissue and protein deficiency reduces the cell's ability to combine the triglycerides with apoprotein. Carbon tetrachloride also exerts its effect through reducing the availability of apoprotein. Disordered carbohydrate metabolism in uncontrolled diabetes leads to excessive peripheral release of fatty acids.

Gross examination of the organs affected by fatty change will show that they are enlarged, yellow and tend to be greasy to touch. Microscopically, the characteristic finding is of vacuoles within the cytoplasm. These may begin as small vacuoles but if the fatty accumulation continues, the vacuoles will coalesce to form larger vacuoles or 'fatty cysts'.

To reiterate, this type of change is entirely reversible if the insult is withdrawn. A binge in the medical school bar on a Friday night may produce fatty change but this will disappear if one is able to abstain for a few days afterwards! Chronic abuse of alcohol may produce sufficient fatty change to interfere with the normal function of the hepatocytes and, in the long term, excessive alcohol consumption may lead to cell death, scarring and cirrhosis, which is not reversible.

There comes a stage at which reversible damage becomes irreversible and cell damage becomes cell death (see Figs 1.2 and 1.7). The cells die or are killed in many ways (though each cell dies only once!). However in each case the final events follow one of the two distinct processes, 'necrosis' or 'apoptosis' (page 19).

NECROSIS

Necrosis is cell death due to lethal injury. Unlike apoptosis the cell death is not an energy dependent active process but is a consequence of sudden changes in the

> ### Key facts
>
> **Causes of fatty change in the liver**
> - Alcohol
> - Protein malnutrition
> - Diabetes
> - Acute fatty liver of pregnancy
> - Congestive cardiac failure
> - Ischaemia/anaemia
> - Drugs: steroids, methotrexate, i.v. tetracyclins
> - Carbon tetrachloride
> - Obesity

Figure 1.7 Nuclear changes in cell death

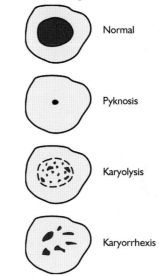

microenvironment abolishing cell function. The changes seen in the tissues are a consequence of denaturation of proteins and release of digestive enzymes which destroy the tissue.

In general terms, the microscopical changes include eosinophilia (red staining on the haematoxylin and eosin stain) of the cytoplasm, pyknosis and disintegration of the nuclei (karyorrhexis) and finally complete dissolution of the nuclei (karyolysis). However, there are different morphological patterns of necrosis under different circumstances. The principal types are:

- coagulative
- colliquative or liquefactive
- caseous.

COAGULATIVE NECROSIS

If you consider Figs 1.8 and 1.9, one is of a normal kidney with normal glomeruli and tubules, while the adjacent picture is from a kidney that has suffered an ischaemic insult and is showing coagulative necrosis. Spot the difference?

The second picture (Fig. 1.9) is essentially the ghost outline of the first! The difference between the two is that the damaged kidney shows loss of nuclei from the cells and the cytoplasm stains a slightly darker pink. This pattern of necrosis is the most common type and occurs in many solid organs like the heart and kidney (Fig. 1.10). The necrosis following a myocardial infarction is therefore of the coagulative type. Strange isn't it?

Figure 1.8 **Normal kidney**

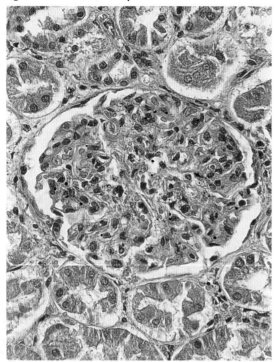

Figure 1.9 **Coagulative necrosis**

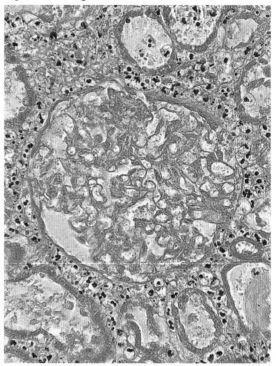

Why should the basic architecture and cellular outline be preserved if the cells are dead?

Perhaps the offending injury not only destroys the vital structural proteins within the membrane, cytoplasm and nucleus but also destroys the enzymes within the lysosomes that would otherwise degrade the cellular and extra-cellular components. The tissue, of course, doesn't remain in that state forever. If you recall the example of myocardial infarction, we stated that polymorphs move in within 24 hours of infarction. These inflammatory cells release enzymes that digest the cellular components and the resulting debris will be removed by phagocytic cells such as the macrophages. It should be clear from this that the appearance of an area of coagulative necrosis will change with time.

COLLIQUATIVE OR LIQUEFACTIVE NECROSIS

The hallmark of this type of necrosis is the release of powerful hydrolytic enzymes that degrade cellular components and extracellular material to produce a proteinaceous soup. Characteristically, it occurs in the brain where it produces a cystic cavity containing fluid and necrotic debris (Fig. 1.11).

Figure 1.10 **Kidney, showing wedge-shaped cortical infarct**

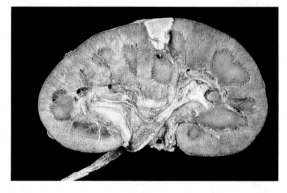

Liquefaction may also be encountered in tissues when there is a superadded bacterial infection. Then, enzymes are released from both the bacteria and the inflammatory cells that have been recruited to fight the infection.

CASEOUS NECROSIS

Caseous necrosis typically occurs in tuberculosis and is so-called because of a resemblance to soft crumbly cheese! The necrotic area is not quite liquid but neither

Figure 1.11 Brain with cerebral infarction

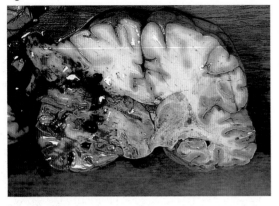

Figure 1.12 Photomicrograph of lymph node with tuberculous granuloma and caseous necrosis (arrowed)

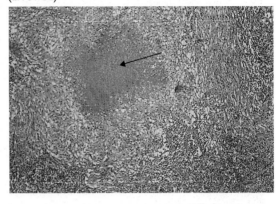

is the outline of the tissue retained as in coagulative necrosis. On microscopical sections stained with haematoxylin and eosin (H&E) (Fig. 1.12), the necrotic area appears homogeneously pink (eosinophilic) with a surrounding inflammatory response involving multinucleate giant cells, macrophages and lymphocytes (see granulomatous inflammation page 116).

It is believed that lipopolysaccharides in the capsules of the mycobacteria may be responsible for this peculiar reaction but the mechanism is unclear.

OTHER TYPES OF NECROSIS

Although these are the main types of necrosis, for completeness, we should briefly mention four others. These are fat necrosis, gangrene, fibrinoid necrosis and autolysis.

Fat necrosis

This type of necrosis is peculiar to fatty tissue and is most commonly encountered in the breast following trauma and within the peritoneal fat due to pancreatitis. Within the breast, trauma may lead to the rupture of adipocytes and release of fatty acids. This will elicit an inflammatory response and the area will become firm due to scarring and forms a palpable lump. Clinically, the lump may be mistaken for a carcinoma and excision and microscopical examination may be required to determine the diagnosis.

In pancreatitis, damage to the pancreatic acini results in the release of proteolytic and lipolytic enzymes, which denature fat cells in the peritoneum and lead to an inflammatory reaction. Calcium is also deposited in the tissues in combination with fatty acids to form calcium soaps. This is a form of dystrophic calcification

Figure 1.13 Coronal computed tomography (CT) following intravenous contrast showing massive splenomegaly with a non-enhancing infarct at the tip of the spleen (red arrows)

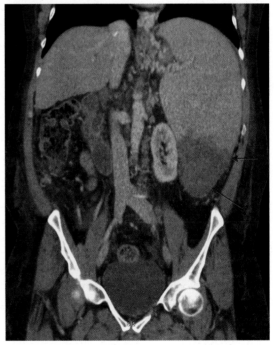

and we will consider calcification again in the section on tissue response to necrosis.

Gangrene

This does not represent a distinctive type of necrosis but is a term used in clinical practice to describe black, dead tissue. It is most commonly seen in the lower limb in patients with severe atherosclerosis, which often causes irreversible ischaemic damage to the most peripheral tissues in the body. If the pattern of necrosis is mainly of the coagulative type, it is referred to as dry gangrene, while the presence of infection with Gram-negative bacteria converts it into a liquefactive type of necrosis, when it is called wet gangrene. It will be apparent from the preceding discussion that the type of necrosis encountered depends on a number of different factors, including the type of tissue involved and the nature of the offending agent. Gas gangrene is the disastrous complication which follows infection of tissue by the Gram-positive organism *Clostridium welchii*, found in soil. The bacterium releases a toxin and also produces gas, which can be felt as crepitation when the affected area is pressed.

Fibrinoid necrosis or fibrinoid change refers to the microscopical appearance seen when an area loses its normal structure and resembles fibrin. It does not have any distinctive gross appearance.

Autolytic change is completely different from the others as it refers to cell death occurring after the person has died. Obviously, the heart stops pumping and all the tissues become irreversibly ischaemic. Enzymes leaking from the cells digest adjacent structures but there is no inflammatory response because the inflammatory system is dead!

Calcification in necrotic tissue

Necrotic tissue may become calcified. When a cell undergoes necrosis, large amounts of calcium enter the cell and this combines with phosphates within the mitochondria to produce hydroxyapatite crystals. Extracellular calcification can also occur, the crystals forming in membrane-bound vesicles derived from degenerating cells. This is the initiation phase. There is then propagation of crystal formation, depending on the local concentration of calcium and phosphate and the amount of collagen present (this enhances calcification). Usually such *dystrophic* calcification is not a problem to the body, but if it affects an important site, such as heart valves, it may affect function (Fig. 1.16). Dystrophic calcification may be useful, as in the microcalcification observed on mammograms; this can alert the radiologist to an early breast cancer (Figs 1.14 and 1.15). Dystrophic should be distinguished from *metastatic* calcification. This is linked to abnormally high serum calcium levels, due perhaps to hyperparathyroidism (increased parathyroid hormone secretion mobilises calcium from the bones), or excess vitamin D ingestion (increased calcium absorption from the gut). Metastatic carcinoma within bones may liberate calcium and result in metastatic calcification, the term metastatic referring to the widespread and scattered nature of the lesions encountered rather than inferring a similar mechanism.

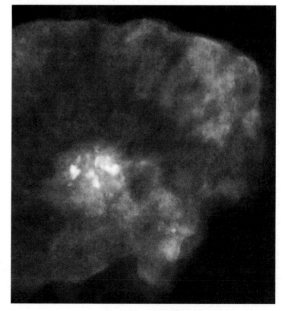

Figure 1.14 X-ray of breast tissue (mammogram) showing a circumscribed abnormality, which is radio-opaque because of dystrophic calcification

---

Key facts

Coagulative and liquefactive necrosis

Coagulative	Liquefactive
Mechanism	
Severe ischaemia destroying proteolytic enzymes	Strong proteolytic enzyme action destroying tissue
Appearance	
Initial preservation of cell outlines and tissue architecture	Loss of cell outlines Tissue becomes cystic or fluid
Occurrence	
Kidney, heart	Brain, bacterial infections

Figure 1.15 Dystrophic calcification in necrotic tumour

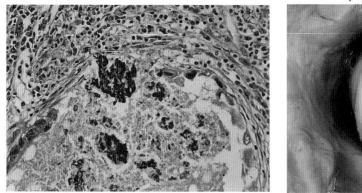

Figure 1.16 Dystrophic calcification in damaged aortic valve, producing stenosis

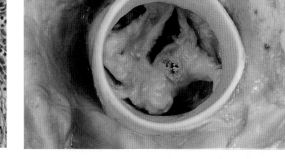

Figure 1.17 Necrosis is a messy business, while programmed cell death (apoptosis) is an ordered event

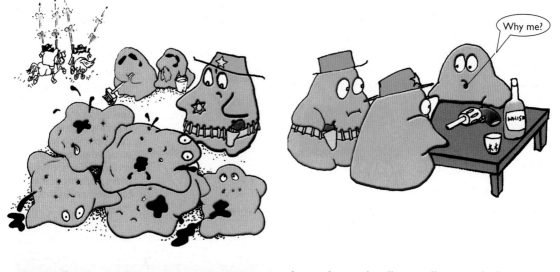

APOPTOSIS AND AUTOPHAGY

Programmed cell death is a planned and co-ordinated mechanism to achieve the death of individual cells and is a process requiring energy input from the targeted cell. The packaged, membrane bound, bundles which are produced are quickly tidied away by nearby cells. On the other hand, necrosis is the result of accidental damage of various types, invariably involves groups of cells and usually generates an inflammatory reaction, tissue damage and often scarring. See Fig. 1.17.

The word 'apoptosis' is derived from Greek and was originally used to describe the falling of individual leaves from a tree. In pathology, it is a specific type of cell death that involves single cells or small groups of cells in a tissue where the other cells are functioning normally. It is one form of programmed cell death (type 1). The other type (type 2) is related to macro-autophagy (Fig. 1.18).

Programmed cell death has an important role in all animals for controlling cell numbers, facilitating tissue modelling and removing damaged cells. It results in the death of the cell. Autophagy, literally self-eating, need not kill the cell but is an essential part of normal cell homeostasis that allows recycling of cell constituents and a source of energy when the cell is starving. Sometimes it can produce cell death and the main differences between autophagic and apoptotic cell death is that apoptosis requires the involvement of a phagocyte to tidy up the cell packages resulting from apoptosis: the 'come and eat me'

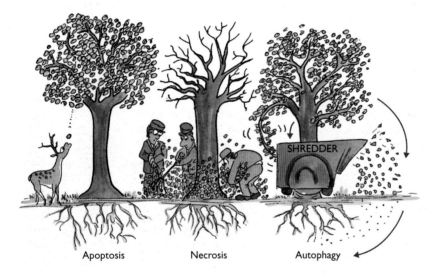

Apoptosis   Necrosis   Autophagy

Figure 1.18 The term apoptosis derives from the Greek for the falling of a single leaf from a tree. Extrapolating the analogy, in this diagram necrosis involves the death of many leaves at once, whereas in the process of autophagy there is death of leaves but their constituents are recycled

component. Autophagy handles things within the cell in three different ways: macro-autophagy, micro-autophagy and chaperone-mediated autophagy (see later) There is much research interest in autophagy and its role or manipulation in the treatment of cancer, muscle disorders and degenerative neurological conditions. At the moment, the most attention is focussed on macro-autophagy (often just called autophagy) because this seems most closely linked to type 2 programmed cell death. Apoptotic and autophagic cell death can co-exist in tissues and be difficult to distinguish (see Table 1.1). An example of this is breast cancer cells being treated with tamoxifen, which show a mixed pattern of electron-microscopically visible changes in the cells. This means that many of the processes in human development and pathology that have previously been ascribed to apoptotic

Table 1.1 Comparison of apoptotic (type 1) and autophagic (type 2) programmed cell death (PCD)

Characteristic	Apoptotic PCD	Autophagic PCD
Involvement of phagocyte	Yes	No
Cell membrane blebbing	Yes	Yes
DNA laddering	Yes	No
Organelles preserved in vacuoles	Yes	No
Cytoskeleton preserved	No	Yes
Caspase dependent	Yes	No

mechanisms may really be autophagic or a mixture; so let's just call it programmed cell death initially.

CAN CELL DEATH BE USEFUL?

The importance of programmed cell death is evident from the earliest stages of the embryo through to the involutional changes of the menopause (Fig. 1.19).

Let us consider the production of a limb with its five digits. To achieve this, tissue growth has to occur by cell division but it is also necessary to produce interdigital cell death. It is either that or ending up as a duck! This type of cell death is genetically controlled. Similarly, there are the stages of metamorphosis which take place to turn a tadpole into a frog. Metamorphosis requires not only mitotic activity and tissue growth but also a large amount of programmed cell death. When a tadpole turns into a frog, the most obvious change is that limbs are formed and the tail is resorbed. During the process of resorption, there is an increase in thyroxine which appears to lead to the activation of collagenases and, hence, destruction of the tail. Here we have an example of how programmed cell death may depend on the production of a hormone with activation of protein enzyme systems to assist the process.

Hormonal effect on cell death is also important in the maturation of the human reproductive system. The reproductive system has an early indifferent phase when it is neither male nor female. The Wolffian duct will differentiate into the epidydimis and vas deferens in the male, while the Müllerian duct forms the uterus and Fallopian tubes in the female. We know from experimental observations that administration of oestrogens at a critical time will feminize the male while administration of testosterone will masculinize the female. In order for that to happen, there has to be regression of the primitive Wolffian or Müllerian structures and this occurs via programmed cell death.

The development of the nervous system is also dependent on programmed cell death. There is an excess of neurons and only those that produce the correct synaptic connections with their target cells survive. The rest, up to 50 per cent of the neurons, die as a result of apoptosis. In gene knock-out mice unable to undergo apoptosis, the cells can be lost via autophagic cell death.

The thymus is large in the fetus and infant but atrophies before adulthood. This involution occurs via cell death which is thought to be steroid sensitive. The steroid hormones are produced in the adrenal gland so that, in this case, one organ is responsible for the

Figure 1.19 **Programmed cell death (apoptosis) at the embryonic stage allows limbs to develop appropriately**

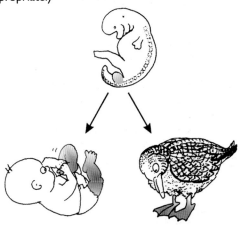

Figure 1.20 **Programmed cell death in the endometrial glands (arrows show apoptotic debris)**

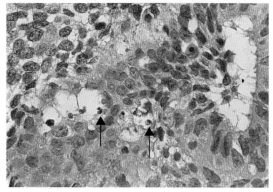

involution of another via its secreted product. This observation is useful in perinatal autopsies for deciding whether the death of a newborn baby is a sudden event or whether it follows several days of problems *in utero*. If the baby has been stressed *in utero*, adrenal steroids will cause premature involution of the thymus so that it is less than half of its normal size. If the baby has been normal *in utero* but has suffered a problem during delivery (e.g. birth asphyxia), then the thymus will be of normal size.

The endometrium is a hormone-dependent tissue that undergoes cyclical changes during the reproductive period as well as involutional changes after the menopause (Fig. 1.20). The oestrogens secreted by the ovary in the early part of the menstrual cycle induce endometrial proliferation and, if pregnancy does not occur, there is programmed cell destruction that results in menstrual shedding. If pregnancy occurs, then there is hyperplasia of the breast in preparation for lactation, which will be followed by physiological atrophy involving apoptosis after weaning. This atrophy is not only due to cell loss but also results from a reduction in cell size and loss of extra-cellular material. After the menopause, the withdrawal of the hormonal influence results in involution of the uterus and ovaries.

Apoptosis plays an important role in the immune system. It is necessary for the selection of specific sub-populations of both T and B lymphocytes and is also important in the destruction of target cells by cytotoxic T cells.

CHANGES IN APOPTOSIS

The original term for apoptosis was 'shrinkage necrosis' as apoptotic cells tend to shrink while necrotic cells initially swell. Apoptotic cells lose their contact with neighbouring cells early on. After 1–2 hours the nuclear chromatin condenses on the nuclear membrane and then the membrane 'packages' these small aggregates of nuclear material to give membrane-bound nuclear fragments. The cytoplasm shrinks and the cell's organelles also become parcelled into membrane-bound vesicles. These are called apoptotic bodies and they contain morphologically intact mitochondria, lysosomes, ribosomes, etc. Finally, these apoptotic bodies are phagocytosed by neighbouring cells or by macrophages. Experimental evidence suggests that an apoptotic cell acquires molecules on its surface which allow neighbouring cells and macrophages to identify it as having committed suicide and hence leads to clearing of the fragments. See Fig. 1.21.

A crucial feature of apoptosis is that the cell's contents are not allowed to leak into the extracellular space, where enzymes may digest adjacent structures, or proteins may stimulate an immune response. Instead, the cell packages itself into small membrane-bound vesicles, which contain functioning mitochondria and other cell organelles. Protein is cleaved by hydrolysis mediated by a series of enzymes called caspases, whose action is mediated by the bcl-2 family of proteins. DNA is broken down into large pieces by endonucleases. Nuclear fragments, together with cell proteins are wrapped in a lipid membrane, which is then marked 'for disposal' by specific markers, such as phosphatidylserine or thrombospondin. These residues can be recognized by macrophages and adjacent epithelial cells, which are then stimulated to phagocytose them and degrade the components in secondary lysosomes. Thus no messy acute inflammatory process is initiated. However, this process requires the expenditure of energy, as with any good garbage disposal system!

Defects in this apoptotic corpse clearance might be associated with the development of auto-immune and inflammatory conditions. The uptake of apoptotic fragments stimulates release of anti-inflammatory mediators and can inhibit secretion of pro-inflammatory mediators (i.e. the opposite to the effect of uptake of necrotic cells).

AUTOPHAGY

Autophagy is about cellular house-keeping. It takes damaged or redundant proteins, organelles, parts of organelles or areas of the nucleus and digests them into their essential constitutents through the action of lysosomal enzymes. Thus, proteins become amino acids and nucleic acids become nucleotides. All this occurs within a membrane bound vesicle where the lysosomal enzymes mix with the substrate. How this vacuole forms is what distinguishes the three types of autophagy (see Table 1.2). In macro-autophagy, the substrates are first packaged in an autophagosome, which has an outer membrane that is not derived from a lysosome. This then joins with a lysosome and the dividing membranes break down allowing the enzymes to reach the substrate. In micro-autophagy, the lysosome itself engulfs the substrate. In chaperone-mediated autophagy, receptors on the surface of the lysosome selectively bind specific substances and allow them to translocate into the lysosomal lumen. Autophagy (Atg) genes identified in yeast are conserved and function in many animals, including mammals.

Autophagy appears to be able both to protect a cell and to destroy it (Fig. 1.22). When nutrients are scarce, digesting intra-cellular macro-molecules can provide the energy to maintain minimal cell functioning. Pathogens

---

Key facts

Factors able to stimulate autophagy
- Starvation
- Oxidative stress
- Irradiation
- Hormonal signals
- Accumulation of mis-folded proteins
- Changes in cell volume

Figure 1.21 Programmed cell death (apoptosis) is an ordered and energy-requiring process that can be stimulated by diverse agents. Once initiated, the process is irreversible. There is no associated inflammation. It can be thought of in three stages: initiation, execution and disposal. The orderly catabolism of the skeleton and packaging of cell components in lipid membranes as the cell disassembles leads to them being phagocytosed and broken down by nearby macrophages or epithelial cells. The cells appear shrunken and condensed under the microscope

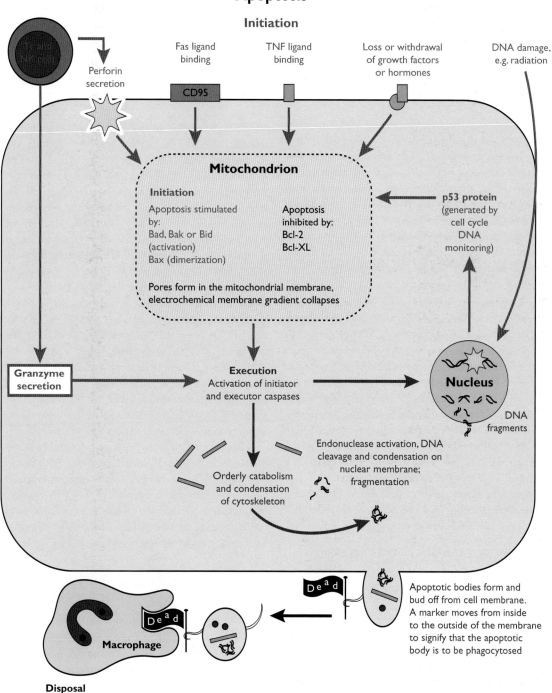

Table 1.2 Comparison of the types of autophagy

Characteristic	Macro-autophagy	Micro-autophagy	Chaperone-mediated autophagy
Occurrence	Stress	Normal physiology	Stress
Sequestering membrane	Non-lysosomal	Lysosomal	–
Receptor-mediated	No	No	Yes
Engulfs organelles	Yes	Yes	No
Digests soluble cytosolic proteins	Yes	Yes	Only KFERQ tagged

KFERQ, the one-letter code for the amino acid sequence Lys-Phe-Glu-Arg-Gln.

and toxins may be segregated and degraded. Abnormal proteins or damaged organelles can be eliminated. All of these can play an important homeostatic role in the early stages of a disease process. Why then is it also a mechanism for killing the cell? The theory is that it protects the cell by removing damaged cell components for as long as it can but if it loses that battle it is best to remove the whole cell; i.e. to order cell death.

SIGNALLING EVENTS IN PROGRAMMED CELL DEATH

Our knowledge has advanced somewhat since the first genetic events in apoptosis were elucidated by the study of the nematode *Caenorhabitis elegans*. We now know that a variety of initiating events can trigger apoptosis, via a final common pathway of caspase activation, leading to endonuclease-mediated cleavage of nuclear DNA and catabolism of the cytoskeleton. In some instances, such as via the action of cytotoxic T cells, the caspases can be activated more or less directly; there is also a so-called 'death receptor' on the cell surface (otherwise known as the fas receptor or CD95) which can stimulate the caspases once activated, for instance by tumour necrosis factor.

More recently, it has become apparent that binding of death ligands on the cell surface can stimulate autophagic cell death as well as apoptotic death.

APOPTOSIS, AUTOPHAGY AND DISEASE

It follows from the previous discussion that a lack of balance in initiating or suppressing programmed cell death can lead to problems.

Apoptosis is an important host defence mechanism against viral infection. When viruses infect cells, they attempt to take over the cell's replication machinery in order to proliferate and spread. Viral antigens are expressed on the host cell membrane and (in concert with CD4$^+$ lymphocytes) CD8$^+$ lymphocytes bind to this and secrete perforin, lysing the affected cell. Alternatively, NK cells recognize the viral antigen and initiate cell lysis. Viruses can sometimes get round this, with anti-apoptotic mechanisms, which come into play when breaks occur in DNA strands as the viral genome incorporates itself into the cell's DNA. Many viruses code for proteins that block apoptosis. Examples include the inactivation of *p53* by HPV16 and Epstein–Barr virus (EBV), which produce molecules that either simulate *bcl2* or block molecules related to the TNF/CD40 pathway.

Too much apoptosis may be also seen if the effector mechanisms malfunction, as is seen in AIDS, when infection of T cells by HIV leads to deletion of the CD4$^+$ population of T cells, wreaking havoc in the immune system due to the loss of its most crucial regulatory cell. Human immunodeficiency virus expresses gp120, which activates the fas ligand on CD4$^+$ cells and leads to apoptosis. CD4$^+$ cells are essential for the generation of memory to intercurrent and opportunistic infections.

It has become clear that apoptosis (or the lack of it) has a role in the development of tumours. Inactivation of the cell cycle regulatory genes (which act as 'quality control officers' on the integrity of the DNA) will permit mutations to be passed to daughter cells by allowing cell replication to take place; usually such cells would be commanded to undergo apoptosis.

TREATING DISEASES BY INTERFERING WITH CELL DEATH

The study of cell death and apoptosis has raised important therapeutic issues, none more so than in the field of oncology. It is now generally accepted that tumour growth is a result of the fine and precarious balance

Figure 1.22 Autophagy: its role in cellular conservation and in cell death
In autophagic cell death, which is often a response to chronic adverse environmental factors such as starvation, the process of lysosomal degradation of cellular components within membrane-bound vesicles has already occurred before cell breakdown. The cells often appear vacuolated under the microscope as they undergo this process

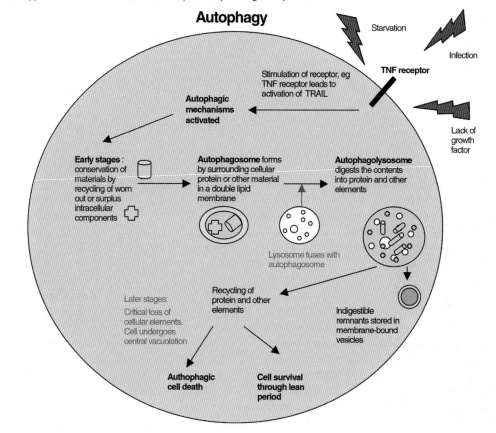

which exists between cell proliferation and cell loss. Tumours that grow fast do so not only by proliferating fast but also by keeping cell death to a minimum.

Cancer treatment involves surgery, radiation and chemotherapy. The latter two act by changing the rate of cell proliferation, and are successful in many types of cancer. The first reported cure with radiotherapy was in 1899 on a basal cell carcinoma of the skin. Therapeutic radiation damages cells by generating ions in the tissue, the most common of which are the oxygen free radicals derived from water. These are the same as those involved in bacterial killing in inflammation (page 101). Indirect biochemical damage includes the peroxidation of molecules (especially lipids), interference with oxidative phosphorylation, changes in membrane permeability and the inhibition of some enzymes. All of these produce necrosis and generate a tissue response

to the damage, and of course normal as well as tumour cells are affected. In addition, radiation damages DNA (as we shall discuss in chapter 2), producing breaks in the strands. These are normally repaired promptly but there may on occasions be errors in the repair, leading to cell death.

There are numerous chemotherapeutic agents with a variety of modes of action. Alkylating agents (e.g. cyclophosphamide and melphalan) form covalent links with certain molecules, the most important of which is the guanine base in DNA. This leads to breaks in the DNA and faulty transcription. Antimetabolites (e.g. cytarabine and methotrexate) resemble naturally occurring substances but are subtly different so that they block an enzyme pathway or damage the macromolecular structure in which they are incorporated. Many are analogues of purine or pyrimidine bases and affect nucleic acid synthesis, while methotrexate interferes with folic acid metabolism, thus blocking DNA and RNA synthesis. Antibiotics useful in chemotherapy (e.g. adriamycin and daunorubicin) often produce a local distortion of the DNA helix that interferes with the function of DNA and RNA polymerases. The vinca alkaloids (e.g. vinblastine) act in a completely different manner and bind to tubulin in the microtubules of the mitotic spindle to block division. The hallmark of both radiotherapy and chemotherapy is that the cell's metabolism becomes irreversibly damaged and the proliferating cell is most likely to perish, i.e. undergo necrosis.

What about apoptosis? Does that have any therapeutic potential? The answer is 'yes'. We are still at an early stage but there is considerable interest in the various cytokines that might be able to promote apoptotic tumour cell death (Fig. 1.23). Cytokines are produced by lymphocytes and macrophages following stimulation and, besides modifying the immune response, may act directly to cause death of tumour cells.

Tumour necrosis factor (TNF or cachectin) is produced by activated macrophages, and its action on tumour cells takes place via various distinct mechanisms. It has a role in inflammation which alters endothelial cells, promoting thrombosis and thus causing ischaemic cell necrosis in the tumour. Although the death of cells in a tumour is rather complex, ischaemia playing a major role, there is evidence that at least some of the cells die as a result of attack by lymphocytes. In experimental models, TNF also causes an increase in apoptotic cell death, which appears to be a direct effect as there is an early rise in the synthesis of RNA in the affected cell. We have already discussed the interaction of the TNF pathway with the fas receptor. Various interleukins appear to produce tumour cell death secondary to stimulation of cytotoxic T cells and NK cells, which then act on the tumour cells to initiate apoptosis.

Interferons, on the other hand, appear to exert their effects by acting in synergy with the above factors. They have been shown to enhance the cytotoxicity of T lymphocytes and NK cells, and they also increase the phagocytic activities of macrophages on tumour cells. They are known (in combination with TNF) to reduce the rate of tumour cell multiplication.

To this we can now add the potential of type 2 programmed cell death (autophagic death). The difficulty is that it is currently impossible to predict whether stimulating or inhibiting autophagy would be most appropriate.

Figure 1.23 Possible means by which the actions of cytokines may inhibit tumour growth

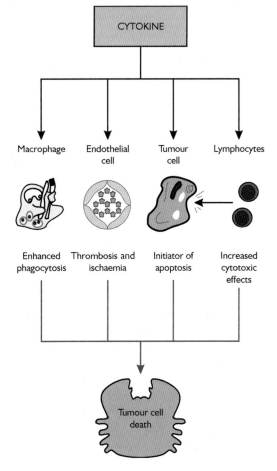

This is principally because of the importance of autophagy in normal cell house-keeping and the fact that stimulating autophagy is not the same as ordering cell death.

In breast cancer, it has been suggested that deletions of one allele of *beclin1* (which interacts with *bcl2*) may contribute to tumour production. *beclin1* is important in autophagy and a *reduction* in autophagy could allow cells to be in a faster synthesis and growth phase and be more likely to acquire useful malignant mutations. At a later stage of tumorigenesis, an *increase* in autophagy could be an advantage to the tumour as it needs to survive stressful conditions when central tumour mass cells are poorly nourished. Other ideas on how autophagy might operate in myopathies, neurodegenerative and infectious diseases are listed in Table 1.3.

Table 1.3 Possible effects of autophagy in various conditions	
Disease	**Change in autophagy**
Cancer: early stage	Inactivation favours tumour growth
Cancer: late stage	Activation allows survival of cells in centre of tumour
Vacuolar myopathies	Inactivation leads to accumulation of vacuoles that weaken muscles
Neurodegeneration: early	Activation helps remove protein aggregates (helpful)
Neurodegeneration: late	Damaged neurons undergo autophagic cell death
Axonal injury	Inactivation prevents removal of damaged organelles and transmitter vacuoles so that neurotransmitters are released in cell and induce apoptosis
Infectious disease	Inhibition facilitates viral infection of cell and allows survival of bacteria

AGEING

Sadly, neither we nor our cells live for ever. Despite the cells' ability to replicate and repair, things do come to an end. So what are the main mechanisms? We have already discussed sub-lethal cell injury and it is thought that progressive accumulation of cellular and molecular damage is what ages our tissues. This is, of course, influenced by both environmental and genetic factors. If environmental insults result in free-radical mediated damage, then the damaged organelles and proteins can accumulate. If there is a genetic defect affecting the ability to repair DNA, then DNA mutations will accumulate. Then the cell's normal functions become impaired and/or they cannot produce new cells.

Replicative senescence is the term describing a cell's inability to divide. Cells do appear to have a finite number of divisions and this may be linked to telomere shortening. Telomeres are at the linear ends of chromosomes and are important for ensuring their complete replication. With each replication, the telomere becomes shorter until the chromosome ends are damaged and this stops the cell cycle. In cells, such as stem cells or germ cells, that need to continue to divide, there is an enzyme called telomerase that can lengthen the chromosomes. This might also be important in some cancers.

Ageing is not just a random process but involves specific genes, receptors and signals. One of the mechanisms involves insulin growth factor 1 (IGF-1) pathways and decreased signalling following reduced calorie intake has been shown to prolong lifespan (but so far only in *C. elegans*).

Figure 1.24 Lipofuscin pigment (arrow) represents worn-out cell components, mainly cell membranes, packaged in lysosomes which accumulate in long-lived cells such as liver

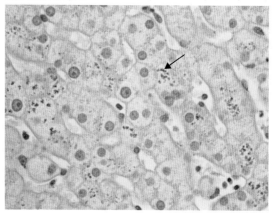

How can you recognize an ageing cell? Table 1.4 lists some of the structural and biochemical changes but probably the most obvious one is the accumulation of the brown pigment, lipofuscin (Fig. 1.24). This is the product of lipid peroxidation and signifies oxidative damage.

Table 1.4 Normal physiological changes with increasing age
Cardiovascular system
↓ Vessel elasticity
↓ Number of heart muscle fibres
↑ Size of muscle fibres
↓ Stroke volume
Respiratory system
↓ Chest wall compliance
↓ Alveolar ventilation
↓ Lung volume
Gastro-intestinal system
↓ Bowel motility
↓ Enzyme, acid and intrinsic factor production
↓ Hepatic function
Urinary system
↓ Glomerular filtration rate (GFR)
↓ Concentrating ability
Nervous system
↑ Degeneration and atrophy of 25–45 per cent of neurons
↓ Neurotransmitters and conduction rate
Musculoskeletal system
↓ Muscle mass
↑ Bone demineralization
↑ Joint degeneration
Immune system
↓ Inflammatory response
Skin
↓ Subcutaneous fat and elastin
↓ Sweat glands
↓ Temperature regulation through arterioles

Key facts

Structural and biochemical changes in cellular ageing

- Reduced oxidative phosphorylation in mitochondria

- Reduced synthesis of nucleic acids, transcription factors, proteins and cell receptors

- Decreased uptake of nutrients

- Reduced repair mechanisms

- Irregular, abnormally lobed nuclei

- Pleomorphic mitochondria

- Decreased endoplasmic reticulum

- Distorted Golgi apparatus

- Accumulation of lipofuscin

- Accumulation of abnormally folded proteins

Figure 1.25 Ageing is normal!

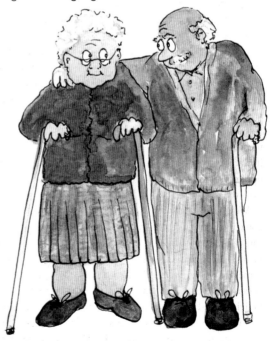

In the post-mortem room we witness the final result of disease, the failure of the body to solve its problems and there is an obvious limit to what one can learn about normal business transactions from even a daily visit to the bankruptcy court.

W. Russell, Lord Brain, 1960

If you look back at page 8, the autopsy report on our patient gave the cause of death as 'myocardial infarction due to coronary artery thrombosis due to coronary artery atheroma'. But what caused the atheroma!? Was it diet or smoking or lack of exercise or genes or a combination? In many situations it is a combination of factors and the person's response that determines any symptoms or signs. Thus, we could list a variety of factors that have contributed to this man's heart attack and could call them 'causes'.

Just as we have chosen a definition for 'disease', we should choose a definition for 'cause', though remembering that there is no single correct answer. Our definition will be 'the cause of a disease is a factor that is clearly associated with the occurrence of the disease and which plays an identifiable role in the initiation of a mechanism(s) that significantly contributes to the manifestation of that disease'. Since multiple mechanisms operate in most diseases, there will be multiple factors involved in causation.

We shall leave the body's response to later sections and concentrate now on a way of classifying the range of causes of diseases. This is inevitably arbitrary but should provide a useful checklist of the broad categories and some specific examples. In simple terms, it is 'intrinsic' versus 'extrinsic', i.e. which factors are personal to the individual and which are acquired from the environment.

Classifying the extrinsic agents is fairly straightforward because we are used to listing them under particular headings (Table 2.1). The 'intrinsic' factors are less simple because our ideas have changed enormously over the last decade as the human genome has been

sequenced. It is tempting now to imagine that every 'intrinsic' factor could be listed under the category of genetic, just as every idea in this book is composed of letters clustered as words and arranged in sentences. However, a book would not be defined as a collection of letters. The science of gene expression and the steps between genotype and phenotype have some gaps left so we shall subdivide the intrinsic factors into genetic, metabolic, cellular and structural. The intrinsic causes will include mechanisms that involve an abnormal response to an extrinsic agent, e.g. the abnormal lymphocyte response in a hypersensitivity reaction is an 'intrinsic cellular' cause that also involves an external factor.

Let us consider the possible mechanisms involved in these varied causes of cell injury and death, bearing in mind that it is not always possible to define the exact site of action of the initial insult. Since the cell membrane, oxidative phosphorylation and DNA are vital to the cell, it is very likely that these will be involved. You will also recall from our earlier consideration of a patient with a myocardial infarct that the final outcome is dependent on the severity and duration of the insult and the metabolic demands of the tissues at the time of the insult.

Physical and chemical agents are well known for causing cell death. We are all aware of the devastating effects of dropping an atomic bomb and the mass destruction caused by chemical warfare. Radiation and chemicals produce cell death by the production of oxygen free radicals, which interfere with DNA structure and replication, resulting in mutations. The effects of these changes may be immediate, or can be subtle, manifesting many years after the initiating event (Figs 2.1 and 2.2).

Electrocution may cause death or severe tissue damage by generating extreme heat, causing severe burns at the entry site and in the tissues (conduction is through ionized fluids within blood and tissues) or by interrupting the normal electrical impulses within the heart

Table 2.1 Classification of extrinsic and intrinsic factors in disease

Category	Agent	Disease example
Extrinsic factors		
Physical	Trauma	Bone fracture
	Radiation	Cancer
	Temperature extremes	Frostbite/electric burn
	Environmental hazards	Drowning
Chemical	Toxic substances	Tobacco lung damage
	Inflammatory substances	Asthma
Biological	Bacteria	Various infections
	Virus	AIDS
	Fungi and parasites	Athlete's foot
	Prions	Creutsfeld–Jacob disease
Nutritional	Various	Malnutrition and some cancers
Intrinsic factors		
Genetic		Sickle cell disease
		Cystic fibrosis
Metabolic		Diabetes
		Gluten induced enteropathy
		Gallstones
Cellular		Autoimmune, e.g. rheumatoid arthritis
		Degenerative and ageing, e.g. Alzheimer's disease
Structural		Congenital, e.g. spina bifida
		Acquired, e.g. atheroma, biliary tract obstruction, osteoarthritis

Figure 2.1 Effects of irradiation, e.g. following a nuclear explosion, can be immediate or delayed

Immediate effects

Death from blast/burn injuries
Acute radiation syndromes:
• Bone marrow depression
• Gastrointestinal tract effects
• Cerebral effects

Delayed malignancies depend on age at time of exposure:

Childhood exposure
• Leukaemias*
• Thyroid cancer
• Breast cancer

Adult exposure
• Leukaemias*
• Lung/breast/salivary gland cancer
• All other cancers increased to some extent

* All leukaemias except chronic lymphocytic leukaemia are increased

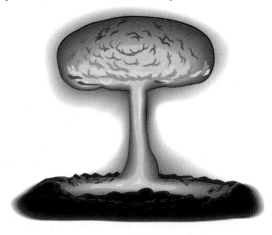

Figure 2.2 Causes of and types of DNA mutation and their consequences

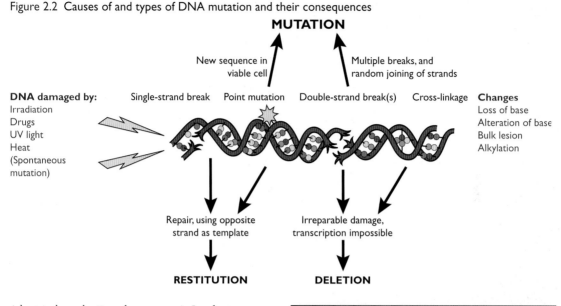

MUTATION

New sequence in viable cell

Multiple breaks, and random joining of strands

DNA damaged by:
Irradiation
Drugs
UV light
Heat
(Spontaneous mutation)

Single-strand break   Point mutation   Double-strand break(s)   Cross-linkage

Changes
Loss of base
Alteration of base
Bulk lesion
Alkylation

Repair, using opposite strand as template

Irreparable damage, transcription impossible

RESTITUTION   **DELETION**

(electrical conduction along nerves). Involuntary muscle contraction may cause the victim to seize and cling to the source of the current (if you come across this situation, turn off the current or knock the patient free with a non-conductive substance before attempting resuscitation!). Electric shocks are useful clinically when a large DC shock, applied to a patient in ventricular fibrillation, may restore the normal rhythm.

Temperature is another important factor. Heat applied to the skin in low doses may induce a coagulative type of necrosis but with intense heat, the tissue may simply vaporize! Those interested in Arctic exploration will be aware of the gangrene induced by extreme cold which is due to a combination of thrombosis in small vessels and ice crystal formation in tissues (frostbite). But how many people realize that hypothermia (a drop in body temperature to less than 35.5°C) may occur in cool but otherwise normal ambient conditions in elderly, immobile or malnourished individuals? Hypothermia is life-threatening in several ways, causing cardiac arrhythmia and death, or a gradual decline in consciousness to coma, often fatal in an isolated elderly person, living alone and not discovered for several days. Hypothermia is characterized by listlessness and confusion. Unconsciousness supervenes at temperatures from 26 to 33°C.

Water, that substance on which all life depends, can be lethal. Drowning is easily understood, but problems with water excretion in a patient with malfunctioning kidneys can also be life threatening.

CLINICAL CASE: FROSTBITE

A 29-year-old skier lost his way after drinking a few beers in a mountain restaurant. He was discovered, unconscious, without a hat, 20 hours later in an exposed location on the mountain face. He had obvious frostbite to his nose and fingertips, manifest as hard white areas. A weak, thready, but regular pulse was present and he was breathing shallowly. He was wrapped in a space blanket and rushed by helicopter to hospital. His rectal (core) temperature was found to be 30°C. He was warmed with blankets and hot water bottles. He suffered a cardiac arrest but was immediately resuscitated. His mild metabolic acidosis was corrected. As he regained consciousness he began to shiver violently and his limbs became reddened and swollen. He tried to raise himself up but promptly fainted. Over the next couple of days his fingertips and nose turned black and the skin began to slough off. At one point it appeared that he would lose the tips of most of his fingers, but after the skin had fallen off only two fingertips were lost and his nose was saved.

WHAT HAS HAPPENED HERE?

Our patient was hypothermic, i.e. his core temperature was less than 35°C (normal temperature 37°C). He contributed to his condition by drinking alcohol (see below). He was not wearing a hat, and 50 per cent of the body's heat loss may be through the head. There is no mention of a face mask, which might have served to warm the freezing air before he inhaled it, losing core heat when the lungs warmed the air prior to exhalation.

The onset of hypothermia is dependent on many factors, including body build, ambient temperature, whether the individual is dry or wet, the presence of protective clothing, whether or not alcohol has been ingested (even small amounts can greatly increase the risk of hypothermia).

Alcohol plus exercise is probably the worst combination, since not only is blood glucose depleted by exercise but the alcohol interferes with the generation of new glucose from body stores by reducing the amount of pyruvate available.

Once he became hypothermic he would have been less able to make rational decisions or take sensible measures such as seeking help, finding shelter or covering exposed areas of his body.

HOW DOES THE BODY RESPOND TO COLD?

Initially the heat gain centre in the hypothalamus directs the body to shiver violently and shut down peripheral blood vessels by vasoconstriction, but if this fails to restore core temperature the cooling of the heart interferes with cardiac output. Below 26°C the cardiac output is too low to sustain life (Fig. 2.4).

Oxygen combines more strongly with haemoglobin at low temperatures, further depleting tissues of oxygen. Anoxic effects on the heart include arrhythmias. Patients whose body temperature is below 30°C are at risk of cardiac arrest and should be monitored by ECG. Respiration is diminished, usually in proportion with tissue requirements but slight CO_2 retention may cause

a respiratory acidosis, compounded by the metabolic acidosis which occurs when lactic acid accumulates as a result of shivering.

WHY DID THE PATIENT FAINT AS HE BEGAN TO RECOVER?

Blood volume falls in the hypothermic patient due to a combination of a 'cold diuresis' which occurs in response to a drop in core temperature and damage to renal tubular epithelium due to cold, preventing sodium reabsorption; this causes a drop in plasma osmolality and water moves out of the vascular compartment into the tissues to balance this. When the patient is warmed and vasodilation occurs the blood volume is insufficient for demand and there is hypotension.

WHAT IS FROSTBITE?

Frostbite is the result of freezing of tissues, which occurs at temperatures below −0.54°C. Before freezing, cooling to less than 12°C causes paralysis of muscles and nerves by interference with the membrane sodium pump. Lack of sodium ions renders nerves and muscles inexcitable. Damage is reversible after a few hours, but not if left longer. If the tissue freezes the tissue proteins become denatured and the cell dies. Vascular endothelial cells are particularly susceptible. When they thaw, plasma leaks out of the small vessels through the damaged endothelium and the retained red blood cells sludge, obstructing the lumen and causing local infarction of tissue.

Although it is dangerous to warm the body of a hypothermic person too quickly, if a patient is suffering only from frostbite it is best to warm the affected area as quickly as possible, so that sludging and infarction is

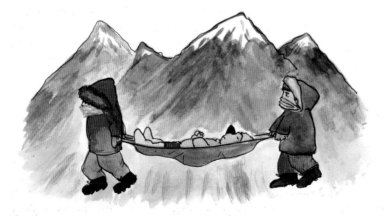

Figure 2.3 Frostbite is caused by the freezing of tissues. Sludging of cells in capillaries causes ischaemic damage. Endothelial cells are vulnerable to both cold and hypoxia; on thawing of the tissues, there is leakage of blood through the damaged vessels and the tissue appears blackened over a larger area than is actually necrotic, so delaying amputation is advised

Figure 2.4 Changes associated with cold and reperfusion

Core

Lungs:
•↓respiration due to ↓oxygen demand from tissues → retention of CO_2 and respiratory acidosis, which is superimposed on lactic acidosis from shivering

Kidneys:
•cold diuresis occurs
•Renal tubular epithelium damaged by cold, fails to reabsorb sodium → ↓plasma osmolality, water →tissues

Vasculature:
•Circulating blood volume reduced
•Oxygen less readily given up to tissues by oxyhaemoglobin at low temperatures

Heart:
•Reduced cardiac output due to ↓blood volume and ↓myocardial contractility
•Risk of arrhythmias
•Risk of cardiac arrest <30°C
•Cardiac output cannot sustain life <26°C

Muscles and nerves:
•Lose excitability due to impaired membrane Na^+ pump
•Severe pain on thawing

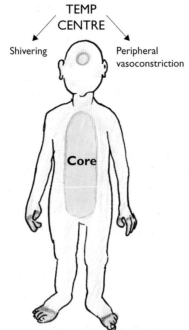

TEMP CENTRE

Shivering — Peripheral vasoconstriction

Core

Peripheries

Peripheries:
<12°C
•Numbness: membrane sodium pump inactivated, nerves and muscles inexcitable
•Capillary endothelium damaged by cold <−0.5°C
•Freezing of tissues damages endothelial cells
•Sludging of cells in blood vessels causes hypoxia or infarction. On thawing, blood and plasma leak into tissues and ↓blood volume

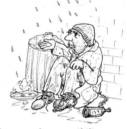

Increased susceptibility to cold if:
•Skin is wet
•Elderly or very young
•Homeless or exposed to the elements
•Alcohol consumed (or other vasodilator)
•Concurrent infection (temperature centre may be compromised)

---

reduced to a minimum due to quick restoration of blood flow. It is harmful to thaw an area of frostbite and then allow it to refreeze, as may happen on a mountainside when colleagues treat the area by warming and then the patient with frostbite is carried back through the same harsh environmental conditions which caused the problem.

Although damage may seem extensive, the actual area of necrosis may be less than it first appears and it may be worth waiting for a few days before amputation of an affected area (Fig. 2.3). The process of thawing out is very painful and requires analgesic support, plus elevation of the affected area to reduce tissue swelling.

Let us discuss in more detail one extrinsic group of causes, one group of intrinsic causes and one which is a combination of the two. We shall consider biological agents (as an extrinsic cause), genetic causes as intrinsic, and hypersensitivity reactions as an abnormal intrinsic cellular reaction to an external agent.

BIOLOGICAL AGENTS AS CAUSES OF DISEASES

This is an enormous topic and could fill many books. Although we would only like to cover some common mechanisms, some short lists of microbes and their relevant diseases are included (see also Figs 2.5–2.8). Two common mechanisms of bacterial disease are toxin production (endotoxin and exotoxins) and direct cell damage.

BACTERIAL ENDOTOXIN

Endotoxin is not secreted by living bacteria but is a cell wall component that is shed when the bacterium dies. The component is called lipid A, which is part of the lipopolysaccharide (LPS) in the outer cell wall of Gram-negative bacteria. It causes fever and macrophage

Table 2.2 Simple summary of the ways of classifying bacteria			
	Gram-positive	**Gram-negative**	**Acid fast**
Examples of aerobic and anaerobic bacteria			
Obligate aerobes	*Bacillus cereus*	*Neisseria*	Mycobacteria
Facultative anaerobes	*Bacillus anthracis* *Staphylococcus*	*E. coli* *Salmonella*	
Microaerophilic bacteria	*Streptococcus*	Spirochaetes	
Obligate anaerobes	*Clostridia*	Bacteroides	
Examples of morphologically distinct Gram-positive and Gram-negative bacteria			
Cocci (spherical)	Streptococci (in chains) Staphylococci (in clusters)	*Neisseria*	
Bacilli (rod-shaped)	*Corynebacteria* *Clostridia* *Bacillus*	*Haemophilus* *Bordetella* *Klebsiella, Proteus,* *Shigella, E. coli,*	
	Listeria	*Vibrio, Salmonella*	
Spiral		*Treponema, Borrelia,* *Leptospira* (spirochaetes). *Helicobacter,* *Campylobacter*	
Pleomorphic		*Chlamydia, Rickettsia* (intracellular obligates)	
Branching	*Actinomyces, Nocardia*		

and B cell activation by inducing host cytokines. Only Gram-negative bacteria have endotoxin, with the one exception of the Gram-positive *Listeria monocytogenes*.

Endotoxin is a potent stimulator of a wide range of immune responses. To the immune system, the recognition of LPS spells danger and warrants an immediate and dramatic response, which is often detrimental to the host itself. Clinically, this manifests as fever and vascular collapse or shock. Macrophages are stimulated by LPS to produce TNF and IL-1 which have many effects including acting directly on the hypothalamus to produce fever (page 109). LPS also stimulates, directly or indirectly, the complement and clotting pathways and platelets to produce DIC (disseminated intravascular coagulation, page 186), thrombosis and shock (page 34). Shock results from increased vascular permeability produced by mediators from mast cells and platelets, combined with TNF and LPS affecting endothelial cells. LPS also stimulates the liver to produce acute phase proteins (page 110) and hypoglycaemia. In Gram-positive organisms, lipotechoic acid within the bacterial wall causes problems similar to LPS in Gram-negative bacteria.

BACTERIAL EXOTOXINS

Exotoxins are proteins released by living bacteria and there are a wide variety with different actions. Neurotoxins act on nerves or end plates to produce paralysis, cytotoxins damage a variety of cells, tissue-invasive toxins are often enzymes capable of digesting host tissues, and pyrogenic toxins stimulate cytokine release and cause rashes, fever and toxic shock syndrome. A very important group are the enterotoxins that act on the gastrointestinal tract to produce diarrhoea by inhibiting salt absorption, stimulating salt excretion or killing intestinal cells. There are two broad categories: infectious diarrhoea and food poisoning with preformed toxin. In infectious diarrhoea, the bacteria proliferate in the gut, continuously releasing enterotoxin. The symptoms do not occur immediately after ingestion but require a day or two for the bugs to become established

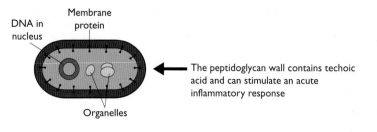

DNA in
nucleus

Membrane
protein

The peptidoglycan wall contains techoic
acid and can stimulate an acute
inflammatory response

Organelles

Gram-positive bacteria stain blue with cresyl violet, which lodges in their thick outer wall. Inside they have a double-layered phospholipid membrane, with membrane proteins, surrounding cytoplasm with organelles and a circular nucleus composed of double-stranded DNA

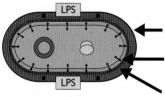

Outer coat contains lipopolysaccharide (LPS), a component of which causes endotoxic shock, fever and diarrhoea. Porin protein ■ allows nutrient transfer

Periplasmic space contains enzymes and proteins in a gel

Thin peptidoglycan coat

Gram-negative bacteria have an extra, double-layered coat that traps cresyl violet before it can reach the peptidoglycan coat (which is thinner than in G+ bacteria). The violet crystals are washed out by alcohol as part of the Gram staining process and the bacterium is visualized using a red counter-stain

Bacterial shapes

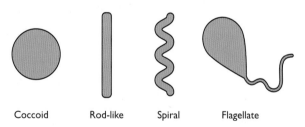

Coccoid   Rod-like   Spiral   Flagellate

Figure 2.5 Gram-positive and Gram-negative bacteria

in sufficient numbers. In food poisoning, the bacteria grow in the food releasing their exotoxin. This acts very quickly after ingestion to produce diarrhoea, abdominal pain and vomiting but the symptoms only last for 24 hours because no new toxin is created.

Bacterial exotoxins may be classified by their site of action:

- extracellular, e.g. epidermolytic toxin *Staphylococcus aureus* that causes scalded skin syndrome
- at cell membrane level (not transported into cell, but causes changes in intracellular cGMP), e.g. *E. coli* heat stable enterotoxin (ST) causing traveller's diarrhoea and *S. aureus* TSST 1 toxin leading to toxic shock syndrome

- on the cell membrane, causing pore formation or disruption of lipid by enzymic activity, e.g. phospholipase C activity toxin *Clostridium perfringens*, spore-forming toxins (thiol-activating haemolysins) such as streptolysin (*S. pyogenes*), pnemolysin (*S. pneumoniae*), listeriolysin (*Listeria monocytogenes*), perfringolysin (*Clostridium perfringens*; gas gangrene), cerolysin (*Bacillus cereus*; food poisoning)
- type III toxins, which act intracellularly by translocating an enzymic component across the membrane (A subunit of domain) which modifies an acceptor molecule in the cytoplasm. These can be grouped by the type of enzymic activity:
  - ADP-ribosylation (cholera, diphtheria, pertussis)

- N-glycosidases (shiga toxin)
- glucosyl transferases (*C. difficile* toxin A and B)
- Zn^{2+}-requiring endopeptidases (tetanus and botulism toxins)

GTP binding proteins are often the target for ADP-ribosylation by type III bacterial exotoxins. These proteins are involved in signal transduction and regulation of cellular function either by cAMP levels or kinase cascades leading to transcription modification. For example:

- G proteins (stimulatory or inhibitory of adenyl cyclase) cholera, pertussis, *E. coli* LT toxin
- elongation factor 2 (translational control); diphtheria toxin
- rho proteins (small G proteins; regulate actin cytoskeleton); inactivated by *C. difficile* A and B toxins and can also be activated by deamination by pertussis necrotising toxin.

The structure of these toxins consists either of A:B5 (enzyme active A subunit and $5 \times$ B subunits required for binding) or A:B type with A (enzyme active) and B (binding) domains on a single polypeptide chain. A:B5 types are seen in cholera and pertussis (whooping cough), *E. coli* LT1 and LT2. A:B types are encountered in diphtheria, botulism and tetanus.

It is fascinating to compare the contrasting actions between two structurally similar neurotoxins produced by members of the same bacterial family, *C. tetani* and *C. botulinum*, which cause tetanus and botulism respectively. These diseases are purely due to toxin-mediated action following infection and are quite different in pathology, yet the molecular action of the two toxins is identical. They are both endopeptidases specific for synaptobrevin, a protein found in the cytoplasm of synaptic vesicles. However, the binding (B) domains of the toxins show different specificities for cell receptors. Tetanus toxin binds to the gangliosides of the neuronal membrane, is internalized and moves by retroaxonal transport from peripheral nerves to the CNS, where it is released from the post-synaptic dendrites and localizes in presynaptic nerve terminals. This blocks the release of inhibitory neurotransmitter, γ-aminobutyric acid to cause unopposed, continuous excitatory synaptic activity, leading to spastic paralysis. Botulism toxin binds ganglioside receptors of cholinergic synapses and prevents release of acetycholine at the neuromuscular junctions, causing flaccid paralysis (Fig. 2.7).

Key facts

Main sources and effects of bacterial toxins

Toxin	Bacteria	Effect
Endotoxin	G-ve lipopolysaccharide	Fever and inflammatory cell stimulation
Exotoxins		
Neurotoxins	*Clostridium tetani*	Disordered neuromuscular transmission
	Clostridium botulinum	(tetanus and botulism)
Enterotoxins (infectious diarrhoea)	*Vibrio cholera, E. coli, Bacillus cereus*	Diarrhoea
Enterotoxins (food poisoning)	*Staphylococcus aureus* *Bacillus cereus*	Diarrhoea and vomiting
Tissue-invasive toxins	*Staphylococcus aureus* *Streptococcus pyogenes* *Clostridium perfringens*	Tissue destruction by enzymes
Pyrogenic toxins	*Staphylococcus aureus* *Streptococcus pyogenes*	Toxic shock syndrome Scarlet fever
Verotoxins	*E. coli* (O157:H7)	Haemolytic uraemic syndrome
Miscellaneous	*Bordetella pertussis* *Corynebacteria diphtheria* *Clostridium difficile*	Whooping cough Diphtheria (heart and nerve damage) Pseudomembranous colitis

Figure 2.6 Cholera toxin permanently activates a Gs protein in the intestinal cell wall. The diagram shows an intestinal cell in the normal state (top) and affected by cholera toxin (below); the diagrams are mirror images with the intestinal lumen in the middle. Cells in the intestinal villus: Na^+ and Cl_2^- absorption is blocked by cholera toxin. Crypt cells: this is the site most affected by cholera toxin. Here Cl_2^- secretion is stimulated. Water passively follows the active ion transport. Dehydration occurs. Although the main Na^+ absorption path (Na^+/H^+ exchange) is blocked by cholera toxin, Na^+ can be co-transported with glucose or amino acids, which is why oral rehydration solutions using glucose are effective in cholera. (Courtesy of Professor Phil Butcher, St George's, University of London)

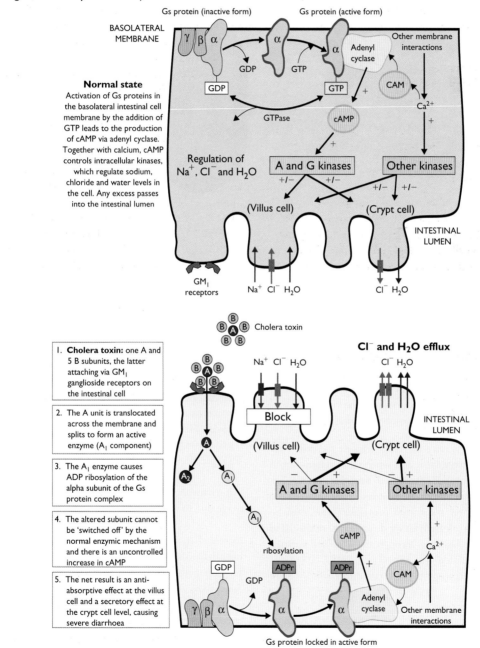

Figure 2.7 Botulinus toxin binds ganglioside receptors of cholinergic synapses and prevents release of acetycholine at the neuromuscular junctions, causing flaccid paralysis

Motor Nerve
Ganglioside receptor blocked
ACH is not released
ACH
ACH
ACH
ACH
Botulinus toxin
ACH receptors
Neuromuscular junction
Muscle not stimulated to contract

DIRECT CELL DAMAGE BY VIRUSES

Microorganisms can also damage cells directly and this is particularly true of viruses. Viruses are obligate intracellular organisms requiring the host cell's machinery for replication (see Figs 2.9–2.11 and Table 2.3). Viruses use three main methods for entering cells:

- translocation of the entire virus through the cell membrane
- fusion of the viral envelope with the cell membrane
- receptor-mediated endocytosis of the virus, followed by fusion with the endosome membrane.

What happens once the virus is inside the cell? First the particle must uncoat and separate its genome from its structural components. It then uses specific enzymes of its own or present in the host cell to synthesize viral genome, enzyme and capsid proteins. These must be assembled and released, either directly (unencapsulated viruses) or by budding through the host cell's membrane (encapsulated viruses).

Viruses can damage the host cell directly in a variety of ways:

- interference with host cell synthesis of DNA, RNA or proteins (e.g. polio virus modifying ribosomes so that they no longer recognize host mRNA)
- lysis of host cells (e.g. polio virus lyses neurons)

Figure 2.8 Sites of action of antibacterial drugs

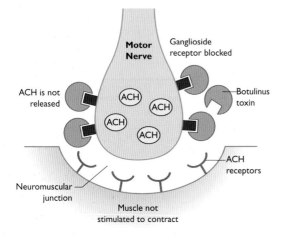

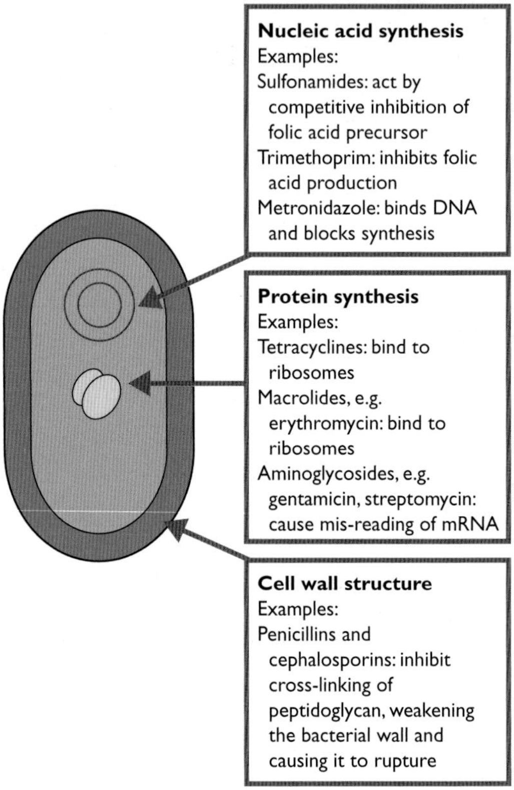

Nucleic acid synthesis
Examples:
Sulfonamides: act by competitive inhibition of folic acid precursor
Trimethoprim: inhibits folic acid production
Metronidazole: binds DNA and blocks synthesis
Protein synthesis
Examples:
Tetracyclines: bind to ribosomes
Macrolides, e.g. erythromycin: bind to ribosomes
Aminoglycosides, e.g. gentamicin, streptomycin: cause mis-reading of mRNA
Cell wall structure
Examples:
Penicillins and cephalosporins: inhibit cross-linking of peptidoglycan, weakening the bacterial wall and causing it to rupture

- inserting proteins into host cell membrane so provoking an immune attack by host cytotoxic lymphocytes (e.g. hepatitis B and liver cells)
- inserting proteins into host cell membrane to cause direct damage or promote cell fusion (e.g. herpes, measles, HIV)
- transforming host cells into malignant tumours (e.g. EBV, papilloma virus, HTLV-1).

Alternatively, the host cell may suffer secondary damage due to viral infection. This may be due to:

- increased susceptibility to infection due to damaged host defences (e.g. influenza viral damage to respiratory epithelium facilitates bacterial pneumonia with *Staphylococcus aureus*, HIV depletes $CD4^+$ T cells, allowing opportunistic infections such as *Pneuomocystis carinii* pneumonia)
- death or atrophy of cells dependent on viral-damaged cell (e.g. muscle cell atrophy after motor neuron damage by polio virus).

Table 2.3 Outline classification of viruses (see also Figs 2.9–2.11)

Nucleic acid	Symmetry	Envelope	Strand	Family	Example
RNA	Icosahedral	No	SS1	Picorna	Polio, coxsackie
			DS	Reo	Rotavirus
		Yes	SS	Toga	Rubella (rubivirus)
				Flavi	Yellow fever
	Helical	Yes	SS1	Corona	Colds
			SS2	Orthomyxo	Influenza A, B and C
				Paramyxo	Mumps, measles
				Rhabdo	Rabies
	Complex	Complex	SS1	Retro	HIV, HTLV
DNA	Icosahedral	No	SS linear	Parvo	Aplastic anaemia
			DS circular	Papova	Papillomavirus
			DS linear	Adeno	Colds
		Yes	DS linear	Herpes	Herpes simplex
					Varicella zoster
					Cytomegalovirus
					Epstein–Barr virus
			DS circular	Hepadna	Hepatitis B
	Complex	Complex	DS linear	Pox	Smallpox

SS, single strand; DS, double strand.

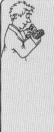

Dictionary

Viral infection can be:

Persistent: virions synthesized continuously, e.g. hepatitis B

Latent: virions temporarily inactive, e.g. herpes zoster in dorsal root ganglia

Abortive: incomplete viral replication

Although the majority of infectious disease is due to bacteria and viruses, there are other categories which are just as important, and which have evolved their own mechanisms for bypassing host defences and causing disease. Briefly, these are the fungi, protozoa, parasites, helminths and prion proteins.

PROTOZOA

Protozoa are free-living, single-celled eucaryotes with nuclei, endoplasmic reticulum, mitochondria and organelles. They ingest nutrients through a cytosome and can reproduce sexually and asexually. Most are able to form cysts when in hostile environments (Table 2.4).

Table 2.4 Examples of protozoa that cause human disease

Organism	Disease
Toxoplasma gondii*†	Cerebral, ocular, lymphoid and lung damage
Plasmodium (falciparum, vivax, ovale and malariae)	Malaria
Leishmania (various)	Cutaneous and visceral leishmaniasis (Fig. 2.12)
Trypanosoma (various)	Sleeping sickness and Chagas' disease
Pneumocystis carinii*†	Interstitial pneumonia
Entamoeba histolytica	Diarrhoea
Giardia lamblia	
Cryptosporidia*	
Isospora*	
Acanthamoeba*	Amoebic meningitis
Naegleri fowleri	
Trichomonas	Vaginal discharge

*People with defective immune systems are more liable to have significant problems with these organisms.
†Problems often relate to reactivation because the immune defences are reduced rather than there being a primary infection.

Figure 2.9 After attaching to the host cell via a receptor, the viral particle enters the cell by fusion of the viral and host cell membranes or by receptor-mediated endocytosis. It then uncoats and releases its nucleic acid. Replication occurs either in the cytoplasm alone, as with most RNA viruses and rare DNA viruses (the pox viruses), or involves both cytoplasmic and nuclear steps. DNA viruses can integrate directly with the host DNA but the only RNA viruses that can achieve nuclear integration are the retroviruses

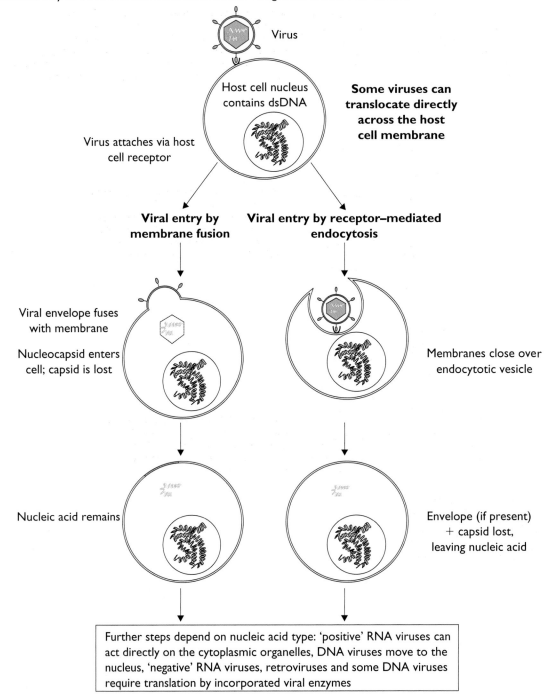

Virus

Host cell nucleus contains dsDNA

Some viruses can translocate directly across the host cell membrane

Virus attaches via host cell receptor

Viral entry by membrane fusion

Viral entry by receptor–mediated endocytosis

Viral envelope fuses with membrane

Nucleocapsid enters cell; capsid is lost

Membranes close over endocytotic vesicle

Nucleic acid remains

Envelope (if present) + capsid lost, leaving nucleic acid

Further steps depend on nucleic acid type: 'positive' RNA viruses can act directly on the cytoplasmic organelles, DNA viruses move to the nucleus, 'negative' RNA viruses, retroviruses and some DNA viruses require translation by incorporated viral enzymes

Figure 2.10 Retroviruses, like DNA viruses, can insert their genes into the host cell DNA, but require an additional step. Their RNA is translated into DNA by reverse transcriptase, supplied by the virus

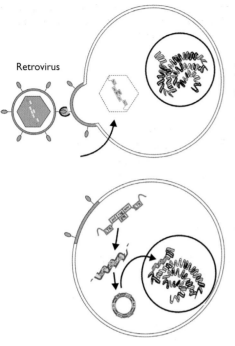

Retrovirus binds to a human surface receptor (e.g. HIV-1 virus binds using its gp120 antigen to human CD4 on T lymphocytes). The viral RNA contains the following genes: *pol* (encodes reverse transcriptase and integrase), *gag* (encodes viral structural proteins), *env* (encodes envelope proteins, including gp120), *reg* (encodes regulatory genes, e.g. *tat, rev*)

The viral and host cell membranes fuse, the viral capsid disintegrates and viral RNA enters the human cell. Viral reverse transcriptase catalyses the production of double-stranded DNA, which enters the host cell nucleus and integrates into host DNA under the influence of integrase

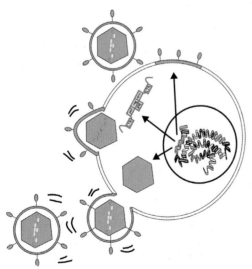

The host cell is induced to manufacture and assemble new virions by long terminal repeat sequences and genes *tat* and *rev*. The new virions peel off an envelope of host cell membrane as they exit

A

Viral particles continually manufactured by host cell. Cell remains intact; virus particles exit, some taking part of the cell membrane as an envelope

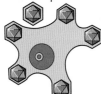

If virus is not cleared by immune mechanisms, replication and inflammation continue, e.g. hepatitis B or C infection may lead to cirrhosis

B

After a transient illness, viral DNA integrates into host nuclear DNA and lies dormant

Viral DNA

C

Infected cell manufactures new viral particles, released by the rupture of the host cell, which is destroyed

← Virus

D

Tumour formation, e.g. hepatitis B virus (hepatocellular carcinoma), Epstein–Barr virus (Burkitt's lymphoma, nasopharyngeal carcinoma, Hodgkin's lymphoma)

E

Reactivation of latent infection in a debilitated or immunosuppressed patient, e.g. herpes simplex (cold sore, genital ulcer), varicella zoster (shingles)

Figure 2.11A–E Possible outcomes in human cells infected by virus in which viral clearance is not achieved by the host's immune mechanisms

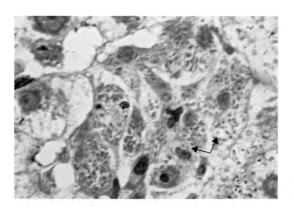

Figure 2.12 *Leishmania,* a parasitic flagellate protozoan (arrows)

HELMINTHS

Helminths or worms can usually be seen by the naked eye. They may be round (nematodes) or flat (platyhelminths). See Table 2.5.

Table 2.5 Examples of helminths that cause human disease

Helminth	Disease
Platyhelminths	
Schistosoma (various)	Schistosomiasis (liver, lung, gut and bladder damage) (Fig. 2.13)
Echinococcus	Hydatid disease
Taenia solium, Taenia saginata and *Diphyllobothrium latum*	Tapeworm infestation from pig, cow and fish
Nematodes	
Necator, Trichuris	Hookworm, whipworm (gut infestation)
Wucheria, Onchocerca	Elephantiasis, river blindness, filariasis

FUNGI

Fungi are eucaryotic cells requiring an aerobic environment. Athlete's foot is a common, but seldom life-threatening, fungal infection. Most fungal infection is relatively rare unless a person is immunosuppressed. See Table 2.6.

Table 2.6 Examples of fungi that cause human disease

Fungus	Disease
Microsporum, Trichophyton (dermatophytes)	Ringworm, athlete's foot, etc.
Histoplasma capsulatum	Pneumonia or disseminated disease
Aspergillus (various)	Pneumonia or disseminated disease (Fig. 2.14)
Candida, Cryptococcus, Coccidioides	Disseminated disease in immuno-suppressed individuals

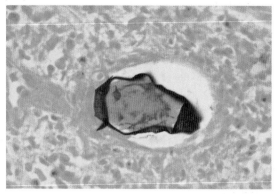

Figure 2.13 Ovum from a schistosome, one of the platyhelminths

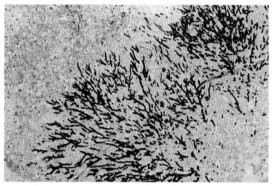

Figure 2.14 *Aspergillus*

SUBCELLULAR INFECTIOUS AGENTS

This is a short section but we should flag up our ignorance concerning certain diseases and some 'infectious' particles. There is great interest in transmissible spongiform encephalopathies which can produce progressive and fatal brain damage in humans (kuru), sheep (scrapie) and cows (bovine spongiform encephalopathy (BSE) or 'mad cow' disease). These diseases are experimentally and naturally transmissible with no viruses or bacteria detectable. Prion proteins have been proposed as the cause. These are naturally occurring proteins in most mammals. Their role is not entirely clear, but it seems that they are important in the differentiation of neurones. Prion proteins may be induced to change shape, either spontaneously (as in sporadic Creutzfeld–Jacob disease (CJD)) or if a mutant or foreign prion protein enters the cell (e.g. variant CJD, thought to be the human equivalent of BSE, caught from infected cattle). The particle is protein without any evidence of nucleic acid. Its neurotoxic effects are thought to be due to abnormal folding, brought about by a mutation of just a few amino acids, which inactivates the normal relationship between the cytoskeletal components and the proteasome. The misfolding seems to be catching, and once it has begun, the normal protein also becomes misfolded. The effects are to cause degeneration of the brain, which develops a sponge-like texture ('spongiform encephalopathy'). The disease is characterized by problems with co-ordination, rapidly progressive dementia and death.

HYPERSENSITIVITY AND AUTOIMMUNE DISEASE

The phenomenon of damage caused by the immune system while trying to combat an insult is referred to as hypersensitivity. As a cause, it is partially 'intrinsic' and partially 'extrinsic'. The precipitating factor may be an external agent but, instead of the immune system coping and restoring the body's homeostasis, the immune response is altered and becomes the 'internal' cause of the disease.

Four main types of hypersensitivity reaction were described by Gell and Coombs, although several types may operate together. Types I–III involve antibodies, type IV involves cells.

The mechanisms involved are:

- release of allergic mediators in type I (anaphylactic) hypersensitivity
- binding of self-reactive antibodies to cells in type II (antibody-dependent cytotoxic) hypersensitivity
- damage to blood vessel walls and tissues by circulating immune complexes in type III (immune complex-mediated) hypersensitivity
- delayed tissue damage due to interactions between sensitized T lymphocytes and other inflammatory cells in type IV (cell-mediated) hypersensitivity.

TYPE I: ANAPHYLACTIC HYPERSENSITIVITY

This is the mechanism behind atopic allergies such as asthma, eczema, hay fever and reactions to certain food. Patients who suffer from this problem have been previously exposed to the allergen and have generated IgE antibodies against it. The IgE antibodies attach to mast

Figure 2.15 Type I hypersensitivity

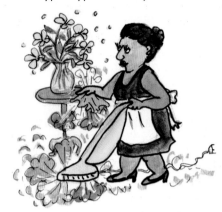

First exposure: nasal and bronchial mucosa exposed to pollen, dust etc.

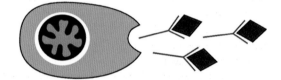

Soluble antigen stimulates production of IgE antibodies

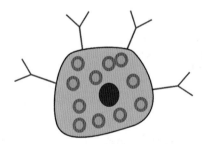

Fc component of IgE attaches to receptor on mucosal mast cell

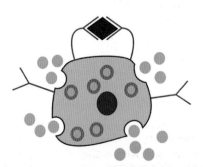

Second exposure to pollen: cross-linking of IgE molecules on mast cell stimulates release of primary and secondary inflammatory mediators

cells via cell surface receptors. A common feature of many allergens is that they have abundant repetition of the same antigenic determinant on their surface. This means that cross-linking of IgE molecules attached to the same mast cell is likely. It is cross-linkage which activates the mast cell.

Re-exposure produces an immediate reaction to the offending agent! The extrinsic allergen (e.g. grass pollen, house dust mite faeces, seafood) binds to IgE on the surface of mast cells in the mucosa of the bronchial tree, nose, gut or conjunctivae, leading to the release of chemical mediators (Fig. 2.15).

Some mediators, such as histamine, are already formed within mast cell granules and the cross-linking of IgE molecules attached to the mast cell surface stimulates the release of the granule contents into the tissues (Fig. 2.16). This is why the effect of antigen exposure can be seen within 5 minutes; the granule contents elicit an inflammatory response which lasts up to an hour.

In the meantime, the cross-linked IgE molecules stimulate the membrane of the mast cell to generate arachidonic acid and its metabolites within its cell membrane. Release of leukotrienes, prostaglandins and platelet activating factor by this mechanism sparks a response which starts 8–12 hours later and may last from 24 to 36 hours.

Generally, the mediators released by these processes act locally but they can also produce life-threatening systemic effects. Effects include constriction of smooth muscle in bronchi and bronchioles, causing wheezing, dilatation and increased permeability of capillaries resulting in localized tissue oedema, increased nasal and bronchial secretions, red watery eyes, skin rashes and diarrhoea. If laryngeal oedema or bronchospasm is severe, death may result from respiratory obstruction.

What can be done about this problem? Antihistamines antagonize the action of histamine and can relieve many of the symptoms. Steroids, which inhibit the leukotriene pathway, can prevent or alleviate the longer term symptoms.

If an 'atopic' patient knows he is likely to encounter an antigen on a particular occasion (e.g. pollen in a hay fever sufferer) he may be able to take drugs which stabilize the mast cell membrane, reducing or preventing its activation.

A course of injections of a very dilute solution of the offending allergen can eventually lead to IgG instead of IgE being generated; since IgG does not stick to mast cells, the problem is avoided. But care must be taken with this approach not to generate anaphylactic shock, a life-threatening complication. In this condition, the patient must be injected immediately, subcutaneously,

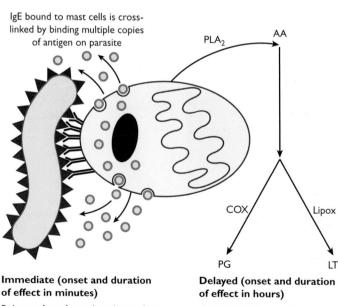

IgE bound to mast cells is cross-linked by binding multiple copies of antigen on parasite

PLA$_2$ AA

COX Lipox

PG LT

Immediate (onset and duration of effect in minutes)

Release of pre-formed mediators from granules, including histamine and lysosyme

Delayed (onset and duration of effect in hours)

Generation of arachidonic acid metabolites

Figure 2.16 Mast cell activation is typically stimulated by IgE antibody cross-linkage as illustrated here, but this is not always necessary. Mast cells can also be directly stimulated by some substances, e.g. mellitin from bee stings or C3a5a complement fragments. PLA$_2$ = phospholipase A$_2$; AA = arachidonic acid, COX = cycle oxygenase; Lipox = lipoxygenase; PG = prostaglandins; LT = leukotrienes.

with adrenaline, which reverses the actions of the mediators causing bronchospasm and oedema. Patients known to be susceptible to this type of response (often to bee stings or peanut protein) carry an 'Epipen' with them, which can deliver a single dose of adrenaline (epinephrine). The action of adrenaline lasts only a finite time, and patients should also be given antihistamine or steroids as back-up.

TYPE II: ANTIBODY-DEPENDENT CYTOTOXIC HYPERSENSITIVITY

In this type of hypersensitivity, antibodies react with antigens *fixed to the surfaces* of various types of body cell to cause damage. The effects can be categorized as complement fixing or functional.

In the complement fixing type, antibodies bind to an antigen, fix complement and so cause the destruction of the target cell (cytolysis, e.g. rhesus disease) or damage the surrounding structures (e.g. Goodpasture's syndrome).

Figure 2.18 illustrates rhesus incompatibility where rhesus antibodies from a Rh− mother cross the placenta to damage the red cells of a Rh+ baby. In Goodpasture's syndrome, antibodies bind to basement membranes in renal glomeruli to damage the surrounding structures and the ability of the kidney to act as a filter.

In the functional type, antibody binding interferes with cell function (often by interfering with hormone receptors, but also with cell growth and differentiation or cell motility). Included in this group are antibodies that block cell function (as in some forms of Addison's disease, in which autoantibodies develop to several adrenocortical proteins) or which stimulate receptor function (as in Graves' disease, causing thyrotoxicosis; Fig. 2.17). Some people split off the last group into a separate hypersensitivity type (type V, stimulatory hypersensitivity).

It is worth remembering that the body is not only on the lookout for foreign organisms, but is generally pretty xenophobic when it comes to cells from another human. Consider, for example, blood transfusion. It is essential that any blood which is transfused into a patient is first cross-matched to ensure that the recipient does not possess antibodies to antigens on the donor red blood cells. This is because the donor red cells will become coated with antibody and/or complement which may promote phagocytosis due to opsonisation, via the Fc or C3b, or fix complement to produce cell membrane damage through C8 and C9 membrane attack complex.

Type II reactions are also involved in some drug reactions (e.g. chlorpromazine-induced haemolytic anaemia and quinidine-induced agranulocytosis). The binding of a drug may alter a normal self antigen and thus something which can no longer be tolerated.

Natural killer cells, which are not restricted by HLA type, can kill through antibody dependent cell-mediated cytotoxicity (ADCC) which may be important for killing large parasites or tumour cells.

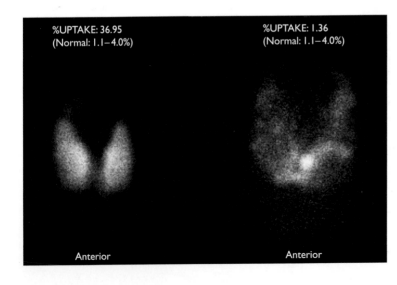

%UPTAKE: 36.95
(Normal: 1.1–4.0%)

%UPTAKE: 1.36
(Normal: 1.1–4.0%)

Anterior

Anterior

Figure 2.17 The scan on the left shows smooth symmetrical enlargement of both lobes of the thyroid gland with markedly increased uptake in a patient with hyperthyroidism related to Graves' disease. Compare the size and uptake with the normal thyroid scan on the right

Figure 2.18 Type II hypersensitivity: rhesus incompatibility

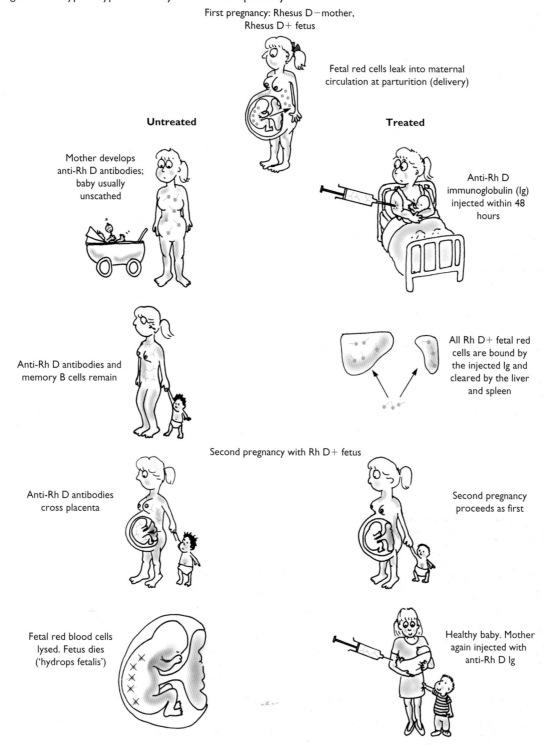

First pregnancy: Rhesus D− mother, Rhesus D+ fetus

Fetal red cells leak into maternal circulation at parturition (delivery)

Untreated

Treated

Mother develops anti-Rh D antibodies; baby usually unscathed

Anti-Rh D immunoglobulin (Ig) injected within 48 hours

Anti-Rh D antibodies and memory B cells remain

All Rh D+ fetal red cells are bound by the injected Ig and cleared by the liver and spleen

Second pregnancy with Rh D+ fetus

Anti-Rh D antibodies cross placenta

Second pregnancy proceeds as first

Fetal red blood cells lysed. Fetus dies ('hydrops fetalis')

Healthy baby. Mother again injected with anti-Rh D Ig

TYPE III: IMMUNE COMPLEX MEDIATED HYPERSENSITIVITY

Like type II, this is an antibody-driven process, but the difference is that antibodies react with free antigen and, under the right circumstances they can form soluble immune complexes which circulate in the blood, giving rise to 'serum sickness'. Immune complexes are only soluble when the ratio of antibody to antigen is roughly equal. Thus the complexes can be insoluble; these forms are usually precipitated at the site where antigen first encounters antibody (known as the Arthus reaction, after an experimental model of the disease which involved injecting pre-sensitized animals with an allergen; the animals developed tissue reactions at the site of injection. Don't confuse this antibody-mediated reaction with type IV, see next section!).

Both the soluble and the insoluble types of complex can activate macrophages, aggregate platelets and initiate the complement cascade. Circulating immune complexes can lodge in the small vessels of many organs to cause a

History   **Nicholas Arthus** (1862–1945)

Nicholas Arthus was a French physiologist who started working on anaphylaxis in 1903. He used subcutaneous injections of horse serum into rabbits and observed the increasing severity of the local response with repeated administrations and also the systemic response if the serum was injected intravenously. He did similar work using snake venoms and recognized that cobra venom produces death through respiratory arrest whereas Russell viper venom causes massive blood coagulation. By using repeated small doses or pre-treating the venom with formalin, he noted that he was able to provide some protection to the animals.

Dictionary

Exogenous antigen: an antigen originating from outside the body

Figure 2.19 Type III hypersensitivity, e.g. farmer's lung (an example of extrinsic allergic alveolitis)

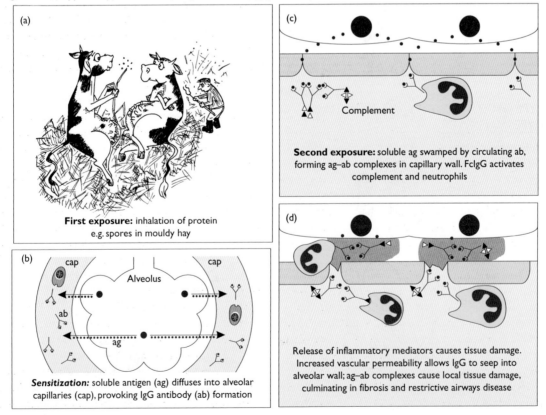

(a) **First exposure:** inhalation of protein e.g. spores in mouldy hay

(b) **Sensitization:** soluble antigen (ag) diffuses into alveolar capillaries (cap), provoking IgG antibody (ab) formation

(c) Complement. **Second exposure:** soluble ag swamped by circulating ab, forming ag–ab complexes in capillary wall. FcIgG activates complement and neutrophils

(d) Release of inflammatory mediators causes tissue damage. Increased vascular permeability allows IgG to seep into alveolar wall; ag–ab complexes cause local tissue damage, culminating in fibrosis and restrictive airways disease

vasculitis (inflammation of the blood vessel wall), principally affecting the kidney (glomerulonephritis), skin and joints. An Arthus-type reaction is encountered clinically in the lung after an exogenous antigen is inhaled and precipitates locally within the alveolar walls.

The inhaled antigens are usually animal or plant proteins and are often associated with specific occupations. The resulting damage to lung alveoli, with repeated episodes of inflammation and scarring, leads to a restrictive form of lung disease called extrinsic allergic alveolitis (Fig. 2.19).

TYPE IV: CELL MEDIATED (DELAYED TYPE) HYPERSENSITIVITY

Unlike the other three forms of hypersensitivity, all of which involve antibody, type IV involves T lymphocytes which, over several hours and days, recruit and activate other T cells and macrophages and produce local tissue damage and granuloma formation. The antigen stimulates T cells to release IL-2, interferon-γ and other cytokines. Recruitment of other cells follows the usual pathways – see Fig. 6.8 on page 145.

This type of hypersensitivity reaction can occur in response to many infective and non-infective causes, such as viruses, fungi, bacteria and insect bites and is often responsible for the contact dermatitis related to simple chemicals. Clinically, it is extremely important in the rejection of transplanted tissue and graft-versus-host reactions.

Hypersensitivity can be useful! The Mantoux test (tuberculin test) takes advantage of this reaction to see whether a person has some T-cell immunity to tuberculosis. This involves injecting a small amount of a (non-infectious) purified protein derivative of *Mycobacterium tuberculosis* into the skin and observing whether a localized red induration occurs over the next 48 hours; T cells and macrophages mount a type IV reaction in a sensitized person. This test is not 100 per cent sure, since some patients with overwhelming tuberculous infection are anergic and show no reaction (Fig. 2.20).

NUTRITIONAL DISEASES

For centuries, the major problems in nutrition were centred around deficiencies. Too little protein resulted in kwashiorkor; too few calories in the first year of life produced marasmus. Other diets lacked one or more vitamins or minerals because the variety of foodstuffs was not available. These problems, sadly, still exist in some developing countries but, in the developed world, malnutrition is more likely to be a consequence of bowel problems, other illnesses or psycho-social issues; while *nutritional imbalance* has become a major public health problem for otherwise healthy people. The key point is that nutritional imbalance for normal adults is a choice, and does not have a biological cause.

The commonest imbalance is ingesting too much. The consequence of excess calorie intake is obesity with its long-term effects on cardiovascular disease, diabetes, osteoarthritis and some cancers. The other most commonly over-ingested substance is alcohol. Chronic alcoholism is now known to produce most of its damage through direct toxic effects rather than secondary to nutritional deficiencies and results in CNS atrophy, cardiomyopathy, peptic ulcers, pancreatitis, liver damage, varices, testicular atrophy and upper gastro-intestinal tumours. We are now becoming much more aware of the effects of other imbalances in our diet. Too much salt worsens hypertension; too much fat increases the amount of atheroma and the risk of heart attack and strokes, certain foods (e.g. smoked foods) may increase gastro-intestinal tumours.

These are lifestyle choices for most people but some are unfortunate and have specific problems with ingesting, absorbing, metabolising or controlling excretion of essential nutrients (see Table 2.7).

These conditions mostly affect general nutrition and this is what you will most commonly see, especially in those with chronic illness. Specific deficiencies are less

Figure 2.20 Type IV hypersensitivity: Mantoux test reaction

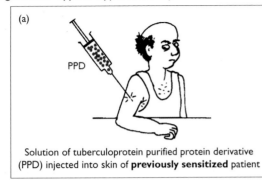

(a)

PPD

Solution of tuberculoprotein purified protein derivative (PPD) injected into skin of **previously sensitized** patient

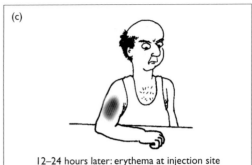

(c)

12–24 hours later: erythema at injection site

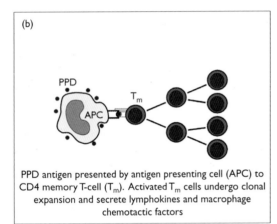

(b)

PPD

APC

T_m

PPD antigen presented by antigen presenting cell (APC) to CD4 memory T-cell (T_m). Activated T_m cells undergo clonal expansion and secrete lymphokines and macrophage chemotactic factors

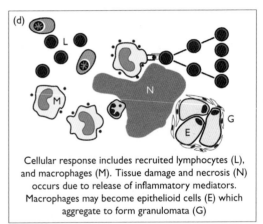

(d)

L

M

N

E

G

Cellular response includes recruited lymphocytes (L), and macrophages (M). Tissue damage and necrosis (N) occurs due to release of inflammatory mediators. Macrophages may become epithelioid cells (E) which aggregate to form granulomata (G)

Table 2.7 Conditions affecting general nutrition	
Mechanism	Example
Reduced ingestion	Psychiatric illness
	Anorexia, e.g. linked to malignancy or chronic illness
	Food allergy
	Gastrointestinal disorders
Reduced absorption	Gut hypermotility
	Inflammatory bowel damage
	Pancreatic or biliary disease
	Achlorhydria
Abnormal metabolism	Malignancy
	Hypothyroidism
	Liver disease
Increased excretion	Diarrhoea
Increased demand	Fever
	Pregnancy and lactation
	Hyperthyroidism

common with iron, folate, vitamin D and vitamin B12 probably being most important. If you are working in areas where nutrition is poor then make sure that you are aware of the clinical effects of all of them (see below Table 2.8).

COELIAC DISEASE: GENETIC PREDISPOSITION AND HYPERSENSITIVITY

Coeliac disease is an example of a genetic *predisposition* to disease. In such patients, inherited characteristics which are dictated by the MHC type I or II molecules on the surfaces of all nucleated cells (type I) or antigen-presenting cells (type II) mean that a person is at increased risk of developing a particular disease. Coeliac patients almost always have either MHC molecules of HLA DQ2 or DQ8 type displayed by their antigen-presenting cells (APC).

Table 2.8 Clinical consequences of malnutrition	
Nutrient deficiency	**Clinical effect**
Calories	Fat loss
	Muscle wasting
	Organ atrophy
	Growth failure in children
Protein (Kwashiorkor)	As above but without fat loss and with oedema and fatty liver
Fat-soluble vitamins	
A	Epithelial changes affecting eyes, skin and viscera
D	Rickets and osteomalacia
E	Neuromuscular degeneration
K	Haemorrhagic disease of newborn
	Effect on anticoagulants
Water-soluble vitamins	
C	Scurvy (bleeding, poor wound healing, bone lesions)
B1 (thiamine)	Beriberi (neural, cardiac and cerebral problems)
B12 (cyanocobalamin)	Pernicious anaemia
Niacin	Pellagra (dermatitis, dementia, diarrhoea)
Folate	
B1, B2 (riboflavin)	Megaloblastic anaemia
	Ocular lesions, glossitis, stomatitis
B6 (pyridoxine)	Infant convulsions, anaemia, dermatitis, glossitis
Iron	Microcytic, hypochromic anaemia
Copper	Nerve and muscle dysfunction
Iodine	Goitre
Zinc	Growth retardation and infertility
Selenium	Myopathy and cardiomyopathy

If gluten molecules enter the lamina propria of the small intestine in an undigested state they may trigger an immune response. Why this should happen has not yet been fully elucidated.

The key to the genetic element is that people with DQ2 or 8 have MHC type II molecules on the surfaces of their antigen presenting cells which can easily bind and display gluten peptides, especially if they have been altered by the tissue enzyme tTG (tissue transglutaminase). The immune response causes enterocyte destruction, local inflammation in the lamina propria and the formation of specific coeliac antibodies. Removal of gluten from the diet is curative and prevents long-term complications of the disease.

Affected people develop coeliac disease when sufficient enterocytes disappear. This causes microscopically visible flattening of the intestinal villi and reduces the available absorptive surface. Patients with coeliac disease suffer from malabsorption of all types of food. Typically osteoporosis may develop, but occasionally osteomalacia, because vitamin D is poorly absorbed.

Treatment is by withdrawal of the stimulus, gluten, and this is usually sufficient to reverse the process. Patients with coeliac disease often suffer from other 'autoimmune' diseases, such as diabetes mellitus (type I) and thyroid diseases. See Figs 2.21 and 2.22, and the clinical scenario.

GENETIC CAUSES OF DISEASE

In considering the Origin of Species, it is quite conceivable that a naturalist, reflecting on the mutual affinities of organic beings, on their embryological relations, their geographical distribution, geological succession, and other such facts, might come to the conclusion that each species had not been independently created, but had descended, like varieties from other species.

Charles Darwin

Since genetic disorders are fundamental to so many diseases, we will illustrate the section on intrinsic causes of disease by using examples of disease mediated via the genes. As with the section on infective agents, this is a massive topic and one that is expanding rapidly.

It is a common misconception amongst medical students that pathology is an exact science. It is sometimes difficult to see why the examination of tissues at

Figure 2.22 Coeliac disease occurs in genetically predisposed individuals who are exposed to gluten molecules that enter the lamina propria in an undigested state. A reaction to gluten in these patients causes enterocyte destruction and local inflammation in the lamina propria. Removal of gluten from the diet is curative and prevents long-term complications of the disease. (APC, antigen-presenting cells; tTG, tissue transglutaminase enzyme; MMP, matrix metalloproteinases; EMA, endomysial antibodies)

Normal duodenum

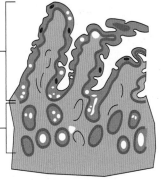

Normal slender villi with few intra-epithelial lymphocytes

Crypt to villus ratio 1:3

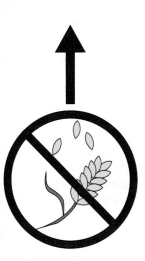

- Coeliac disease is initiated at any age by the inappropriate absorption of whole gluten molecules.

- Lamina propria macrophages engulf gluten, become activated and secrete IL-15. This makes enterocytes display a 'stress-protein' on their surfaces, to which intraepithelial natural killer (NK) cells bind, inducing apoptosis.

- Lamina propria APC also engulf gluten and present peptides to CD4+ cells via MHC II molecules. Some gluten peptides, deamidated by tTG prior to engulfment, fit grooves in MHC type II molecules encoded by the MHC genes in DQ2 or DQ8+ individuals.

- CD4+ cells are activated and stimulate humoral (B cell, antibody) and cell-mediated (CD8+ T cell) responses. CD8+ cells cause enterocytes to undergo apoptosis.

- Anti-gliadin and anti-tTG antibodies are secreted – mainly IgA type, but also IgG, useful for diagnosis. About 4 percent of coeliac patients lack IgA.

- Activated T cells secrete IFNγ, which induces macrophages and fibroblasts in the lamina propria to secrete MMP. These damage basement membrane and other proteins and evoke an inflammatory response.

Gluten induced enteropathy (coeliac disease)

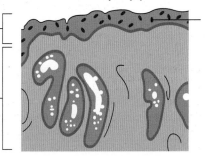

Near total villous atrophy

Lymphocytes

Crypt elongation inflammation in lamina propria (LP) and increased lymphocytes in the surface epithelium (arrow)

Clinicopathological case study   coeliac disease

Clinical

A slightly built 25-year-old woman consulted her family doctor. She complained of tiredness and breathlessness on exertion, worse over the last 6 months. On examination, she was of medium height (1 m 65 cm), low weight (50 kg) (Fig. 2.21) and had pale, mucous membranes. Her doctor pointed out some bruising over her shins; she did not recall the injury but commented that she had bruised easily over recent months.

Pathology

Pallor and symptoms suggest anaemia. Iron deficiency due to menorrhagia is the most common cause of anaemia in a young woman, but bruising would be unusual.

Investigations were as follows

Hb: 9.6 g/dL (N 11–13.5)
MCV: 86 fL (N 78–95)
WCC: 3.8 × 10^9/L (N 3–5.5)
Platelets : 330 × 10^{12}/L (N150–400)
Red cell folate: 152 μg/L (N150–750)
Vitamin B12: 68 ng/L (N 150–1000)
Iron: 13 μmol/L (N 14–30)
INR: 2.5 (N 0.8–1.1)

Microcytic anaemia is the hallmark of iron deficiency and macrocytic anaemia typically indicates folic acid and/or vitamin B12 deficiency. This patient has a low serum iron and low normal red cell folate and her anaemia is normocytic, which means that the average red cell size is normal.

Prolonged prothrombin time, measured as the INR (internal normalized ratio), is likely to be due to decreased vitamin K causing a deficiency of clotting factors (see Table 2.8).

Provisional clinical diagnosis: malabsorption, probably due to coeliac disease (gluten induced enteropathy)

The incidence of coeliac disease in the UK is approximately 1:300 people; Ireland has the highest rate at 1:100 people. Many patients have subclinical disease.

Management and progress

She was referred for investigation at the gastroenterology clinic in her local hospital. The results of the investigations were as follows:

Subtotal villous atrophy with crypt hyperplasia and increased intra-epithelial lymphocytes is the typical microscopical appearance in coeliac disease, due to increased destruction of enterocytes by a T-cell mediated reaction (Fig. 2.22).

- upper GI endoscopy and duodenal biopsy macroscopically normal, but biopsy showed subtotal villous atrophy and increased intraepithelial lymphocytes
- serology for anti-gliadin and other coeliac-disease-related antibodies was positive
- bone density scan showed early osteoporosis.

Anti-tTG and IgA anti-endomysial antibody is positive in 95 per cent untreated coeliacs. Anti-gliadin antibodies are also often positive but can be less specific. Two to four per cent of coeliac patients are IgA deficient, so IgG antibodies are also tested for. The mild osteoporosis noted on the bone density scan was due to vitamin D malabsorption, with resultant poor calcium absorption.

The suspected diagnosis of coeliac disease (gluten-induced enteropathy) was confirmed and she was advised to exclude wheat from her diet (a gluten-free diet). She felt symptomatically improved after 1 month.

A gluten-free diet is difficult to sustain in Western countries: wheat is present in bread, cakes, biscuits and sauces. Any trace is sufficient to spark a recrudescence of disease. Social occasions are fraught with embarrassment and difficulty.

After 6 months she returns to the clinic. She is bored of the gluten-free diet. She feels well and is putting on weight. She requests a return to a normal diet.

Repeat duodenal biopsy after 6 months showed greatly improved microscopic appearances, which were almost normal.

She is warned to remain on a strict gluten-free diet, to prevent long term sequelae.

Short-term problems due to coeliac disease include vitamin deficiencies, growth retardation (in children), steatorrhoea, malnutrition and anaemia and osteoporosis. These are relatively quickly improved on a gluten-free diet.

The duodenal biopsy may take up to 1 year to return to normal (but just days to show subtotal villous atrophy again after a gluten challenge!).

Long-term problems include an increased incidence of malignant gastrointestinal tract tumours, e.g. coeliac patients are at 50–100 times the normal risk of developing malignant lymphoma and there is a moderately increased risk of small and large bowel adenocarcinoma and squamous carcinoma of oesophagus. It appears that the increased risk can be averted by adherence to a gluten-free diet.

Other members of her family are screened for occult coeliac disease.

The prevalence of coeliac disease in relatives is as follows:

- first-degree relatives, 10–15 per cent
- HLA identical siblings, 30 per cent
- Dizygotic twins, 25 per cent
- Monozygotic twins, 70–100 per cent

There are strong associations between HLA DQ2 and DQ8 and coeliac disease. Most coeliac patients inherit a particular HLA type, which renders them more likely to develop the disease (see Fig. 2.22).

Figure 2.21 Body mass index is calculated as follows: weight(kg)/height(m)^2. Values from 18.5 to 25 are healthy. Our coeliac patient's BMI is 18.3, so she is fractionally underweight

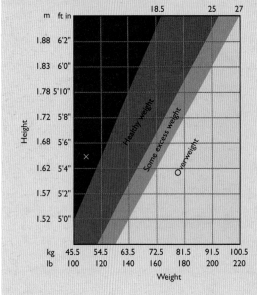

post-mortem, both grossly and microscopically, cannot give a precise answer. Yet a short time in a laboratory will reveal that the terms 'possibility' and 'probability' are well known to the pathologist. If you encounter a patient with metastatic tumour in the liver, it is *possible* that the primary tumour may have arisen in the nose, but it is much more *probable* that it arose in the colon! The study of genetics involves appreciating how the inheritance of genes produces diseases so that the *probability* of a particular individual developing a disease can be calculated.

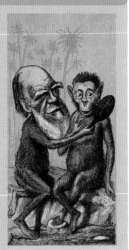
Most of us take our existence for granted but life really is a source of constant wonder and it has occurred against probability. Let us begin when there was no life on Earth. At some stage, molecules must have come into existence that were capable of self-replication and these molecules multiplied. If you have two molecules, one that manages to replicate and make copies without any mistakes while the other makes a lot of mistakes each time it is copied, then the correctly copied molecule is more likely to increase in number. Ironically, the molecule that copies perfectly will never change and it will still be the same molecule after 1 year, after 50 years and after a billion years. If a random mistake happens in the copying then there is the opportunity for change; possibly for the better, probably for worse. This is the basis for evolution recognized by Darwin in 1838. The other important factor is that there should be a 'struggle for survival', an evolutionary pressure that gives an advantage to the molecules or animals best adapted to the prevailing conditions.

MENDEL AND HIS PEAS

The probability of inheriting characteristics from parents was studied by Gregor Mendel. Mendel took garden peas with contrasting characteristics, seven to be exact, and bred from the plants which differed in only one characteristic. For the sake of discussion, let us consider violet and white flowers. He crossed plants with violet flowers with those bearing white flowers to produce the next generation, called the F1 generation. He found that the F1 generation plants all had the same colour flowers. Let us say that they were all violet. The F1 plants were then self pollinated (inbred) to produce the next generation, called F2. Interestingly, there were three plants with violet flowers for every one plant with white flowers. He took this one step further and self pollinated the white plants which gave rise to an F3 generation of plants that all had white flowers. Self-pollination of the violet plants produced an intriguing result; some plants produced only violet plants while others produced a mixture of white and violet plants in the ratio of 1 to 3 (Fig. 2.24). As Mendel correctly deduced, although the violet plants in the F2 generation all looked the same, they had different inheritance factors. He postulated that each plant must possess two factors which determine a given characteristic, such as colour of the flower. If two plants are crossed, each will contribute one factor to the next generation and it is purely random

Figure 2.24 Mendelian inheritance

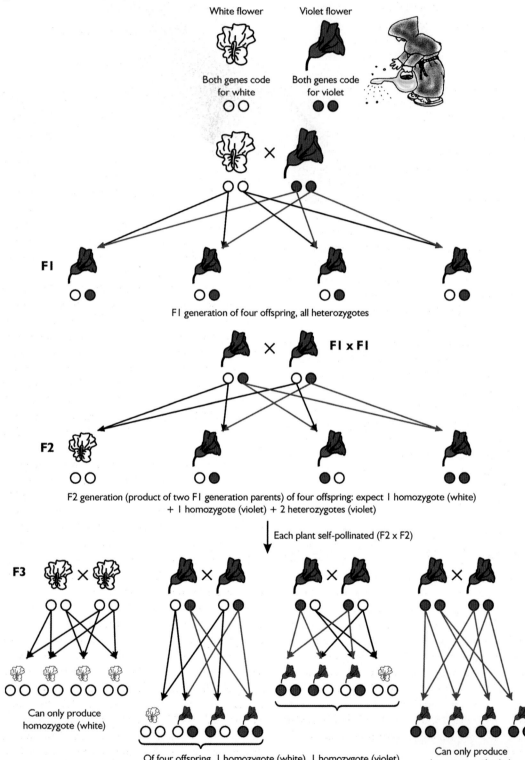

as to which factor is passed on. This is the law of segregation, also known as Mendel's first law. We now know that these 'factors' are genes on chromosomes which are paired and the two genes on the two chromosomes are alleles of each other. In Mendel's experiment, violet is the dominant allele and white is the recessive allele. The F1 generation has one white plant, which is homozygous for the white allele, one violet plant which is homozygous for the violet allele and two violet plants which are heterozygous, i.e. they have one white and one violet allele but the violet one dominates. In simple examples like this, one allele dominates; i.e. if the plant has at least one violet allele then all the flowers will be violet. Sometimes the situation is more complicated as there will be variable penetrance; i.e. the 'dominant' allele only dominates in a percentage of cases. It was later appreciated by Morgan (1934) that cell differentiation might depend on the variation in the action of genes in different cell types. In the later part of the nineteenth century, DNA, RNA and histones were discovered and it was originally believed that the histone proteins were genes. However, in 1944, Avery, MacLeod and McCarty recognized that DNA was the structural component of the gene. In 1953, Watson and Crick elucidated the double helical structure of DNA which provides the basis for its ability to replicate.

Obstetrics forms a major part of the medical curriculum, and during your training, you will meet pregnant women who are naturally concerned about their unborn baby. Let us briefly consider a clinical scenario to illustrate a possible problem you might encounter.

CLINICAL CASE: TURNER'S SYNDROME

A 34-year-old woman was seen in the ante-natal clinic complaining of abdominal pain and 'spotting' of blood. This was her first pregnancy and examination revealed a uterus of approximately 20 weeks' size. The gestation should have been 22 weeks according to her estimated date of delivery. The doctor failed to hear a fetal heart sound and he arranged an ultrasound scan of her abdomen. This revealed an intrauterine death and evacuation of the fetus was carried out. Post mortem examination of the aborted fetus was carried out to elucidate the cause and the pathology report is illustrated on the next page.

Let us consider some of the questions you may be faced with in clinical practice:

- What are the commonest genetic diseases?
- How can you diagnose them?
- Who should have their genes examined?

WHAT ARE THE COMMONEST GENETIC DISEASES?

INCIDENCE

Table 2.9 lists the incidence per 1000 live births of the commonest genetic disorders. It is helpful to subdivide them into abnormalities of chromosomal structure or number. The single-gene disorders are due to abnormalities of structure, which will be inherited in a Mendelian fashion. Abnormalities of chromosomal number are not normally inherited.

There are several points to highlight. The first is that the incidence relates to live births, which means that genetic abnormalities causing intrauterine death will be under-reported. This principally influences the figures for the chromosomal abnormalities, as their incidence in spontaneous abortions and stillbirths is 50 per cent while the incidence in live births is 6.5 per 1000. In spontaneous abortions with chromosomal abnormalities, around 50 per cent will have a trisomy, 18 per cent will be Turner's syndrome (XO) and 17 per cent will be triploid.

The commonest condition is X-linked red–green colour blindness which, fortunately, is only a very minor handicap (and is not an excuse for avoiding histology sessions!). Klinefelter's syndrome is due to an extra X chromosome in males (47,XXY). Affected individuals are generally of normal intelligence and are tall with hypogonadism and infertility. XYY syndrome also produces tall males. They may have behavioural problems, especially impulsive behaviour.

In familial hypercholesterolaemia patients have increased plasma low-density lipoprotein (LDL) levels and a predisposition for developing atheroma at an early age which gives them an 8-fold increased risk of ischaemic heart disease. The primary defect is a deficiency of cellular LDL receptors so that the liver uptake is reduced and plasma levels are two to three times normal. Around 30 different mutations of the LDL receptor gene have been identified. About 1 in 500 people are affected and they are heterozygotes that have half the

Pathology report

Name: Fetus of A. Smith
Consultant: Mr. I. M. Obs
Date of operation: 12.5.97
Gestation: 20 weeks

External examination:
The body was that of a female fetus and external measurements were consistent with a gestation of 18 weeks. There was generalized subcutaneous oedema and a cystic hygroma (benign cystic tumour of lymphatic vessels) was noted in the posterior aspect of the neck. The placenta was pale and bulky.

Internal examination:
The organ weights were consistent with a gestation of 18 weeks. The main abnormality was in the cardiovascular system. The left ventricle was small and the aorta proximal to the ductus arteriosus was narrowed – a severe infantile coarctation.

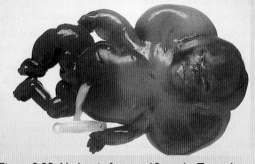

Figure 2.25 Hydropic fetus at 18 weeks: Turner's syndrome (Courtesy of R. Scott, UCLMS)

Special investigations:
Placental tissue was sent for cytogenetic analysis. Chromososmal analysis revealed the karyotype 45,X confirming a monosomy X, i.e. Turner's syndrome.

Condition	Estimated frequency/1000 live births	Abnormality
Red–green colour blindness	80*	X
Total autosomal dominant disease	10	AD
Dominant otosclerosis	3	AD
Klinefelter's (XXY)	2*	N
Familial hypercholesterolaemia	2	AD
Total autosomal recessive disease (Fig. 2.26)	2	AR
Trisomy 21 (Down's)	1.5	N
XYY	1.5*	N
Adult polycystic kidney disease (Fig. 2.27)	1	AD
Triple X syndrome	0.6†	N
Cystic fibrosis	0.5	AR
Fragile X-linked mental retardation	0.5*	X
Non-specific X-linked mental retardation	0.5*	X
Recessive mental retardation	0.5	AR
Neurofibromatosis	0.4	AR
Turner's syndrome (XO)	0.4†	N
Duchenne muscular dystrophy	0.3*	X
Haemophilia A	0.2*	X
Trisomy 18 (Edward's)	0.12	N
Polyposis coli	0.1	AD
Trisomy 13 (Patau's)	0.07	N

Table 2.9 Common genetic disorders

AD, autosomal dominant; AR, autosomal recessive; X, sex-linked disorder; N, disorder of chromosome number.
*Per 1000 male births.
†Per 1000 female births.

normal number of LDL receptors. One in a million people are homozygotes and they usually die from cardiovascular disease in childhood.

Adult polycystic kidney disease is due to a defect on the short arm of chromosome 16 that is inherited in an autosomal dominant fashion. Both kidneys are enlarged with numerous fluid filled cysts and may weigh a kilogram or more (normal = 150 g). The patients develop symptoms of renal damage and hypertension in their third or fourth decade.

Triple X syndrome produces tall girls who may have below average intelligence and, although gonadal function is usually normal, there may be premature ovarian failure. Fragile X syndrome was first described in 1969 and is now recognized as the second commonest cause of severe mental retardation after Down syndrome. Affected males have a reduced IQ, macro-orchidism and a prominent forehead and jaw. Heterozygote females can show mild retardation but counselling is difficult because not all female carriers show the chromosomal abnormality on testing. Turner's syndrome (monosomy X, i.e. 45,X) is a common cause of fetal hydrops and spontaneous abortion. About 95 per cent of affected pregnancies will abort. Those surviving to delivery will be less severely affected and generally show short stature, webbing of the neck, normal intelligence, infertility, aortic coarctation and altered carrying angle of the arm (cubitus valgus).

Although we have listed the common genetic disorders and their karyotype, this does not answer the question: 'How are they caused?' This is really two questions:

- How does the genetic abnormality produce disease?
- How does the genetic abnormality arise?

HOW DOES THE GENETIC ABNORMALITY PRODUCE DISEASE?

From our list so far, we have only explained the pathophysiology of familial hypercholesterolaemia. Now we shall discuss the recent discoveries that have increased our understanding of cystic fibrosis. Patients with cystic fibrosis present in infancy with pancreatic insufficiency, malabsorption and lung damage. This is an autosomal recessive disease and occurs in about 1:3000 live births with about 60000 affected people worldwide. Approximately 1:25 people are heterozygotes. The pathological manifestations result from thickened secretions that lead to obstruction, inflammation and

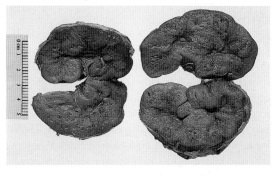

Figure 2.26 Autosomal recessive polycystic kidney disease. Smaller normal kidneys are included for comparison: 37 weeks' gestation (Courtesy of R. Scott, UCLMS)

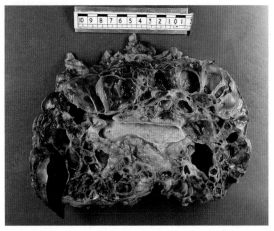

Figure 2.27 Adult autosomal dominant polycystic kidney disease. Gradually cystic dilatations of renal tubules and collecting ducts accumulate and distend the kidney, causing pressure atrophy of the renal tissue

scarring. The tenacious secretions are an indicator of a fundamental problem in water and electrolyte handling. This has been recognized for a long time and used as a diagnostic test, the sweat test that looks for elevated levels of sodium in the sweat.

The reason for the increased electrolytes in sweat is that there is defective, cyclic-AMP mediated regulation of chloride channels. The gene has now been identified on the long arm of chromosome 7 (7q31) and called the cystic fibrosis transmembrane conductance regulator (CFTR). The CFTR gene codes for a protein of 1480 amino acids and the structure of this protein is similar to the family of ATP-binding proteins. It is not clear yet whether the CFTR protein transports chloride directly or regulates chloride indirectly via another protein, but it is clear that a change in CFTR protein would affect electrolyte transport.

Over 1400 mutations have been identified in the CFTR gene; however, in about 70 per cent of cases of cystic fibrosis, there is a homozygous mutation referred to as the Delta F508 mutation (ΔF508-CFTR). In 90 per cent, at least one of the alleles is mutated (heterozygous mutation). This is a deletion in the codon at position 508 that leads to loss of a phenylalanine molecule in a highly conserved region of the CFTR protein. This is thought to alter the folding of the protein. The abnormal protein that is produced is unable to respond to cyclic AMP. Other, less common, mutations lead to complete absence or reduced amount of the protein or one that has reduced capacity to secrete chloride. In the pancreas and lungs, this leads to reduced chloride and water secretion so the mucus is thick. In the sweat test, the sweat glands secrete water and chloride normally but the secretory coil does not respond to β-adrenergic stimulation and does not reabsorb the chloride ions, hence allowing increased chloride and sodium in the sweat.

HOW DOES THE GENETIC ABNORMALITY ARISE?

We need to consider abnormalities of chromosome number separately from abnormalities in chromosome structure or single-gene disorders, as different mechanisms operate.

Abnormal chromosome number

This occurs because of problems at the anaphase stage of meiosis leading to unequal sharing of the chromosomes so that one daughter cell will have an extra chromosome (trisomy) while the other is missing a chromosome (monosomy) (Fig. 2.28). A pair of chromosomes or sister chromatids may fail to separate, so-called non-disjunction, or there may be delayed movement (anaphase lag) of chromosomes so that one is left on the wrong side of the dividing wall. The cause is unknown but the incidence increases with maternal age as we discuss when considering Down syndrome (page 72). It may also be associated with irradiation, viral infection or familial tendencies. Polyploidy means that the cell contains at least one complete extra set of chromosomes.

Most commonly, this is one extra set, i.e. 69 chromosomes, or triploidy. Affected fetuses usually die *in utero* or abort in early pregnancy. It can result from fertilization by two sperm (dispermy) or from fertilization in which either the sperm or ovum is diploid because of an abnormality in their maturation divisions.

Abnormal chromosome structure

Abnormalities in chromosome structure occur when chromosomes are inaccurately repaired after breaks have occurred. Chromosomal breakage can happen randomly at any gene locus but there are some areas that are particularly liable to breakage. The rate of breakage is markedly increased by ionizing radiation, certain chemicals and some rare inherited conditions. Structural abnormalities, such as translocations, deletions, duplications and inversions (see Fig. 2.29), occur when two break points allow transfer, loss or rearrangement of chromosomal material.

Single-gene disorders

Single-gene disorders can also result from structural abnormalities involving minute areas of the chromosome. These are produced by the same mechanism, i.e. breakage resulting in deletions, etc. Alternatively, single-gene disorders are due to a point mutation at the gene site. Point mutations are usually spontaneous and of unknown cause, but are probably mostly due to copying errors. Substitution of one base within a codon may lead to a different amino acid being inserted into the protein and major pathological effects, e.g. sickle cell disease. However, this is not inevitable because there are only 20 amino acids but 64 possible codons (4 × 4 × 4), which is the basis of degeneracy of the genetic code. For example, an mRNA sequence of GAA or GAG will code for alanine, thus some point mutations can alter the codon but have no effect on the amino acid sequence. Approximately 25 per cent of point mutations have no effect.

As well as coding for amino acids, codons also act as start and stop instructions. Messenger RNA employs UAA, UAG or UGA as stop codons. If a point mutation produces a stop codon, then the amino acid chain will terminate too early and this is the effect of about 5 per cent of point mutations. The ultimate problem is a frameshift mutation where gain or loss of one or two bases produces a nonsense message because it alters every codon.

Figure 2.28 Abnormal chromosome numbers may arise because of non-disjunction during anaphase II

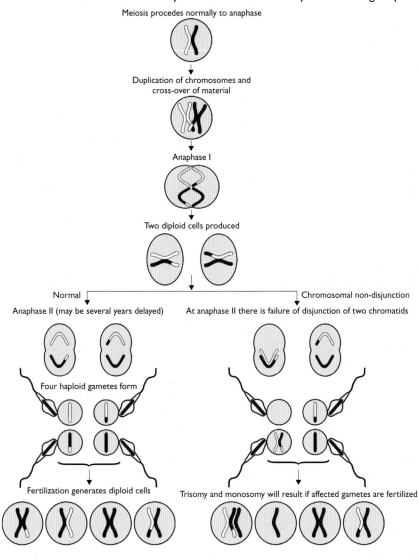

Meiosis procedes normally to anaphase

Duplication of chromosomes and cross-over of material

Anaphase I

Two diploid cells produced

Normal

Anaphase II (may be several years delayed)

Four haploid gametes form

Fertilization generates diploid cells

Chromosomal non-disjunction

At anaphase II there is failure of disjunction of two chromatids

Trisomy and monosomy will result if affected gametes are fertilized

By way of illustration, take a look at the following sentences:

SHE HAD ONE MAD CAT AND ONE SAD RAT

SHE HAD ONE **B**AD CAT AND ONE SAD RAT

THE MAD BAD CAT ATE THE ONE SAD RAT

THE MAD **SHE** CAT ATE THE ONE SAD RAT

THE MAD **HEC ATA TET HEO NES ADR AT**

- The first sentence is the normal code.
- The second has a point mutation without a frameshift so there is a 25 per cent probability that it will not have any effect.
- The third sentence has a length mutation, possibly a translocation.
- The fourth sentence is a mutation of the third where SHE represents a premature stop codon.
- The fifth sentence changes the sex of the cat and makes nonsense.

MULTIFACTORIAL DISORDERS

Every new patient is asked about their 'family history', the idea being that if their parents and siblings suffer from a particular disease then they are at increased risk. Unfortunately, for most diseases it is not known how

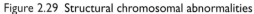

Figure 2.29 Structural chromosomal abnormalities

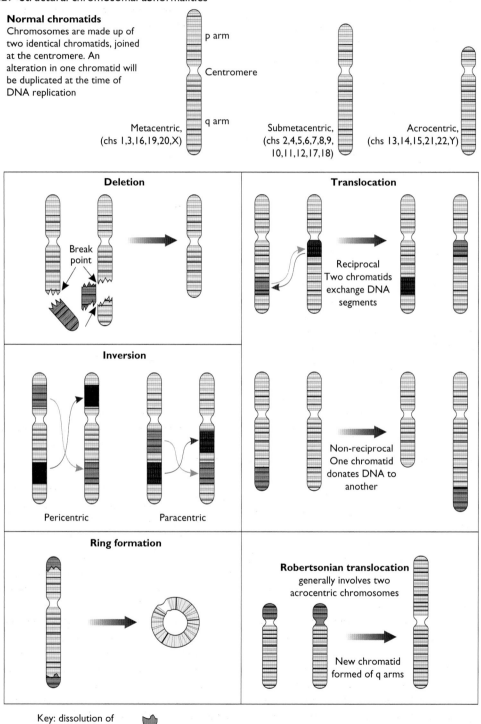

Normal chromatids
Chromosomes are made up of two identical chromatids, joined at the centromere. An alteration in one chromatid will be duplicated at the time of DNA replication

p arm

Centromere

q arm

Metacentric, (chs 1,3,16,19,20,X)

Submetacentric, (chs 2,4,5,6,7,8,9, 10,11,12,17,18)

Acrocentric, (chs 13,14,15,21,22,Y)

Deletion

Break point

Translocation

Reciprocal Two chromatids exchange DNA segments

Inversion

Pericentric

Paracentric

Non-reciprocal One chromatid donates DNA to another

Ring formation

Robertsonian translocation
generally involves two acrocentric chromosomes

New chromatid formed of q arms

Key: dissolution of redundant chromosome

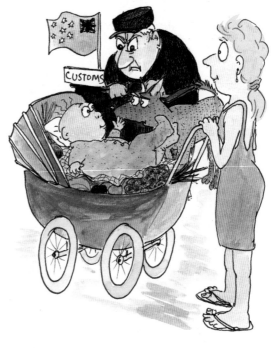

Fig 2.30 Because genetic disease may be difficult to identify, some countries take stringent protective measures to prevent the introduction of harmful genetic material

great that increased risk may be because the inheritance does not follow simple Mendelian principles but is multifactorial. It is likely that there will be a variety of genes involved which interact with a number of environmental factors. Research into multifactorial disorders adopts a similar approach to single-gene problems. First, it is necessary to identify the diseases with a significant genetic component by comparing the incidence in family groups with the general population. This genetic contribution is termed heritability and some examples are listed below.

The next step is to look for genetic, biochemical and immunological features that affected individuals have in common. It is well established that certain HLA types are associated with particular diseases and this may be helpful in counselling affected families. For example, in a family with ankylosing spondylitis, a first-degree relative has a 9 per cent risk of developing the disease if HLA-B27 positive but less than a 1 per cent risk if HLA-B27 negative.

The ultimate goal is to identify the gene or genes and the environmental factor(s), so that those at particularly high genetic risk could attempt to avoid the relevant environmental hazard. At a simple level, this would mean giving vitamin supplements to pregnant women at risk of producing babies with neural tube defects, or advising potential 'arteriopaths' to modify their diet and not smoke.

Diabetes is a disease with a wide geographic variation in which a genetic predisposition and environmental factors seem to interact to produce the clinical manifestations of pancreatic islet cell damage. It is associated with HLA and two haplotypes are particularly associated with the disease, DR4-DQ8 and DR3-DQ2, which are present in 90 per cent of children with type 1 diabetes. It is

clear, however, that the environment plays a significant role, with viruses the major culprit. Enteroviruses, rotaviruses and, in particular, rubella appear to be the principal candidates.

HOW CAN GENETIC DISORDERS BE DIAGNOSED?

NON-INVASIVE TESTS

Fortunately, the majority of pregnancies progress without any problems to produce a normal healthy baby after approximately 40 weeks' gestation. It would be unreasonable to subject all pregnant women to the stress and possible hazards of the many investigations that are available to detect fetal abnormalities. In recent years, the quality of ultrasound scanning has achieved a standard that makes it useful for detecting internal and external fetal malformations as well as giving accurate information on the rate of fetal growth through head circumference and body length measurements. In practice, early ultrasound (at 8–10 weeks) can be used to date the pregnancy and identify anencephaly. Neural

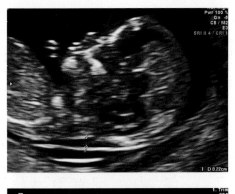

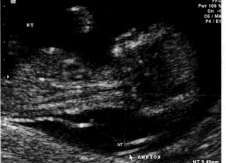

Figure 2.31 The nuchal translucency (NT) thickness (+....+) is measured using ultrasound at the 11–13 weeks stage of pregnancy. NT is subcutaneous fluid which normally collects at the back of a baby's neck. Increased NT thickness indicates an increased risk of Down syndrome. The low-risk scan shown on the left equates to <1/300 chance, whereas the high-risk scan on the right indicates a chance of >1/300 of having Down syndrome. To measure the NT a magnified true sagittal image preferably showing the nasal bone (red arrow) in profile should be obtained. This bone may be absent in Down syndrome, but this may not become clear until later scans (e.g. at 18 weeks). Women with high-risk pregnancies are offered diagnostic tests such as chorionic villus sampling (CVS) or amniocentesis, procedures that are invasive tests carrying a 0.5–1% risk of miscarriage. If the chromosomes are normal, other causes for elevated NT readings may include cardiac anomalies, diaphragmatic hernia and genetic syndromes. (Courtesy of Dr Kerry McMahon, Consultant in Women's Diagnostic Imaging, Queensland X-ray)

tube, cardiac and skeletal abnormalities are best identified on ultrasound done at between 17 and 20 weeks. The tests mentioned so far are non-invasive and no risks have been identified to either mother or baby. Recently, ultrasound scanning has proved useful in detecting the increased nuchal fold thickness of fetuses with Down syndrome; this can then be confirmed by chorionic villus sampling or amniocentesis (Fig. 2.31).

INVASIVE PROCEDURES

One of the simplest tests is to measure the mother's serum α-fetoprotein (AFP) concentration. Ultrasound is very good at picking up neural tube defects, hence this test is useful mainly for small defects that are missed. It is measured at about 16–18 weeks' gestation and will be raised in 90 per cent of mothers bearing children with open neural tube defects and 95 per cent of anencephalic cases. Obviously, this means that 5–10 per cent of cases will remain undetected so it is essential to offer more sensitive techniques to mothers at particularly high risk. AFP is also increased in multiple

pregnancies, threatened abortions and a variety of fetal malformations. Its level is lowered in Down syndrome.

Screening for fetal well-being has developed rapidly over the last decade and many centres use a 'triple test' for Down syndrome. This includes AFP, hCG (choriogonadotrophic hormone) and oestriol. Such screening tests are particularly useful in detecting Down syndrome in younger women who do not have any particular risk factors for fetal abnormalities.

Amniocentesis can be performed at between 15 and 16 weeks' gestation and involves removing about 20 mL of amniotic fluid, which contains small numbers of amniotic cells that can be cultured. The fluid can be tested for AFP and acetylcholinesterase activity to detect neural tube defects or more specialized tests for detecting rare inborn errors of metabolism. The cells are cultured and used for karyotypic (chromosome) analysis.

Fetoscopy which involved introducing a scope into the amniotic cavity has also been used to perform fetal blood sampling and for therapeutic procedures such as intrauterine transfusion. It does have the risk of inducing an abortion.

METHODS OF GENETIC ANALYSIS

CYTOGENETIC ANALYSIS

The human nucleus contains 23 pairs of chromosomes, 22 pairs of autosomes and one pair of sex chromosomes. It has been apparent for some time that certain diseases are associated with specific chromosomal abnormalities and it is logical to divide these into those affecting the *autosomal chromosomes* and those affecting the *sex chromosomes*. As we shall see, these groups can also be divided into abnormalities affecting *numbers* of chromosomes and those affecting the *structure* of chromosomes.

At metaphase, the two chromatids of each chromosome are joined by a centromere and the long arm is termed 'q' and the short arm is 'p'. There is a convention for reporting karyotypes so that the total number of chromosomes is given first followed by the sex chromosomes. Examples are illustrated in Table 2.10.

The child with mosaicism has two genetically different cell types distributed in its tissues. These are not distributed evenly and some affected individuals may demonstrate only a normal phenotype in their peripheral blood lymphocytes. Therefore, it may be necessary to culture from other organs, such as skin, to confirm a suspected abnormality. Patients with mosaicism are generally less severely affected than those with the full

Dictionary

Mosaicism: The presence of two or more cell lines that are both karyotypically and genotypically distinct but are derived from the same zygote

disorder. This makes prenatal counselling difficult if mosaicism is detected in a fetus, as the clinical effects could be mild. There is also the complication that any mosaicism detected in chorionic villus samples may only indicate an abnormal genotype in some placental cells and the fetus need not be affected.

Chorionic villus sampling has some advantages over amniocentesis in that it can be performed at between 8 and 12 weeks' gestation so that a diagnosis can often be made by 12–14 weeks' gestation when termination is easier. It also provides material suitable for DNA analysis which is necessary when the genetic changes are too small to be seen on light microscopical chromosomal preparations. It does have a greater risk of miscarriage, however.

FLUORESCENCE *IN SITU* HYBRIDIZATION

Recent advances in molecular biology have led to novel technologies for the assessement of chromosomes and

Table 2.10 Examples of karyotypes

Chromosomes	Result
46XY	Normal male
46XX	Normal female
47XXY	Male with Klinefelter's syndrome
If there is a change in chromosomal number, then the affected chromosome is indicated with a + or −, e.g.	
47 XX + 21	Female with Down syndrome
If there is a structural rearrangement, the karyotype indicates the precise site affected and the nature of the abnormality, e.g.	
46 XX del 7 (p13-ptr)	Deletion of the short arm of chromosome 7 at band 13 to the end of the chromosome
46 XY t (11;14) (p15.4;q22.3)	A translocation between chromosome 11 and 14 with the break points being band 15.4 on the short arm of chromosome 11 and band 22.3 on the long arm of chromosome 14
Mosaicism indicates that two different cell lines have derived from one fertilized egg and the karyotype specifies both cell lines	
46 XX/47 XX + 21	Down's mosaic
46 XX/45 X	Turner's mosaic

genes. One such technique is fluorescence *in situ* hybridization (FISH) (Fig. 2.32). This technique has been used extensively in research as well as in clinical diagnosis. The idea behind the technique is very simple. DNA probes labelled with fluorescence dyes are hybridized to the chromosomes to reveal their structure and number. An advantage of this method is that, unlike classical karyotyping, it can also be used on interphase nuclei. This is particularly important for diagnosis in certain tumour types, e.g. leukaemias, where metaphase chromosomal spreads are difficult to obtain. Comparative genomic hybridization (CGH) is yet another adaptation of the FISH technique which allows a global view of DNA copy number changes within a single hybridization. This has opened up avenues not only in tumour research but also in assessing genetic alterations in a clinical setting.

Dictionary

Haploid: cells have only one set of chromosomes, i.e. 'n', as occurs in gametes

Diploid: cells have normal number of chromosomes, i.e. 46 = '2n', as in all somatic cells

Polyploid: cells have extra sets of chromosomes, i.e. 'xn'

Aneuploid: cells have an abnormal number of chromosomes but not an exact multiple of the haploid 'n' state

DNA ANALYSIS

First, let us remind ourselves of some basic facts about DNA (deoxyribonucleic acid). DNA consists of two anti-parallel strands which have a backbone of deoxyribose sugars from which project purine and pyrimidine bases (Fig. 2.33). The sequences of these bases determines the genetic code. It is estimated that there are approximately 6 billion bases in the human genome. The purine bases are adenine (A) and guanine (G) and the pyrimidine bases are cytosine (C) and thymine (T). The two strands form a right-handed double helix with about 10 nucleotide pairs per helical turn. They are linked through these purine and pyrimidine bases with G always pairing with C and A pairing with T. This point is fundamental to the use of probes for analysing DNA.

Figure 2.32 Fluorescence *in situ* hybridization (FISH) for HER2 gene which resides on chromosome 17. The green dots represent probes on chromosome 17 (two dots for the two chromosomes) and the red dots represent increased copy numbers of the HER2 gene (amplification: there should only be two dots but in this case, there are multiple dots)

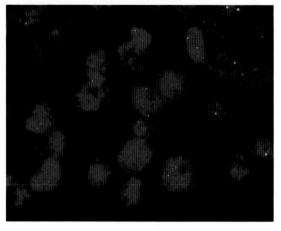

The binding of complementary purine and pyrimidine bases also allows DNA to act as a template for the production of mRNA. This process is called transcription. The mRNA moves to the cytoplasm, attaches to a ribosome and is then used for protein production. This is termed translation and involves binding of transfer RNAs (tRNA) carrying a specific amino acid. The amino acids then combine to form a polypeptide chain and are released (see Fig. 2.34). RNA differs from DNA in three respects: it is a single-stranded molecule, it contains ribose sugar instead of deoxyribose and the base thymine (T) is substituted by uracil (U).

There have been three major advances that have made DNA analysis possible: the ability to cut DNA, the ability to sort the resulting fragments and the ability to amplify pieces of DNA. Certain bacteria can produce enzymes that are capable of cutting DNA at specific sites and only at those sites. These enzymes are called restriction endonucleases and the DNA fragments are known as restriction fragments. Different bacteria produce enzymes that cut DNA at different sites. How is this useful in diagnosis? If you consider the sentences below, there are two identical sentences.

The capacity to blunder slightly is the real marvel of DNA; without this special attribute, we would still BE anaerobic bacteria and there would BE no music.

Figure 2.33 Structure of DNA, showing the bases

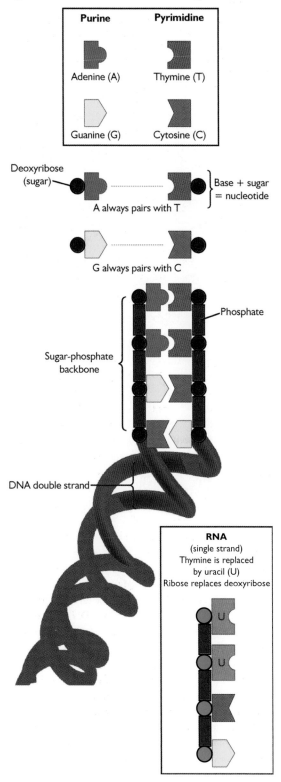

The capacity to blunder slightly IS the real marvel of DNA, without this special attribute, we would still be anaerobic bacteria and there would be no music.

One has been cut whenever a 'be' appears and the other whenever 'is' appears. You can see that the fragments produced are of different lengths. In the first case, there are three fragments with the smallest composed of 'no music'. In the second case, there are two large fragments. The same principle applies to the endonucleases. Once fragments of different sizes are produced, they are run on an electrophoretic strip, which separates the fragments according to their size, and then 'stained' with a DNA probe. The details of these electrophoretic methods are not important, suffice it to say that the method used for DNA fragments is called Southern blotting, after its inventor, and the corresponding technique for RNA is northern blotting. The technique for analysis of proteins is called western blotting. There is no eastern blotting! The binding of the probe to its complementary sequence is called hybridization. The DNA probe or oligonucleotide is a short length of DNA whose nucleotide sequence is known. These are labelled, for example with a radioactive element or fluorescence dye, so that their position on an electrophoretic strip can be identified. Their importance lies in their ability to bind only to a specific section of the patient's DNA, i.e. to a piece with an identical sequence of complementary bases.

This use of restriction endonucleases relies on the enzyme digesting at exactly the point that mutates to cause the disease. Often we do not know the precise mutation responsible for an inherited disease, but it may be possible to identify which section of DNA it is in by comparing the DNA of affected family members with healthy family members. The human genome has approximately 6 billion bases, so how do we start looking for differences? We can look for restriction fragment length polymorphisms (RFLP). These are variations in DNA fragment lengths that can be produced by using a restriction endonuclease and probe appropriate for detecting a particular disease. For example, the DNA from family members with Huntington's disease was investigated with an enormous range of enzymes and probes. It was discovered that digestion with an enzyme called Hind III, combined with hybridization with a probe called G8, identified variations in the short arm of chromosome 4 which segregated with the disease. What is the principle behind this technique? It relies on variations in the genetic code that influence restriction endonuclease digestion but do not cause any clinical problems. We have

Figure 2.34 Gene expression: transcription and translation

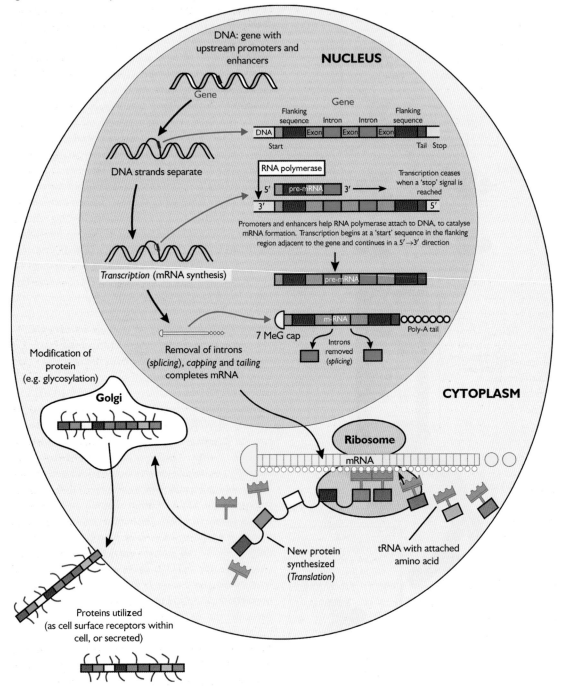

already seen that a change of just one base causes sickle cell disease, so why do other common mutations have no effect? It is because only about 10 per cent of DNA codes for proteins while the rest has no clearly defined function. The coding regions (structural genes) are fairly constant from person to person and mutations in these regions generally cause disorders. The non-coding regions can vary from person to person and this diversity is useful for producing the 'DNA fingerprint'. Although the coding regions (genes) are clearly important, the non-coding or 'junk DNA' is increasingly being recognized as also playing an important role in disease, and hence in the future will play a bigger role than just as 'markers' in DNA finger printing.

If a mutation has occurred in a non-coding region that is fairly close to the gene responsible for a disease, then it will be inherited with the disease gene. Obviously, the same mutation must not have occurred near to the normal gene or no difference will be detected. Provided that an enzyme exists which digests at the altered non-coding area, then the disease gene can be tracked. There is the inevitable problem of new mutations or cross-over of chromosomal material that might 'unlink' the mutant non-coding region from the disease gene, but this technique is useful for counselling families for future pregnancies *after* an affected child is born.

So far, we have only mentioned the use of oligonucleotide probes as 'stains' for the altered fragment produced by restriction endonuclease digestion. They can also be used on DNA without digestion to demonstrate deletions that are too small to see on light microscopical chromosomal preparations. Haemophilia A, Duchenne muscular dystrophy, α-thalassaemia and some cases of β-thalassaemia can be detected in this way.

Their most sophisticated use, however, is for 'staining' the gene that causes the disease. Provided that the same genetic change is always responsible for the disease, then this approach can be used without the need for family studies. In sickle cell disease, an oligonucleotide probe has been produced that detects the normal β-globin gene sequence and another probe detects the mutant sickle gene. Each probe binds only to its specific complementary nucleotide sequence so the 'normal' probe binds to the normal gene, the 'sickle' probe binds to the mutant gene and, in heterozygous people, both probes will bind – one to each chromosome 11. How do the oligonucleotide probe sequences differ? Since we know that sickle cell disease involves a change from GAG to GTG, then the probes must be:

normal probe   xxxxxxCTCxxxxxx
sickle probe   xxxxxxCACxxxxxx

POLYMERASE CHAIN REACTION

One of the problems of analysing DNA by the means so far described is that a relatively large amount of material is required. An ingenious technique which harnesses DNA's normal role, to act as a template for producing complementary DNA or RNA strands, has been developed. It is called the polymerase chain reaction (PCR). It is without doubt one of the most significant technological advances of the twentieth century. The method involves amplifying a specific segment of DNA through successive rounds of replication.

This amplified segment, which must contain the area suspected of containing the mutant code, is then cut with the appropriate restriction enzyme and run on an electrophoretic agarose gel. It is not necessary to use a specific probe to stain the digested fragments because it is the relevant area that has been amplified. Instead the DNA bands themselves can be viewed under ultraviolet light after staining with ethidium bromide. This is much faster than using autoradiography and can provide a result within 2 days of taking the sample. PCR is also used in forensic work to produce the well known 'DNA fingerprint' from small samples of blood, semen or hair left at the scene of the crime.

WHO SHOULD HAVE THEIR GENES EXAMINED?

FAMILY HISTORY

It is not difficult to appreciate that those who have a family history of a disease may need testing. It is not quite that simple though as one needs to be sure what is meant by a 'positive family history'. One also needs to decide which of the enormous range of diseases are due to a genetic abnormality that can be transmitted to the offspring. This requires careful observation of the incidence of a disease in the general population and within a family group. Many disorders, however, are multifactorial in nature, with both genetic predisposition and environmental agents influencing the outcome. We will illustrate the importance of family history by considering the example of sickle cell disease.

SICKLE CELL DISEASE

Patients with this recessive haemoglobin disorder may present clinically with abdominal pain, joint pains, cerebral symptoms, renal failure and cardiac failure, which result from thrombotic and ischaemic damage (Fig. 2.35). This occurs because the red cells 'sickle', so altering their shape and occluding capillaries. The red cells have an abnormal haemoglobin which, under hypoxic conditions, polymerizes and alters the cell's shape.

Figure 2.35 Pelvic X-ray showing avascular necrosis of the right femoral head in a patient with sickle cell disease

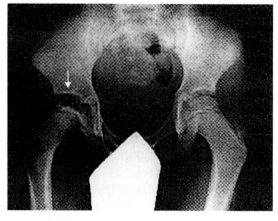

Figure 2.36 Possible outcomes for the offspring of two people with sickle cell trait. N, normal gene; S, sickle cell gene

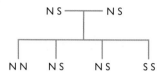

In 1949, Pauling analysed the haemoglobin from patients with sickle cell anaemia and discovered that its mobility on electrophoresis differed from normal haemoglobin. He called it haemoglobin S (Hb S). Later, family studies suggested that the gene for sickle cell haemoglobin was an allele of the normal gene on chromosome 11 for the β chain of the haemoglobin molecule, that is, an alternative gene at the same locus on the chromosome. The difference between the normal haemoglobin gene and the sickle cell gene is a change in one base pair; GAG becomes GTG. This causes valine to replace glutamic acid in position 6 of the β chain. That's it, a point mutation changing just one nucleotide leads to the translation of one different amino acid, which entirely changes the property of the protein!

Fortunately, genes are paired and people who are heterozygous (i.e. one normal allele, one sickle cell allele) do not usually have any problems unless they become unusually hypoxic (e.g. at surgical operation). They have a mixture of the normal and abnormal haemoglobin.

For practical purposes, we can regard sickle cell disease as an autosomal recessive disorder. How should we counsel a healthy pregnant woman who has a family history of sickle cell disease? The problem lies in deciding which members of the family are carriers of the gene because two people with sickle cell trait (heterozygotes) are likely to produce one healthy child, one sick child and two carriers (Fig. 2.36).

Carriers of the sickle cell gene can be identified by adding a reducing agent to the blood *in vitro* which

induces the red cells to sickle. More recently, techniques have been developed to analyse the DNA itself. This is particularly useful in prenatal diagnosis for testing the fetus before it has switched on to full production of the β chains. It is not possible to detect the abnormal β chains in fetal red blood cells because the fetus is relying on haemoglobin produced from α and γ chains, i.e. HbF. However, it is possible to remove a small piece of placenta (chorionic villus sampling) for DNA analysis relying on the point mutation to alter the binding of specific oligonucleotide probes or interfere with restriction enzyme digestion.

OTHER HAEMOGLOBINOPATHIES

Sickle cell disease is not the only haemoglobinopathy, although it is one of the commonest. Haemoglobinopathies can be due to an abnormal chain being present or one type of chain not being produced. Haemoglobin is composed of two pairs of (i.e. four) polypeptide chains, each of which is linked to a heme group. The heme group is a protoporphorin molecule chelated with iron and able to carry oxygen. For the moment, we shall concentrate on the polypeptide chains. The normal chains are called alpha (α), beta (β), gamma (γ) and delta (δ). All normal haemoglobin has one pair of a chain combined with a pair of another type of chain. Hence there is haemoglobin A ($\alpha_2\beta_2$), haemoglobin A2 ($\alpha_2\delta_2$) and haemoglobin F ($\alpha_2\gamma_2$) HbF predominates in the fetus and HbA predominates in the adult. See Fig. 2.37.

Besides sickle cell disease, the other major group of haemoglobinopathies are the thalassaemias. In thalassaemias, the chains are normal in structure but not enough are produced. This condition is common in people originating from the Mediterranean, Africa and Asia and is due to a wide variety of underlying genetic changes. The severity of the person's symptoms depends on the chain involved and whether they are homozygous or heterozygous for the abnormality. All normal haemoglobin has alpha chains so complete absence of alpha chains is

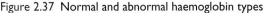

Figure 2.37 Normal and abnormal haemoglobin types

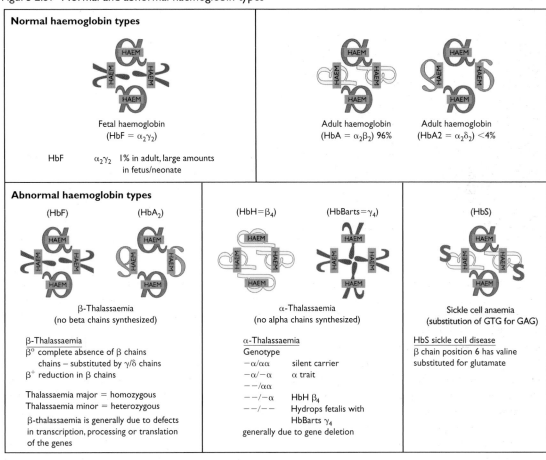

Normal haemoglobin types

Fetal haemoglobin
(HbF = $\alpha_2\gamma_2$)

Adult haemoglobin
(HbA = $\alpha_2\beta_2$) 96%

Adult haemoglobin
(HbA2 = $\alpha_2\delta_2$) <4%

HbF $\alpha_2\gamma_2$ 1% in adult, large amounts
in fetus/neonate

Abnormal haemoglobin types

(HbF)   (HbA$_2$)

(HbH=β_4)   (HbBarts=γ_4)

(HbS)

β-Thalassaemia
(no beta chains synthesized)

α-Thalassaemia
(no alpha chains synthesized)

Sickle cell anaemia
(substitution of GTG for GAG)

β-Thalassaemia
β^0 complete absence of β chains
   chains – substituted by γ/δ chains
β^+ reduction in β chains

Thalassaemia major = homozygous
Thalassaemia minor = heterozygous

β-thalassaemia is generally due to defects
in transcription, processing or translation
of the genes

α-Thalassaemia
Genotype
$-\alpha/\alpha\alpha$ silent carrier
$-\alpha/-\alpha$ α trait
$--/\alpha\alpha$
$--/-\alpha$ HbH β_4
$--/--$ Hydrops fetalis with
         HbBarts γ_4
generally due to gene deletion

HbS sickle cell disease
β chain position 6 has valine
substituted for glutamate

---

incompatible with life and an affected fetus will be oedematous (hydropic). In the absence of any alpha chains, the other chains do their best to produce a haemoglobin molecule by combining together as HbBart's (γ_4) and HbH(β_4). This is the position with deletion of all four genes and, predictably, the severity decreases with the addition of each α chain (see Fig. 2.37). This group of conditions is called alpha-thalassaemia.

Around 95 per cent of adult haemoglobin is HbA composed of alpha and beta chains, so the other important disease is beta-thalassaemia with absent or reduced beta chains and attempts to compensate by producing HbA$_2$ and HbF using gamma and delta chains respectively.

The main clinical problems in thalassaemia are due to haemolysis of the red cells with the abnormal haemoglobin. These cells have a reduced life span and are removed in the reticuloendothelial system, particularly the spleen and marrow. Here the red cell components are broken down for reuse or excretion. The iron is stored in the tissues as ferritin and haemosiderin and, if excessive, can cause tissue damage called haemochromatosis. The protoporphyrins are degraded to produce bile pigments and any excess gives the patient a yellow tinge to their skin and sclerae, i.e. jaundice.

MATERNAL AGE

Separate from the desirability of testing the genes of people with a strong family history of a particular disease, is the need to consider the increased risk in pregnancies in older women. There is a dramatic increase in the number of chromosomally abnormal fetuses in women over the age of 35 years. This affects a wide variety of disorders with the commonest being Trisomy 21 or Down syndrome (Fig. 2.38).

Figure 2.38 Incidence of Down syndrome with increasing maternal age

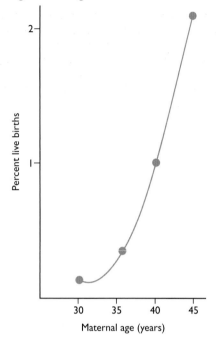

People with Down syndrome are mentally retarded, may have congenital heart disease and an increased incidence of infections and leukaemia. In 1959, Lejeune and his colleagues showed that these patients have an extra chromosome 21. This most commonly arises because of non-disjunction of chromosome 21 during meiosis in one of the parents, so that either the egg or the sperm carries two copies of chromosome 21. In about 5 per cent of cases, there is a translocation of chromosome 21 to 14 and occasionally translocations of chromosome 21 to chromosome 22, or 21 to 21.

For Down syndrome, the risk is 10 per cent when the mother is the carrier of the translocation and 2.5 per cent if the father is the carrier. Obviously, it is important to investigate the parents of children with such inherited disorders to look for balanced translocations, although non-disjunction is the commonest cause.

Dictionary

Translocation: the transfer of part of one chromosome to another chromosome

About half of fetuses affected by Down syndrome do not survive to term. The incidence in live births is 1 in 650, but that is an average figure for all ages. The risk at maternal age 30 is 1 in 900, which doubles by age 35, stands at 1 in 100 at age 40 and 1 in 40 at age 44. This age distribution makes it sensible to screen women over 35 years by examining chromosomes cultured from amniotic cells and measuring α-fetoprotein levels which are *lowered* in Down syndrome. (Note that they are *raised* in many other abnormalities, e.g. neural tube defects.)

MOLECULAR FAMILY PLANNING

With the advent of modern molecular biology techniques combined with *in vitro* fertilization, 'designing' babies has become a reality in the last few years. Several companies have publicized that they can now perform sex selection by means of sperm sorting. Briefly, owing to differences in nuclear morphology and genetic content of spermatozoids harbouring X or Y chromosomes, they may be sorted by DNA analysis with fluorescence *in situ* hybridization (FISH) and then separated by flow cytometry. Currently, it has been widely tested in animals and it is claimed that this technique has a specificity of up to 90 per cent . Other method is based on *in vitro* fertilization coupled with biopsy and genetic analysis of the polar body.

Currently, in most of the Western countries, sex selection is only accepted for a medical reason, such as the prevention of certain (X-chromosome linked) genetic disorders that are serious, untreatable and prematurely fatal (i.e. Duchenne muscular dystrophy or Lesch–Nyhan syndrome or some forms of inherited Alzheimer's disease).

New technologies allow quite a range of genetic abnormalities to be assessed prior to implantation when IVF is being done. This raises ethical issues of potential eugenic practices and debate on whether more minor problems (e.g. hereditary deafness) would be a reason for not implanting the fertilized egg.

As an amusing digression, it is interesting that several disputable methods for 'designing babies' have been publicized. Most of them have no scientific basis. Included in this category are special diets, complicated coital and post-coital practices, as well as the 'Selnas Method', which has received great popularity in Europe. This method requires knowledge of mother's age, blood group, and menstrual history and the proponents claim that using this information, it is possible to 'conjure up the dates in the year when intercourse will result in a baby of the couple's choice'. So far, no papers describing the efficacy of these techniques have been reported in peer-reviewed journals.

FAMILY HISTORY OF CANCER

This is covered in detail in the Part 4 on neoplasia. Where there is a strong family history of cancer, it may be necessary to screen for mutations in specific genes in order to counsel the patients regarding risk to themselves or their family members. Examples include BRCA1/2 mutations in breast and ovarian cancer.

Those of us who have the duty of training the rising generation of doctors must not inseminate the virgin minds of the young with the tares of our own fads. It is for this reason that it is easily possible for teaching to be too 'up to date'. It is always well, before handing the cup of knowledge to the young, to wait until the froth has settled.

Sir Robert Hutchison, 1925

PART 2

Defence against disease

Introduction: The role of epidemiology
in disease   77

Chapter 3: The body's response to
infection   79

Major routes for the
transmission of infection   79
What are the body's natural
defences against infection?   79
How do microorganisms
evade our defences?   81
Are some people more
susceptible to infection
than others?   83
Antibiotic resistance   83
How can we prevent or
overcome bacterial resistance?   85
How do viruses develop
resistance to antiviral agents?   87

Chapter 4: The acute inflammatory
response   89

What is inflammation?   89
What is the difference between
acute and chronic inflammation?   90
What happens to the patient
with acute inflammation?   90
Mechanisms for bacterial killing   101
The systemic effects of
inflammation   109

Clinicopathological case study:
lobar pneumonia   114

Chapter 5: Chronic and granulomatous
inflammation, healing and
repair   115

Chronic inflammation   115
Granulomatous inflammation   116
Tuberculosis   117
Sarcoidosis   121
Other types of chronic
granulomatous disease   122
Macrophages   122
Wound healing and repair   124
Healing by primary and
secondary intention   126
Bone healing   131
What can go wrong with the
healing processes?   134
Clinicopathological case study:
alcoholic liver disease   137

Chapter 6: The immune defence
against infection   139

The lymphatic system in
inflammation   139
The adaptive immune
response   143
Tolerance   155
Autoimmune disease   155
Immunization   159

INTRODUCTION

THE ROLE OF EPIDEMIOLOGY IN DISEASE

Defence against disease is essentially the art of survival. It is not only the response to a dangerous microbe but also about ensuring that the body is kept healthy with the right supply of nutrients and avoidance of toxic agents. Malnutrition is a disease that we defend against by eating a balanced diet. As we learn more about the factors influencing cardiovascular atheroma formation and some gastrointestinal tumours, we could include diet as one of the defences against cancer and heart attacks. Putting sun tan lotion and a hat on will reduce the risk of sun-induced skin cancers. Having warm clothes and shelter will prevent hypothermia in cold climates.

You will appreciate that defence against disease goes beyond merely considering the tissue defences protecting us from microbes. However, much of the contribution of medicine to improving people's health over the last century has been due to advances in understanding and treating infections, so we will devote this section to that topic. Later sections discuss both the causes and defences involved in cardiovascular disease and cancer.

We have learned already about how disease can come about. Obviously the body has defence mechanisms tailored to deal with many of the insults we have discussed in Part 1. Before we even consider these though we should appreciate the great contribution made in the 1800s by Dr John Snow in identifying the role of water in spreading disease. His work led to one of the first environmental measures taken to prevent the spread of infection. Since then, epidemiological studies have identified the causative agents responsible for many diseases.

JOHN SNOW AND THE BROAD STREET PUMP

It would be quite possible to go through the entire medical curriculum without ever hearing the name of John Snow (1813–58). He was a man of simple habits and seemed to lack the charisma which is vital in attracting attention on the world stage. Yet his contributions to medicine were certainly 'world class'. If you think that epidemiological studies might be dull, Snow's biography is well worth a read. It demonstrates eloquently how they can have a truly dramatic impact on public health. Snow is perhaps best remembered for having anaesthetized Queen Victoria in 1853 and 1857, giving credibility to the use of pain relief during childbirth! But it is his contribution to the understanding of cholera that is relevant here. Snow's link with cholera evolved over a number of years. His first encounter with the disease was in Newcastle upon Tyne during the epidemic of 1831–2, when he had just started his medical training. It was during the next cholera epidemic of 1848–9 that he made his seminal contribution. By now Snow was in London and here he began to unravel the mode of transmission of the disease. Snow's work was a masterpiece in epidemiological investigation. He meticulously mapped the houses in which new cases of cholera were being diagnosed and observed a marked difference in the incidence and mortality of cholera in the south of London (8 deaths per 1000 inhabitants) compared to other areas (1–4 deaths per 1000 inhabitants). This led him to hypothesize that cholera was spread by water. He identified the public pumps from which the families living in the affected and unaffected areas drew their water. He noticed that there were surprising sites of sparing within otherwise heavily affected areas. His suspicion that the infection was in the water supply grew when he found that those living in the spared areas worked at a local brewery and received free beer, which was made with water from a source away from that supplying their homes. Even before the identification of bacteria, he postulated that the transmission was the result of a *living* organism that had the ability to multiply. Snow is of course remembered for urging that the handle be removed from the pump that supplied contaminated water in Broad Street in London during the epidemic of 1854. This led to a dramatic decrease in new cases in the area. Snow postulated that social conditions and hygiene were of paramount importance in the spread of infection. Although there was no medical treatment for cholera, it became apparent that the way to stop an epidemic was through good sanitation and good hygiene.

It follows from this that our first line of defence against infection is the prevention of the multiplication and spread of organisms. Open sewers, overcrowded living conditions, contaminated drinking water, poor food storage and preparation, inadequate personal hygiene and unprotected sexual contact are a recipe for disaster. This is not a text on public health medicine or politics, so we will not dwell on these points. But remember that each year in Asia, Africa and Latin America, roughly four to six million people die from diarrhoea and one to two million die from malaria. One third of the world's population is sub-clinically infected with tuberculosis and three million die from TB each year; twelve million people are infected with HIV worldwide. All these problems are more likely to be solved by engineers and politicians than by the latest advances in molecular biology!

Figure 1 Deaths from cholera (–) in Broad Street, Golden Square, London, and the neighbourhood, 19 August to 30 September 1854. Water pumps are shown. John Snow realized that deaths were clustered around the Broad Street pump. Families working for the local brewery received free beer in preference to water and did not catch cholera! (Reproduced with permission from Wellcome Library, London)

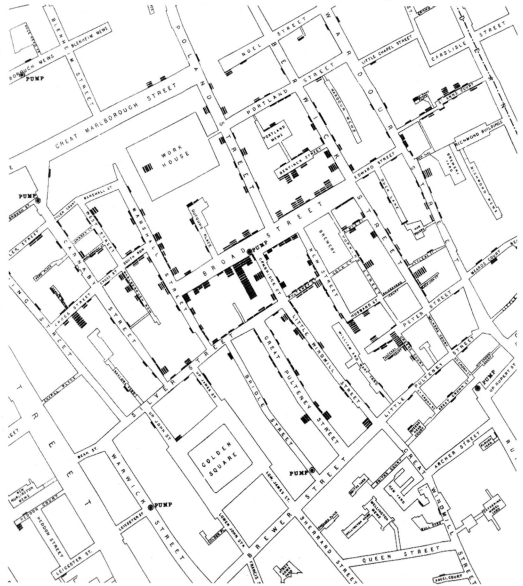

CHAPTER 3

THE BODY'S RESPONSE TO INFECTION

MAJOR ROUTES FOR THE TRANSMISSION OF INFECTION

Infections start from a reservoir of some kind, which acts as a source of pathogens. The commonest source of human infections is infected humans, although some diseases involve animal reservoirs or soil organisms.

It is not difficult to work out the main routes of spread from one infected human to another. Bugs in one person's respiratory tract are coughed out as aerosols, become air-borne and are inhaled by other people. A simple bus journey is laden with opportunities for bacteria and viruses to visit new human hosts. Direct mucosal contact is important in sexually transmitted diseases (HIV, herpes simplex, hepatitis B, papilloma virus, chlamydia, gonorrhoea and syphilis) and viruses infecting salivary glands (herpes and mumps).

Gut pathogens are excreted in the faeces and can re-enter the same or another gut via faecal contamination of water or food (faeco-oral route). Contamination of food is due generally either to lack of human hand-washing or failing to cover food to protect it from flies.

There is a much more sinister group of arthropods than the simple fly with dirty feet. These are insects that are themselves infected with an organism which they transfer by injection into humans (for example, malaria and yellow fever). This is one means by which blood-borne spread can occur. An insect sucks up infected blood from a human or animal and transfers it to another human or animal when it next bites. In some instances (e.g. malaria) the insect is an essential component because part of the infective agent's life cycle takes place within its body. Humans traditionally fear rats, possibly because of their historical links with bubonic plague. But, like flies, they are relatively innocent, being mere vehicles for the ticks which live on their bodies and which carry the bug (*Yersinisa pestis*) to the human.

Comparable methods of spread are via hypodermic needles shared by drug addicts (e.g. hepatitis B) or through use of contaminated blood products (e.g. HIV and hepatitis C in haemophiliacs).

Before we consider how the body can respond to disease we should consider its natural defences. For practical purposes the defences of the body can be separated into three components: structural barriers, innate immunity and adaptive immunity. This is a rather artificial separation. As we will see, these three components are intimately linked and act together in many instances to protect the body. Let us start with the structural barriers.

WHAT ARE THE BODY'S NATURAL DEFENCES AGAINST INFECTION?

The body is covered by epithelium, inside and out. The skin, with its stratified squamous epithelium topped with a waterproof layer of keratin, covers the outside. It contains some large holes, leading to areas covered by more permeable epithelium. From the top down these are the eyes, nasal cavity, mouth, anus, urethra and vagina, and each one has its own defence system (Fig. 3.1).

The eye drops its portcullis and floods the moat at the slightest provocation, because it is determined to repel invaders before they can produce any tissue damage. The main parts of the eye must be transparent and able to transmit light without distortion. A scarred cornea can render the eye useless so anything worse than a little inflammation of the conjunctiva can be devastating. So the eye's defences include a nerve reflex to close the eyelids as danger approaches, and a lacrimal gland to secrete tears to wash away particles, chemicals and bugs in a matter of seconds. In addition, tears contain lysozyme, an enzyme capable of degrading bacterial cell walls. If you have ever had even the smallest scratch to the surface of your eye, you will know that the flow of tears and the desire to keep the eyelids closed keeps going until the epithelial covering is re-established. Fortunately, this generally takes less than 24 hours.

Figure 3.1 Natural defences against infection

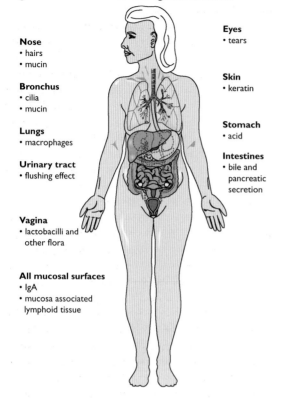

Nose
• hairs
• mucin

Bronchus
• cilia
• mucin

Lungs
• macrophages

Urinary tract
• flushing effect

Vagina
• lactobacilli and
  other flora

All mucosal surfaces
• IgA
• mucosa associated
  lymphoid tissue

Eyes
• tears

Skin
• keratin

Stomach
• acid

Intestines
• bile and
  pancreatic
  secretion

The nose can be considered with the respiratory tract, since both are covered predominantly by respiratory epithelium. This is characterized by the presence of mucus-secreting cells and cilia. Cilia are tiny hair-like structures that beat in a synchronous fashion to move particles up the respiratory tract. A layer of mucus lines the respiratory tract, providing a barrier against infectious agents and trapping inhaled particles. The mucous layer acts as a conveyor belt propelled by the underlying cilia. This is the muco-ciliary clearance mechanism and it is severely damaged by smoking. The airways also have a nervous mechanism of defence in coughs and sneezes, which forcefully expel unwanted material. This is good for the individual but potentially hazardous for those in the vicinity, as it is a super method of spread for air-borne bugs. If microbes get past the muco-ciliary defence, there is a second line of defence involving the macrophages in the alveoli; often termed the sentries of the lung.

The mouth and anus form the ends of the gastrointestinal tract and both are protected by non-keratinizing stratified squamous epithelium and a layer of mucus from local glands. The mouth has teeth and an enzyme (amylase) both of which, it could be argued, have a

defensive role but their main purpose is clearly related to digestion. There are similar dual-purpose roles for the hydrochloric acid and enzymes in the stomach or the secretions of the small intestine; their main role is digestive but they may also be harmful to many microorganisms. The gut, like the respiratory tract, has a layer of protective mucus. Immunoglobulins are specifically made for the lining of the gut and disable many bacteria and other organisms ingested with food. The gut, of course, is not sterile. It is colonized by a range of bugs that often live in peaceful co-existence unless something upsets the balance. This commonly occurs when a course of antibiotics destroys one type of bacterium, so allowing another to over-proliferate and cause problems, so-called antibiotic-associated or pseudomembranous colitis. *Clostridium difficile* is a bacterium that proliferates under these circumstances and secretes a toxin to produce bloody diarrhoea.

The urinary tract is normally protected by a one-way flow of urine from kidney to urethra, along tubes lined by a multilayered transitional epithelium. There is no mucus barrier here but it should not be needed, as the urine formed in the kidney is sterile. Its defences are the high volume of urine flushing the system, the physical barrier of the empty urethra and the natural variation of the pH of the urine. Women have a short urethra and are more liable than men to urinary tract infections, which often occur after sexual activity. This can cause perineal bacteria to be massaged up the urethra into the bladder ('honeymoon cystitis'). The urine may have an acidic or alkaline pH, favouring the growth of some bacterial strains over others. Hopefully, natural variations in the urinary pH will prevent a particular bacterium from becoming established and proliferating. Diabetics can have particular problems if the urine contains glucose, which will nourish bacterial growth.

The genital tract of the female starts its defences with the vagina, which is lined by non-keratinizing stratified squamous epithelium and mucus and friendly colonies of Doderlein's bacillus, a lactobacillus that metabolizes glycogen to lactic acid to produce a pH5 which inhibits colonization by most other bacteria. Unfortunately, glycogen is only present when the vaginal epithelium is stimulated by oestrogens, between puberty and the menopause. At other ages, the vagina is alkaline and liable to infection with pathogenic staphylococci and streptococci. The main defence, however, is the mucus, lysozyme and ciliary action in the normal cervix. The uterus and tubes are specialized for their reproductive role but it is possible that the monthly shedding of the endometrium may be a useful defence against infection. The stereocilia in the Fallopian tubes, while wafting the ovum down, produce currents that may help to prevent bacteria from ascending.

Should the first line of defences fail, the body has a regular guard of armed and dangerous cells and molecules, whose brief is to resist attack (innate immunity). This army comes swiftly to the defence within seconds and minutes of damage occurring.

The innate immunity guard consists of neutrophil polymorphs and macrophages, which immobilize and engulf damaging agents, complement proteins, which attract inflammatory cells to the site of damage, molecules related to blood clotting and factors released from a variety of cells, which assist in the inflammatory response. We will hear more of these when we come to discuss acute inflammation in chapter 4.

Because bugs sometimes manage to break through the first and second line defences, we need another line of defence involving the inflammatory response and the immune system, so-called adaptive immunity. These are specific defences, which take time to develop, but because they are targeted specifically at the causative agent they generally cause less in the way of 'collateral damage' as they exert their effect than the innate defence mechanisms. T and B cells work to produce agents specifically against particular intruders. There are exceptions though (see tuberculosis later!).

HOW DO MICROORGANISMS EVADE OUR DEFENCES?

Entry through intact skin is most easily achieved if there is an animal vector designed for the purpose. Many microorganisms associate with biting insects that pierce human skin and so provide a route into the human body. The rabies virus relies on larger animals such as infected dogs or bats to bite humans and then on its acetyl choline-binding receptor to enter a neuronal cell. HIV, once in the blood (e.g. on a contaminated needle), binds helper T cells via the CD4 receptor, which binds to gp120 antigen on the viral surface. In these examples, the microorganism itself does not have special characteristics for skin penetration but some, such as the helminth larvae of hookworm or schistosoma, have lytic proteases to allow them to digest and burrow through intact skin.

Some viruses start out with a 'key to the door' in that they have receptors which bind specific molecules on the host cell surface, which allow them to gain entry.

A good example of this is the rhinovirus, which binds ICAM-1 on mucosal cells.

Protective coverings as in bacterial spores, protozoan cysts and thick-walled helminth eggs can evade the digestive tract's acid and enzymes (Fig. 3.2). Some parasites' eggs (e.g. *Giardia*) actually need stomach acid as a stimulus to cause them to hatch into the trophozoites that infect the intestine. Many of the non-enveloped viruses (hepatitis A, rotavirus, reovirus and Norwalk agents) are resistant to digestive juices and bacteria can 'hide' in food to avoid the acidity. *Helicobacter pylori* is the only pathogen that survives in the stomach acid. It does this by producing a urease that converts urea to ammonia and, thereby, changes the pH of its microenvironment.

The respiratory tract's mucociliary defence may be impaired by the host's own actions if they smoke or aspirate stomach acid. Neuraminidase-producing microorganisms may degrade the mucin layer and toxins produced by *Haemophilus* and *Bordetella* can paralyse mucosal cilia. Even if the mucociliary mechanisms are working well, some viruses can still avoid being expelled by having specific methods for adhesion to the epithelial surface, such as haemagglutinins on influenza virus. Once the defences are damaged, for example by a bad cold or flu, bacterial pneumonias are common.

Many microorganisms avoid our second line of defences by not attempting to pass through the epithelial surface but being content to grow on the top. Skin fungi (dermatophytes, e.g. *Candida*) and skin viruses (papilloma viruses causing warts) live in the superficial layers. Gut pathogens, such as *Vibrio cholera*, multiply in the mucus layer releasing exotoxins that cause watery diarrhoea. Some bacteria cause us harm without even entering the body if they produce exotoxins that contaminate food (e.g. staphylococci, see page 34).

So the first line of defence has been breached but the immune system and inflammatory mechanisms should still be able to defend us; shouldn't they? Thankfully, they normally do but the microbes have some clever tricks to avoid them.

First the immune system must spot the invader so the invaders change their surface antigens by shedding the antigens, changing the antigens during an infection or having numerous antigenic variants so that infective episodes do not produce useful immune memory. The next phase is killing the bugs by phagocytosis, complement-mediated lysis, antibody-mediated mechanisms or neutrophil activity. Yes, you've guessed. Somewhere there is a bug that will have evolved a way round each of these and a few examples are given in Table 3.1.

Figure 3.2 Bacterial protection against attack

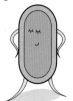 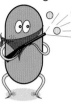 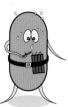 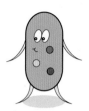 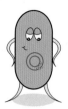

| Thick, sometimes waxy, outer capsule | Exotoxin production | Endotoxin production when bacterium lysed | Enzymes, may also digest connective tissue for ease of spread | Acquisition of DNA conferring antibiotic resistance |

Table 3.1 Mechanisms used by microbes to evade the immune system

Mechanism	Example
Shedding of antigens	*Schistosoma mansoni*
Changing antigens during infection	*Neisseria* altering pilins African trypanosomiasis
Many antigenic variants so no protective cross-immunity	Rhinovirus Influenza virus
Resistance to phagocytosis	Carbohydrate capsules of *Pneumococcus*, *Meningococcus* and *Haemophilus*
Interference with antibodies or complement	Protein A molecules of *Staphylococcus* blocking Fc portion of immunoglobulin Digestion by proteases of *Neisseria*, *Streptococcus* and *Haemophilus*
Resistance to complement-mediated lysis	K antigens on some *E. coli*
Resistance to macrophage killing	*Legionella*, *Mycobacterium* and *Toxoplasma* inhibit acidification
Inaccessible to immune system	Gut luminal proliferation of *Clostridium difficile* Papillomavirus or fungi in superficial layer of skin Direct viral transfer between adjacent cells
Specific damage to immune cells	*Pseudomonas* secretes a leucotoxin to kill neutrophils
Mimicry of host antigens	Group A streptococci and myocardium
Interference with MHC presentation of antigens	Herpes simplex inhibits peptide transporter CMV blocks MHC I presentation and expresses MHC I mimic
Bind to and inhibit cytokines	Vaccinia virus produces soluble interferon receptor
Immunosuppression	HIV, Epstein–Barr virus

By now you will have realized that in any war, a lot of innocent bystanders get hurt. The bugs need to survive, replicate and be shed to find new hosts. The normal flora or commensals manage this without causing damage but the pathogens are greedy, have more weapons and provoke a conflict with the inflammatory and immune cells. Damage to the host cells occurs because of competition for nutrients, release of inflammatory mediators and toxic substances by the host's inflammatory cells, production of substances by the microbes that damage the host's tissues and direct cellular damage by bugs.

ARE SOME PEOPLE MORE SUSCEPTIBLE TO INFECTION THAN OTHERS?

Since the antiseptic treatment has been brought into the full operation, and wounds and abscesses no longer poison the atmosphere with putrid exhalations, my wards, though in other respects under precisely the same circumstances as before, have completely changed their character: so that during the last nine months not a single instance of pyaemia, hospital gangrene or erysipelas haws occurred in them. As there appear to be no doubt regarding the cause of this change, the importance of the fact can hardly be exaggerated.

Joseph, Lord Lister (1827–1912), British surgeon

Let us consider a normal healthy individual; this person is not malnourished, not on immunosuppressive drugs nor just recovering from an operation. From a bug's point of view, what are the possible routes into the body? The surface of the body is covered by skin which, as we have discussed, has holes in it. Most of the holes lead down into sweat ducts, hair shafts and other skin appendage structures that still have an epithelial lining although a more delicate one. Bugs can live down these holes without causing particular problems unless the environment is upset by something which disturbs the delicate balance between host and bug. This occurs for example in scarring acne when the composition of the sebaceous gland secretion is altered, leading to blockage of the neck of a hair follicle, proliferation of bacteria behind the blockage, and the destruction of the follicle's epithelial line of defence to provoke inflammation in the surrounding skin.

In fact, skin is built to take knocks and we are all liable to develop small cuts and grazes on a frequent basis. We know that when this defence is down we must be extra-vigilant and keep the area clean and dry and do what mother says and resist picking at the delicate protective layer of scab which forms at the site of damage. This becomes even more important when the skin contains a large wound, as may follow a surgical operation. This is the time when bacteria have a really good chance of successfully invading a human body, because they have a band of helpers. These are the doctors and medical students who move rapidly from one patient to the next in the post-op surgical wards generously ensuring that all patients have the opportunity to acquire each other's skin flora.

The combination of overcrowding (i.e. many sick people living in a closed environment), difficulty with personal hygiene (just try having a bed bath!) and unprotected (non-sexual!) contact with a large number of strangers describes both a post-op surgical ward and a bacterium's idea of heaven. Add to this the likelihood of acquiring a bacterium which has been around in hospital for a while, and has learned a few tricks in terms of antibiotic resistance (see later), and an already weakened patient can have a big problem.

Diabetics are particularly prone to skin infections because, if their blood glucose levels are hard to control, all their body fluids can be high in glucose, and this provides an excellent culture medium for bacteria. Often diabetics have poor circulation due to vascular disease so bacteria can flourish relatively undisturbed by any immune response. The problem may be compounded by traumatic damage to the skin if they also have a loss of sensation due to diabetes-induced peripheral nerve damage meaning that they might not feel, for example, the early stages of blisters or small abrasions.

ANTIBIOTIC RESISTANCE

Since the discovery of penicillin and sulfonamides in the first half of the twentieth century we have been able to treat many bacterial infections. However, superbugs have begun to emerge, resistant to many antibiotics. The first reports are now emerging of a strain of MRSA (methicillin-resistant *Staphylococcus aureus*) which is resistant to all known antibiotics. Drug-resistant tuberculosis is increasingly a problem (see page 117). We know that the same genes which encode the various

Figure 3.3 **Transformation**

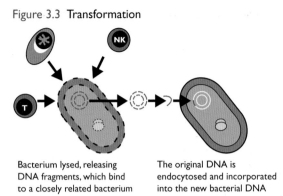

Bacterium lysed, releasing DNA fragments, which bind to a closely related bacterium

The original DNA is endocytosed and incorporated into the new bacterial DNA

resistance factors can be found in several unrelated classes of bacteria. How do the bugs transmit resistance to each other?

Resistance involves the transfer of genes. This can be achieved in four four main ways:

- transformation
- transduction
- conjugation
- transposon insertion.

TRANSFORMATION

Naked DNA fragments are released from a bacterium as it is lysed. These fragments then bind to the cell wall of another bacterium, are taken in and become incorporated into the recipient's DNA (Fig. 3.3). Sounds simple but generally only occurs between closely related bacteria with similar DNA (i.e. extensive homology) and suitable binding sites on the cell wall.

TRANSDUCTION

Bacteria themselves can be infected by viruses, called bacteriophages (Fig. 3.4). These viruses bind to specific receptors on the bacterial surface and then push a tube through the wall and inject the viral nucleic acid. The virus (bacteriophage) can take over the bacterial cell's replication mechanism in the same way as viruses replicate in human cells. New capsid proteins, nucleic acid and enzymes are produced and assembled so that, when the bacterial cell lyses, the phages are released. This is what occurs with virulent phages but there are also temperate phages which can insert their DNA into the host's DNA and lie dormant for long periods. Eventually, these little time bombs go off and replicate and lyse the

host cell in similar fashion to virulent phages but the fact that they have inserted into the bacteria's DNA is relevant to our discussion of transfer of resistance.

Generalized transduction involves virulent phages taking over the bacterial cell and accidentally packaging some bacterial DNA fragments instead of viral nucleic acid into one of the daughter phages. The mutant daughter phage will inject this bacterial DNA into the next cell it tries to infect and the bacterial DNA may incorporate into the host cell DNA (comparable to the changes in transformation). The host cell survives happily because no viral nucleic acid is injected and it may gain useful resistance or virulence factors, depending on the source of the fragment of bacterial DNA.

Specialized transduction utilizes temperate phages. When the phage DNA in the host genome (prophage) is reactivated, it is spliced out of the bacterial chromosome, replicated, translated and packaged into a capsid. The splicing may include taking some bacterial DNA immediately adjacent to the prophage and this will be incorporated into daughter phages. If the bacterial DNA confers resistance or virulence, this is a powerful method for sharing the information and it is called 'lysogenic conversion'. The genes for exotoxin production by *Corynebacteria diphtheriae*, *Vibrio cholera* and *Streptococcus pyogenes* (scarlet fever) can spread in this way.

CONJUGATION

Conjugation is the major mechanism for transfer of antibiotic resistance and involves the exchange of plasmids. Plasmids are pieces of circular double-stranded DNA, separate from the chromosome, which carry a variety of genes, including some for drug resistance and some coding for the enzymes and proteins needed for conjugation. These are called self-transmissible or F plasmids and bacteria can be F+ or F− depending on whether they contain the plasmid.

Bacterial sex involves a specialized sex pilus protruding from the surface of an F+ bacterium. This binds to and penetrates the cell membrane of an F− bacterium and a single strand of the F plasmid DNA passes from one cell to the other (Fig. 3.5).

The former F− cell is now F+ and has the information for resistance and for conjugation with other cells. The plasmid DNA is not totally fixed but can acquire additional bacterial genes if it integrates into the bacterial chromosome in a similar fashion to a temperate bacteriophage, i.e. when it is spliced out of the host

Figure 3.4 Transduction: bacterial DNA is transmitted via bacteriophages, of which there are two main types, virulent and temperate phages

A **virulent phage** injects its DNA into a bacterium and utilizes the bacterial replication equipment to form further phage particles

The bacterial DNA becomes fragmented and a portion may be incorporated into newly formed phages, which are released as the bacterium lyses

A **temperate phage** injects its DNA into a bacterium; this becomes incorporated into the bacterial DNA and remains there until a stimulus to reproduce is received

Then the phage DNA is translated and often accidentally incorporates some of the adjacent bacterial DNA within the genome of the new phages, due to inaccurate splicing. The bacterium disintegrates as the phages are released

Stimulus to reproduce

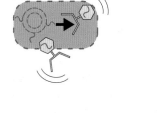

DNA encodes protein confering antibiotic resistance

The next bacterium to be invaded by a bacteriophage receives DNA from another bacterium. If it is lucky, this will confer on it an advantage, such as antibiotic resistance

chromosome it includes some of the adjacent bacterial DNA and is called an F prime (F′) plasmid. An alternative is that the bacterial chromosome with the incorporated plasmid is all transferred to the F− cell during conjugation.

Plasmids encode medically important enzymes, such as penicillinase, and virulence factors, such as exotoxin and fimbriae.

TRANSPOSONS

Transposons are also DNA fragments that can carry genes for resistance and virulence, but differ in that they can insert into host DNA which is dissimilar (i.e. lacks homology) and so can spread resistance across

bacterial genera. They can insert into phages, plasmids and bacterial DNA (Fig. 3.6).

HOW CAN WE PREVENT OR OVERCOME BACTERIAL RESISTANCE?

Life is a struggle for survival and the animal, plant or microorganism best adapted to a particular environment is most likely to flourish. Humans can have an enormous impact on the environment and we must use this ability with care. In this context, we are concerned that we might alter the microbes' environment so as to give the resistant bacteria a survival advantage. If everyone was taking a particular antibiotic, only microbes resistant to that drug would survive and so that specific environmental niche would become populated with resistant bugs and the antibiotic would be useless. This is the fear with tuberculosis as the incidence of dormant multiple drug-resistant tuberculosis increases. Of course, we don't have everyone on the same antibiotic and we have to hope that the non-resistant bugs will predominate when the antibiotic is stopped.

Problems occur when antibiotics are widely used, particularly in a hospital setting, and the resistant bug gains a clear advantage. We shall consider methicillin-resistant *Staphylococcus aureus* (MRSA) as an important example of how man and microbe each develop strategies to defy the other. *Staphylococcus aureus* is a Gram-positive coccus that was originally sensitive to penicillin. By the 1950s, the bug had developed enzymes (β-lactamases) to destroy penicillin. Man then produced a penicillin analogue called methicillin with a side chain which reduced lactamase binding to the enzyme. Further drug development led to the widely used flucloxacillin, so Man had the upper hand until the late 1970s and early 1980s, until *Staphylococcus aureus* strains resistant to multiple antibiotics, including methicillin and gentamycin, emerged. These bugs are an enormous problem in hospitals, particularly on surgical wards where wound infections are a major concern. The only effective drug against such staphylococci is vancomycin which is somewhat toxic and requires intravenous administration. The recent identification of vancomycin-resistant enterococci in a patient with MRSA sets the scene for the nightmare scenario where resistance to vancomycin may be transferred from the enterococci to the MRSA, both of which may be found in the gut or surgical wounds. A truly 'superbug' MRSA would then be unstoppable. It is just a matter of time since nothing we have done with antibiotics suggests we can contain such an event!

Figure 3.5   Bacterial conjugation

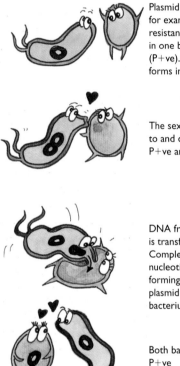

Plasmid determining, for example, penicillin (P) resistance, is present in one bacterium (P+ve). A sex pillus forms in the P+ve cell

The sex pillus extends to and connects the P+ve and P−ve bacteria

DNA from the plasmid is transferred. Complementary nucleotides are added, forming a complete plasmid in each bacterium

Both bacteria are now P+ve

Figure 3.6   Transposon insertion

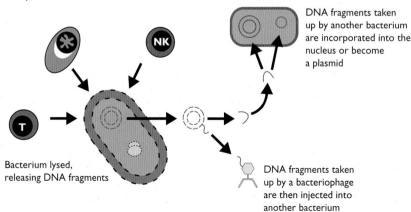

DNA fragments taken up by another bacterium are incorporated into the nucleus or become a plasmid

Bacterium lysed, releasing DNA fragments

DNA fragments taken up by a bacteriophage are then injected into another bacterium

There are three main strategies for trying to avoid or overcome bacterial resistance:

- control of antibiotic use
- modification of existing antibiotics or development of new antibiotics capable of bypassing the bacterium's method of resistance
- use of combinations of antibiotics employing different mechanisms.

The best approach is preventative. If antibiotics are used less and are only used appropriately, then resistant strains are less likely to evolve. This means that there should be great caution about using antibiotics as growth promoters in animal feeds for fear that this will result in resistant bugs which may be transferred to humans. In humans, antibiotics should not be used unnecessarily and care should be taken to avoid incomplete treatment. Incomplete treatment is a problem in tuberculosis where lengthy treatment with multiple drugs may be necessary to eradicate the organisms but patient compliance may be poor. Incomplete treatment will allow the most resistant bug to survive, regrow and spread to other susceptible individuals. Multiple drug resistant TB strains now represent more than 20 per cent of cases in parts of New York and are now being found in mainland Europe and the UK. Common sense also demands that, particularly in hospitals, transfer of bugs from one patient to another must be minimized and this requires special attention to disinfection of endoscopes, bronchoscopes, etc. which cannot be autoclaved.

The second strategy involves developing new drugs or modifying existing ones. The idea is that once the mechanism for bacterial resistance is understood, it should be possible to redesign the molecule to get around the problem. We have already mentioned the example of methicillin with its side chain to prevent it from binding to the enzyme β-lactamase. Another example involves the tetracyclines which have little effect on bugs that have developed a highly efficient mechanism for excreting the drug from the bacterial cell through specific 'efflux proteins'. A new group of tetracyclines called glycylcyclines have an altered side chain that prevents their excretion via efflux proteins.

The third approach is to use combinations of antibiotics. Sometimes the combinations have been developed empirically but some combinations have been specifically designed to overcome resistance. This is the case with clavulanic acid which is only a weak antibiotic but binds irreversibly to many β-lactamases and so can protect β-lactam antibiotics from destruction. This is used clinically as Augmentin which is a combination of amoxycillin and clavulanic acid.

HOW DO VIRUSES DEVELOP RESISTANCE TO ANTIVIRAL AGENTS?

Viruses also become resistant to anti-viral agents through the selection of naturally occurring mutants, which have amino acid changes at the active site or binding site of the anti-viral agent. This is only normally seen in immuno-compromised hosts where the number of viral particles (viral load) is high, thus increasing the chances of a natural mutant occurring. Viruses have small genomes (HIV = 9 kb, herpes = 500 kb, bacteria = 3 Mb, human = 4000 Mb), so the chance of a mutant occurring is dependent on the number of virions and the size of the genome. HIV is a good example of this both in terms of drug resistance and immune evasion.

The first part of HIV replication is the conversion of its RNA genome into DNA prior to integration into the host cell chromosome as proviral DNA. This reaction is unique to retroviruses and is mediated by the virally encoded RNA-dependent DNA polymerase: reverse transcriptase (RT). RT is the target for the anti-viral AZT drug used in the treatment of AIDS. AZT is an analogue of thymidine with an azide group at the 3' OH group of the ribose moiety. When incorporated into DNA by RT, AZT causes chain termination and stops DNA synthesis and halts the viral life cycle. Fortunately, AZT has higher affinity for RT than for cell-encoded DNA polymerases, hence its selective toxicity. AZT-resistant HIV mutants have amino acid substitutions in the active site, so AZT no longer binds. The RT of HIV does not possess any proofreading activity seen in cellular DNA polymerases and has an error rate of 10^{-4}; i.e. makes a mistake every 10 000 bases, which is about once every time a genome is copied. Thus, if 10^8 virions were made, there would be a chance for each base to be changed in the viral progeny (genome size = 9000 bases). During HIV infection, about 10^9 virions are made and destroyed by the immune system every day, so it is easy to see that a random mutation in the active site of RT is highly likely. Use of AZT selects out the resistant mutant which continues to replicate and spread within the body; thus, AZT resistance can emerge readily in a few months or less. Combined anti-HIV chemotherapy is now used that includes several anti-RT compounds and a protease inhibitor because it is much less likely that any one virus will acquire mutations in two or three separate sites to affect the binding and activity of all of the inhibitors. HIV also uses this natural mutation rate to its advantage to change the amino acid sequences of its exterior glycoprotein (gp120) which binds the cell CD4 receptor. The V3 region of gp120 shows epitope changes in isolates from the same patient infected with HIV and these have been shown to permit escape from a cytotoxic T cell immune response. Thus, RT error rate provides a mechanism for generating immune escape mutants and drug resistance.

It is hardly surprising that infection is still a challenge and the next chapter is devoted to inflammation, which includes conditions of infective and immune aetiology.

CHAPTER 4

THE ACUTE INFLAMMATORY RESPONSE

No natural phenomenon can be adequately studied in itself alone, but to be understood must be considered as it stands connected with all nature.

Sir Francis Bacon (1561–1626)

WHAT IS INFLAMMATION?

It is a mechanism by which the body deals with an injury or insult. Tissue injury stimulates inflammation. Causes of tissue damage were discussed chapter 2. When living tissue is damaged, a series of local processes are initiated in order to contain the offensive agent, to neutralize its effect, to limit spread and hopefully to eradicate it. As part and parcel of this process, there is initiation of healing and repair of the injured tissue. Inflammation, healing and repair are like the black and white stripes of the zebra; in order truly to understand the zebra, one cannot study the stripes in isolation. In the same way, the processes of healing and repair have to be addressed in their relationship to the process of inflammation.

The circulatory system is of fundamental importance in the inflammatory response. In general terms, the offending agent, whatever it may be, causes a change in the microvasculature of the injured area leading to a massive outpouring of cells and fluid. This collection of cells and fluid is known as the inflammatory exudate, and within this exudate, we find ingredients that are needed to combat the offending agent and to begin the process of healing and repair. However, this is only half the story. It is romantic to imagine an army being sent to deal with an invading force and to restore the peace and tranquillity to the area. Life is not quite so simple; there is a price to be paid for war! The ugly side of it ranges from cosmetic problems, such as keloid scars, to life-threatening illnesses, like autoimmune diseases.

Many of John Hunter's experiments are absolutely fascinating as well as crazy and amusing, but more of that later, so keep reading!

History   John Hunter (1728–1793)

John Hunter, surgeon to St. George's Hospital from 1768 to 1793, was interested in inflammation and repair. He was an incredible man whose aim was the total understanding of mankind! Hunter was born in Scotland on 14 February 1728, the last of ten children. He spent the first 20 years there and his childhood has been described as 'wasted and idle'. This is because he '…wanted to know all about the clouds and the grasses, and why the leaves changed colour in the autumn…'. Hunter's inquisitiveness and fascination with nature stood him in good stead when he began to unravel the mysteries of the human body. His book, *A Treatise on the Blood, Inflammation, and Gunshot Wounds*, is a monument to his thoroughness and powers of observation in delineating the processes of disease. Hunter was one of the first to observe that inflammation was not a disease but a response to tissue injury.

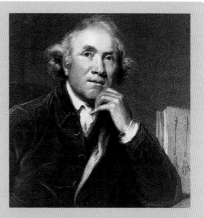

Figure 4.1 John Hunter (1728–93)
© CORBIS

Anyone who has had a boil or any other skin infection, will be familiar with the four cardinal signs of inflammation: rubor (redness), calor (heat), tumour (swelling) and dolor (pain). A Roman physician, Cornelius Celsus, first described these in the first century AD. To this a fifth sign was later added, *laesio functae* (loss of function); however, this is not a necessary accompaniment of the inflammatory process.

So what is the pathophysiology behind these clinical signs?

MICROVASCULATURE

The microvasculature plays a central role in inflammation and the *redness* is caused by vasodilatation. This is important for increasing the flow of blood to the affected area and, hence, delivering cells and plasma-derived substances needed for combat. Vasodilatation also produces the *heat*. The *swelling* results from increased permeability of vessel walls leading to the outpouring of fluid and cells, the inflammatory exudate. In some circumstances, the swelling may cushion the affected part and lead to immobilization (*loss of function*). The sign that is the most difficult to explain is *pain*. This probably arises from the combination of stretching of tissue by exudate and the action of some of the chemical mediators involved in inflammation.

But what are the underlying mechanisms of this process? In broad terms, there are two aspects to consider:

- the cells of inflammation
- the chemical mediators.

CELLULAR MEDIATORS

The principal cells of inflammation are the polymorphonuclear leucocytes or granulocytes (which include neutrophils, eosinophils and basophils) and the lymphocytes, plasma cells and macrophages (Table 4.1). A Russian microbiologist, Elias Metchnikoff, working at the Pasteur Institute in Paris in 1884, demonstrated that leucocytes phagocytose bacteria and concluded that the purpose of the inflammatory response was to bring phagocytic cells to the area to kill the organisms. Inflammatory cells descend on a focus of tissue damage in 'waves'; the first cell type recruited is the neutrophil polymorph (an 'acute' inflammatory cell), which is followed by macrophages, lymphocytes and plasma cells ('chronic' inflammatory cells). Later, the tissue generates new blood vessels and fibrous scar tissue as reparative work begins.

THE CHEMICAL MEDIATORS

In 1927, Sir Thomas Lewis identified histamine, present in tissue mast cells, as a mediator of acute inflammation. Since then a vast array of mediators have been identified, but not all have a proven role *in vivo*. They may be derived from the plasma, the participating inflammatory cells or from the damaged tissue itself.

The cell-derived products include:

- vasoactive amines
- cytokines and growth factors
- arachidonic acid derivatives (eiocosanoids)
- platelet activating factor
- lysosomal enzymes
- oxygen-derived free radicals
- nitric oxide.

The plasma derived mediators include:

- the kinin system
- the coagulation and fibrinolytic system
- the complement system.

Some are important in the amplification of the inflammatory response; others play their role in the elimination of the offending agent. The mediators and their roles in inflammation will be discussed in more detail later.

WHAT IS THE DIFFERENCE BETWEEN ACUTE AND CHRONIC INFLAMMATION?

Acute inflammation, generally, is of short duration, lasting from a few minutes to a few days and the cellular exudate is rich in neutrophil polymorphonuclear leucocytes with some macrophages arriving after the initial insult.

Chronic inflammation may last for months or years and the chief cells involved are lymphocytes, plasma cells and macrophages (see page 116).

The inflammatory process, whether acute or chronic, may be modified by a whole host of factors such as the cause of the damage, the nutritional status of the patient, the competence of the patient's immune system and intervention with antibiotics, anti-inflammatory drugs or surgery.

WHAT HAPPENS TO THE PATIENT WITH ACUTE INFLAMMATION?

The patient with a boil on the bum will be less impressed than we are with the inflammatory processes

Table 4.1 Cells involved in inflammation (see Figs 4.3 and 4.4)

Cell category	Cell type	Origin	Per cent white cells	Major function
Circulating cells				
Granulocytes (polymorphonuclear leucocytes)	Neutrophils	Bone marrow	75	Acute inflammatory cell involved in bacterial killing and phagocytosis. Granule contents for increasing vascular permeability, chemotaxis, killing organisms and digesting extracellular matrix
	Eosinophils	Bone marrow	1	Acute inflammatory cell particularly common in allergic and parasitic conditions. Granules include major basic protein
	Basophils	Bone marrow	<1	Circulating cells that give rise to **mast cells**. Granules include histamine
Lymphocytes	T cells	Lymphoid organs and thymus	20	Various subtypes involved in antigen recognition and presentation, cell killing and regulation of immune responses (e.g. helper, suppressor and natural killer cells)
	B cells	Lymphoid organs and bone marrow		On antigen stimulation, proliferate and give rise to specific **plasma cells**, which synthesize specific immunoglobulins
Macrophage system	Monocytes	Bone marrow	4	Migrate into tissues to be **macrophages** capable of phagocytosis, cytokine production and antigen processing and presentation
Non-circulating cells				
Kupffer cells (liver sinusoids) Macrophages (bone marrow, spleen and lymph nodes)				Fixed phagocytic cells lining sinusoids and filtering large molecules/particles from blood or lymph
Megakaryocytes in bone marrow				Produce platelets which contain serotonin, platelet-derived growth factor, etc. Also important in haemostasis
Hepatocytes				Produce proteins important in: • clotting and fibrinolytic system • complement system • kinin system • acute-phase proteins

taking place (Fig. 4.2). He will be well aware that the boil exhibits the cardinal features of pain, swelling, redness and heat! He may regard the fact that the injury has caused microvascular changes via mediators, leading to cellular and humoral factors accumulating at the site of injury, as of less importance than the burning question, 'What will happen next?'

There are several possibilities. The inflammatory and healing process may restore the tissue to its normal state, with nothing to suggest that anything has been amiss. Healing may take place but leave a scar. The injury and the inflammation may grumble on for a long time or the injury, particularly if infected, may completely overwhelm the body and lead to death. This last outcome

Figure 4.2 Possible outcomes following acute inflammation

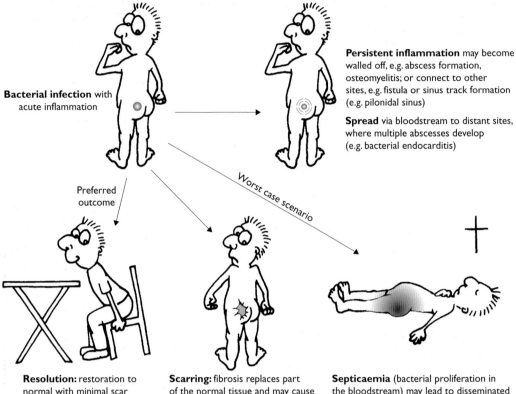

Bacterial infection with acute inflammation

Persistent inflammation may become walled off, e.g. abscess formation, osteomyelitis; or connect to other sites, e.g. fistula or sinus track formation (e.g. pilonidal sinus)

Spread via bloodstream to distant sites, where multiple abscesses develop (e.g. bacterial endocarditis)

Preferred outcome

Worst case scenario

Resolution: restoration to normal with minimal scar formation (e.g. surgical scar)

Scarring: fibrosis replaces part of the normal tissue and may cause deformity (e.g. traumatic skin wound with soft tissue injury)

Septicaemia (bacterial proliferation in the bloodstream) may lead to disseminated intravascular coagulation or shock; death may occur (sequel to many overwhelming infections, e.g. bronchopneumonia)

is especially likely where inflammatory defences are deficient, such as in AIDS, cancer patients treated with cytotoxic drugs or patients receiving immunosuppressive drugs for auto-immune disease or following organ transplantation. The final outcome depends on the interactions between the various processes involved in inflammation. Just as the zebra is neither black with white stripes nor white with black stripes, so it is the combination of the various inflammatory components that determines the texture of the whole.

Now that we have the overall concept of inflammation and its clinical relevance, we must look more closely at the complex cellular and molecular events of this process. We shall first examine the changes in the microvasculature.

VASCULAR CHANGES

We are indebted to Julius Conheim (1839–84) for investigating the pathophysiology of inflammation. He was a German pathologist, a pupil and later assistant to the 'father' of cellular pathology, Rudolf Virchow. He delineated the vascular changes of inflammation using living preparations of thin membranes, such as the mesentery, and demonstrated the vasodilatation and the subsequent exudation of fluid. His experiments with frog mesentery beautifully demonstrated that injury produced vasodilatation resulting in more blood entering the tissue but sometimes a slower flow of blood in capillaries. This allows white cells (leucocytes) to attach to the vessel wall (margination) and then move across the wall to the extravascular compartment (diapedesis or emigration).

Before we consider the causes of altered vascular permeability, it is worth revising the normal physiological factors that control the movement of fluid across a small vessel wall and into the extravascular tissues.

Fluid flows away from areas of high hydrostatic pressure and towards areas of high osmotic pressure (Fig. 4.5). Thus, fluid leaves from the arterial end of the capillary network and is reabsorbed at the venous end (a), with

Figure 4.3 Haemopoietic and lymphoid cells originate in the bone marrow and usually circulate in the blood, lymphoid organs or tissues as indicated. pmn, neutrophil polymorph; eo, eosinophil; mast, mast cell; baso, basophil; mono, monocyte, which becomes mac, macrophage in the tissues; dend APC, dentritic antigen-presenting cell; rbc, red blood cell

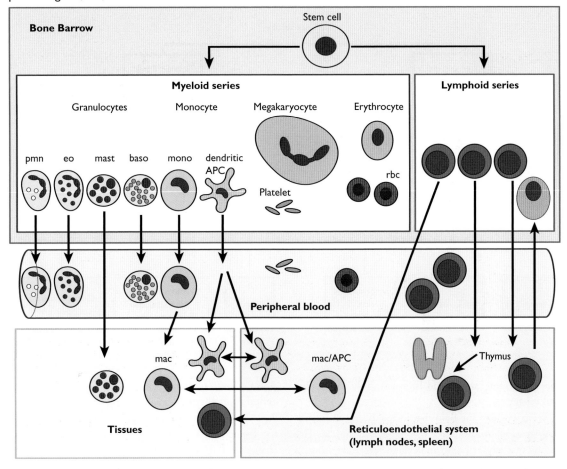

any excess being removed via lymphatics. A rise in hydrostatic pressure within the vessel without changes in permeability will increase leakage of fluid out of the vessel but it will have no protein in it (b). However, if the permeability of the vessel wall increases, then fluid can move more readily and protein molecules may also leak across. Movement of protein molecules will alter the osmotic pressure gradient, such that less fluid is reabsorbed into the blood at the venous end of the capillaries and tissue fluid will increase (c). In areas of inflammation there is usually a rise in hydrostatic pressure and an increase in vascular permeability (d).

This is an appropriate time to introduce a number of new words. An exudate is the fluid within the extravascular spaces which is rich in protein and hence

has a specific gravity of greater than 1.020. On the other hand, a transudate has a low protein content and specific gravity of less than 1.020. Oedema simply refers to the presence of excess fluid within the extravascular space and body cavities and may be an exudate or transudate. Pus can be thought of as a special kind of exudate, a purulent exudate. Besides protein-rich fluid exudate, it contains dead or dying bacteria and neutrophils. The consistency of the pus depends on the amount of digestion by neutrophil enzymes and the colour depends on the type of organism and the presence of neutrophil-derived myeloperoxidase, which imparts a yellow-green colour. Exudates generally contain fibrinogen which is converted to fibrin through the action of tissue thromboplastin. The fibrin forms a mesh

Figure 4.4 Origins of important meditaors of inflammation

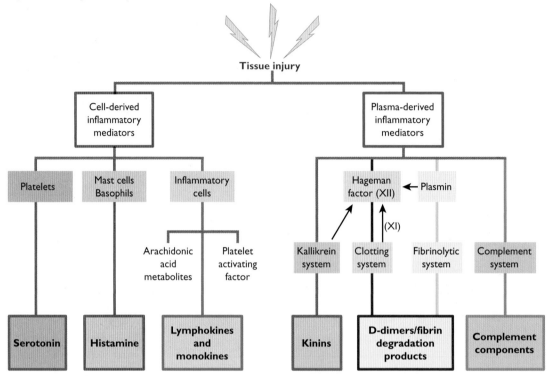

for cells to migrate on and later a scaffold for healing and repair.

If we examine the fluid that forms during an inflammatory reaction, we find that it is an exudate. This means that large protein molecules have leaked out of the microvasculature. What is the mechanism of the increased permeability? Most vessels are lined by endothelium which is termed 'continuous'. In the endocrine organs, intestines, liver and renal glomeruli, the endothelium is normally more permeable because it contains 'windows', hence the name fenestrated endothelium, while in the spleen, liver and bone marrow the endothelium is discontinuous. What happens following injury has been elegantly demonstrated using simple experiments involving the intravenous injection of Indian ink (Fig. 4.6). The ink will remain within the vascular compartment except in the liver and spleen where the discontinuous endothelium allows ink to escape. If a mild injury is produced (e.g. by using heat), the damaged area will turn black. Microscopical examination would reveal that the ink particles have crossed the endothelial layer and are trapped at the basement membrane. Injection of

a vasoactive substance, histamine, would cause the endothelial cells of the small venules to contract, creating gaps through which the ink molecules could pass. In reality, the situation is more complicated as the vascular changes will depend on the severity of the insult.

Three types of vascular response have been demonstrated, although they generally overlap in real situations:

- the immediate–transient response
- the immediate–persistent response
- the delayed–persistent response (Fig. 4.7).

The immediate–transient response

This occurs immediately following injury, reaches a peak after 5–10 minutes and ceases after 15–30 minutes. This response can be produced by histamine and other chemical mediators and is blocked by prior administration of anti-histamines. The leakage occurs exclusively from small venules which develop gaps between the endothelial cells as these cells contract. This occurs after nettle stings or insect bites.

Figure 4.5 Factors affecting the movement of fluid across vessels

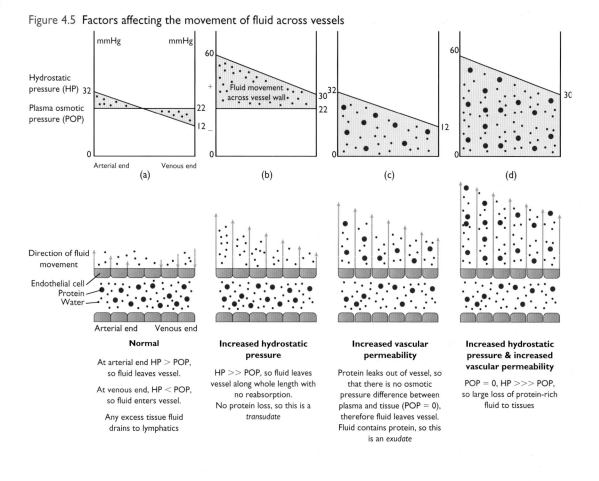

Normal

At arterial end HP > POP, so fluid leaves vessel.

At venous end, HP < POP, so fluid enters vessel.

Any excess tissue fluid drains to lymphatics

Increased hydrostatic pressure

HP >> POP, so fluid leaves vessel along whole length with no reabsorption.
No protein loss, so this is a *transudate*

Increased vascular permeability

Protein leaks out of vessel, so that there is no osmotic pressure difference between plasma and tissue (POP = 0), therefore fluid leaves vessel. Fluid contains protein, so this is an *exudate*

Increased hydrostatic pressure & increased vascular permeability

POP = 0, HP >>> POP, so large loss of protein-rich fluid to tissues

Figure 4.6 Vascular endothelium is continuous everywhere except the liver and spleen; here the endothelium is fenestrated. Because of this, an intravenous injection of Indian ink will lead to the accumulation of ink particles in the liver and spleen. However, if endothelium elsewhere is damaged, e.g. by heat, gaps appear between the endothelial cells and ink particles can leak out of circulation at these sites

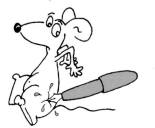

Ink is injected intravenously

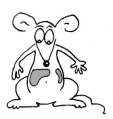

Ink escapes in organs with discontinuous endothelium

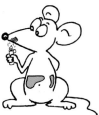

or if the endothelial cells are damaged

The immediate–persistent response

This results from severe injury such as burns, where there is direct damage to endothelial cells. The leak starts immediately and reaches a peak within an hour.

As the endothelial cells are damaged and may even slough off, the leak will continue until the vessel has been blocked with thrombus or the vessel is repaired. Unlike the previous example, it can affect any type of vessel.

Figure 4.7 Types of vascular response

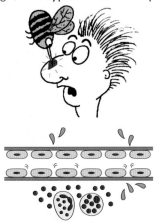

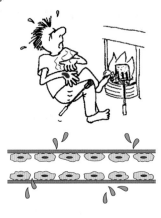

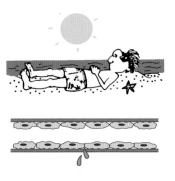

Immediate-transient response:
Immediate onset, peaking in 5–10 minutes and lasting from 15 to 30 minutes. Small blood vessels are affected. The temporary damage is caused by histamine, bradykinin, nitric oxide, complement (C5a), leukotrienes (e.g. LTB₄), platelet-activating factor (PAF). Causes include nettle sting, insect bite

Immediate-persistent response:
Caused by direct endothelial cell injury, arises immediately, peaking in about 1 hour and lasts until the vessel is plugged by thrombus or repaired. Any vessel type may be involved, the mechanism of injury being due to bradykinins, nitric oxide, complement, leukotrienes (e.g. LTB₄), platelet-activating factor (PAF), and potentiated by prostaglandins. Causes include severe direct injury, such as burns. Takes days to recover, as endothelium must regenerate

Delayed-persistent response: Caused by more subtle endothelial cell injury; arises in 18–24 hours and progresses for up to 36 hours (sometimes longer). Capillaries and venules are affected. Causes include sunburn, DXT (radiotherapy), bacterial toxins

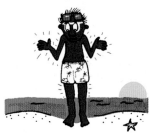

The delayed–persistent response

This is a very interesting type of response, familiar to anyone who has over-indulged in a tropical holiday after a period under the clouds of English skies. There is an interval of up to 24 hours before the leak starts from sun-damaged capillaries and venules. Small aggregates of platelets and endothelial cells are seen in some capillaries and it seems that the endothelial cells are damaged directly.

We shall next look at the cellular component of the inflammatory response.

CELLULAR EVENTS

The principal cells of the acute inflammatory response are the neutrophils and macrophages. However neutrophils circulate in the blood and have to be recruited to the site of injury so the first cells involved are those found within the tissues, the tissue macrophage and the mast cell. Following injury, and in response to certain signals, the neutrophils migrate out of the vessels, the number recruited depending on the type of injury.

For example, infections with bacteria attract more acute inflammatory cells than purely physical injuries. After the neutrophils, a second wave of cells arrives, the macrophages. These are derived from monocytes which circulate in the blood. The movement of leucocytes out of the blood vessels and their role in combat can be divided into discrete steps. These are:

- margination
- adhesion
- emigration
- chemotaxis
- phagocytosis and degranulation.

Margination and adhesion

When haemodynamic changes take place in the vasculature during inflammation, white cells fall out of the central axial flow and line themselves up along the wall (a little reminiscent of the school disco!). This is a result of rolling of leucocytes on the endothelial surface. There are specific complementary 'adhesion molecules'

Figure 4.8 Polymorph movement across blood vessels in acute inflammation is mediated by adhesion molecules and then follows a chemotactic gradient to the source of the inflammatory response

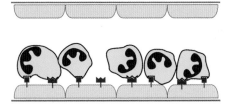

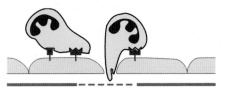

(a) Laminar flow: Polymorphs normally lie in the central stream, but the flow rate slows in acute inflammation and they 'fall out' of the axial stream towards the margin. IL-1, TNF and endotoxins upregulate E-selectin on the lining endothelial cells. The polymorphs bind these loosely and *roll* along the endothelial surface.

(b) Next the endothelial cells express integrins (e.g. ICAM-1), which bind tightly to LFA-1 on the polymorph, tethering it to the wall. These are also induced by acute inflammatory mediators. Polymorphs and other inflammatory cells migrate into the extravascular space by extending a pseudopodium into the junction between endothelial cells. They dissolve the basement membrane with proteases.

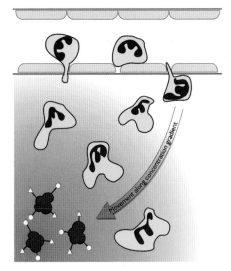

(c) The polymorph migrates between endothelial cells and the defect in the basement membrane seals behind them. Some red cells follow, but in acute inflammation there is generally little extravasation of red cells unless there has been vascular damage. The polymorph then moves along a chemotactic gradient set up by chemokines (which attach to matrix proteins in the soft tissues) to the inflammatory stimulus. Other inflammatory cells, particularly macrophages and eosinophils, use the same principles.

Figure 4.9 Photomicrographs illustrating margination (a) and emigration (b)

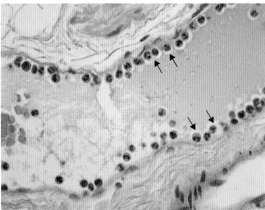

(a)

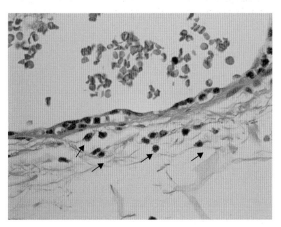

(b)

which stick leucocytes to endothelial cells and the number of these molecules on the cell surfaces is increased by inflammatory mediators. There are two main groups involved in the attraction and binding of neutrophils and macrophages. First, within minutes, P-selectin is upregulated on the endothelial cell of the blood vessel and then within 1–2 hours of injury, E-selectin is upregulated on the surface of the endothelial cell. Their complementary binding molecules, glycoproteins called Lewis X or A, are present on the leucocyte surface. These paired molecules only bind loosely and the leucocyte rolls along the blood vessel wall, slowing as it encounters each E-selectin molecule. The next pair of molecules, ICAM-1 on the endothelium and LFA-1 on the leucocyte, bind together like 'lock and key' arresting the rolling leukocyte on the endothelial surface.

Table 4.2 Adhesion moleules (see Figs 4.8 and 4.9)

Family	Some family members	Principally expressed on	Main function
Integrins	b1 family, e.g. VLA-4 b2 family, e.g. LFA-1	Lymphocytes and monocytes	Mediates immune and inflammatory responses including binding immunoglobulin superfamily molecules on endothelial cells to provide firm adhesion to vessel wall prior to migration
Immunoglobulin superfamily	ICAM-1, -2 and 3, VCAM-1	Endothelial cells, lymphocytes and monocytes	As above by binding to integrins
Selectins	E-selectin L-selectin	Endothelium Lymphocytes, polymorphs and monocytes	Initial phase of leucocyte adhesion to vessel wall
	P-selectin	Platelets and endothelial cells	
Cadherins	B, E, M, N, P, R, T	Range of tissues	Homophilic calcium-dependent cell–cell adhesion, e.g. at sites of desmosomes and adherens junctions. Not specifically involved in inflammation

ICAM-1, intercellular adhesion molecule 1; LFA-1, leucocyte function-associated antigen 1; VCAM-1, vascular cell adhesion molecule 1; VLA-4, very late antigen 4.

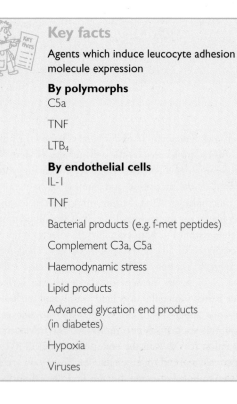

Key facts

Agents which induce leucocyte adhesion molecule expression

By polymorphs

C5a

TNF

LTB$_4$

By endothelial cells

IL-1

TNF

Bacterial products (e.g. f-met peptides)

Complement C3a, C5a

Haemodynamic stress

Lipid products

Advanced glycation end products (in diabetes)

Hypoxia

Viruses

These molecules have to be induced, which takes about 6 hours. Resting endothelial cells and leucocytes express very few adhesion molecules but some inflammatory mediators increase leucocyte expression of LFA-1 (e.g. complement fragments (C5a) and leukotrienes (LTB$_4$)), while other mediators enhance endothelial ICAM-1 expression (e.g. interleukin-1 and bacterial endotoxin). This adhesion is of great importance and people with a genetic deficiency of these adhesion molecules suffer from repeated bacterial infections.

Our knowledge of adhesion molecules is expanding rapidly. Broadly, there are four families, three of which are involved in inflammation; the integrins, the immunoglobulin gene superfamily and the selectins (the last family is the mucin-like glycoproteins, which are found on many cell surfaces and in the extracellular matrix, and which bind CD44 on the surfaces of leucocytes). Some (but not all) of their family members are listed in Table 4.2. Their expression changes during inflammation so that different types of cells adhere at different stages. Some of these molecules have been termed addressins because they act as address labels to allow cells to leave the circulation in a specific tissue.

This is particularly important in the recirculation and 'homing' of lymphocytes which is discussed on page 139.

Emigration and chemotaxis

Once the cells have firmly adhered to the endothelium, they form foot-like processes termed pseudopodia that push their way between the endothelial cells. This occurs in response to the binding of ICAM-1 (which triggers the leucocyte to flatten against the endothelial surface) and the presence of molecules called chemokines, which lie on the endothelium and the extracellular matrix and bind leucocytes, the binding process stimulating the formation of pseudopodia and movement towards the point of binding. Eventually, the leucocyte lies between the endothelial cell and the basement membrane where it releases a protease to digest the basement membrane, which allows it to reach the extravascular space. Neutrophils, basophils, eosinophils, macrophages and lymphocytes all use this route. Red blood cells may also pass through the gaps, but only as passive passengers.

The cells are able to move towards a chemical signal and this specific movement is termed chemotaxis. (Note that this is different to chemokinesis, which is an increased and accelerated *random* movement.) The Boyden chamber is a popular system for demonstrating chemotaxis. It consists of two chambers separated by a micropore filter. The cells go into one chamber and the putative chemical mediator is placed in the other. If cells move from the first to the second chamber, then chemotaxis is demonstrated. The compounds that have been suggested as chemotactic agents can be considered as exogenous or endogenous. The former include bacterial products such as f-met peptides, unmethylated nucleotides, lipopolysaccharide (LPS, also known as bacterial endotoxin) and bacterial proteoglycans, plus dsDNA from some viruses. Endogenous chemotaxins include fragments of the complement system (the most potent is C5a), products of arachidonic acid metabolism (e.g. prostaglandins and leukotrienes, particularly LTB_4) and cytokines such as IL-8.

How does it work? Well, like so many cellular stimuli, the first stage depends on the chemotactic agents binding to specific receptors (G-protein coupled receptors) on the leucocyte cell membrane. This leads to an increase in ionized calcium within the cytoplasm. Movement is achieved by the polymerization, coupling and decoupling of actin, which is calcium-dependent.

Leucocyte activation

There has been much interest in recent years over how white blood cells of all types are activated. Several classes of surface receptor exist and promote their effects via a variety of signalling pathways. The effects of leucocyte activation are their migration along chemotactic pathways, their arming (production of increased lysosomal granules and their contents in the cases of macrophages and neutrophils) and increased activity, e.g. increased phagocytic activity in neutrophils and macrophages. Recent interest has centred on a family of toll-like receptors, which recognize a variety of microbial constituents and can generate an inflammatory response which is appropriate to the initiating organism. Signalling by toll-like receptors can activate transcription factors such as NF-κB and signalling pathways such as MAP kinase.

PHAGOCYTOSIS

Once the neutrophils and macrophages have arrived at the site of injury, they ingest the debris and bacteria, a process termed phagocytosis. This requires a number of distinct steps: the material has to be recognized as foreign or dead, it has to be engulfed and ingested and finally, it has to be killed or degraded.

Not all of the processes by which neutrophils and macrophages differentiate between normal tissue and foreign or dead tissue are known, however it is clear that bacteria coated with certain substances are ingested more readily. The factors which coat bacteria are called opsonins and the process is termed opsonization. This is derived from the Greek word 'opson' meaning 'relish', i.e. getting ready for eating. There are two major opsonins, for which the phagocytes (usually neutrophils and macrophages) have specific, high-affinity, receptors:

- immunoglobulin (IgG), which binds to FcγRI (receptor for constant portion of IgG) (see page 147)
- C3b component of complement, which binds to CR1 (complement receptor 1) (see page 46).

There are several minor opsonins, such as mannose binding lectin, fibronectin, fibrinogen and C-reactive protein, all of which are present in the plasma and can coat particles such as invading microorganisms (Fig. 4.10).

After the opsonized fragment attaches to the receptor, the cell puts out a pseudopodium. This extension of

Figure 4.10 Phagocytosis by macrophages and neutrophil polymorphs is more efficient if the microbe is opsonized by antibody or complement. However, this is not essential and either cell can recognize foreign particles and engulf them. Factors which assist recognition include lectins, e.g. mannose, present on many organisms but not on mammalian cells. The macrophage scavenger receptors, which bind modified LDL , can bind to some microbes.

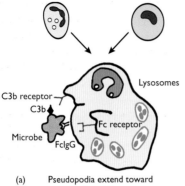

Macrophages and polymorphs are the main phagocytes

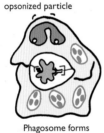

(a)   Pseudopodia extend toward opsonized particle

(a) Binding foreign material:
Microbes which are opsonized by C3b or antibody are easily bound via C3b receptors and FcγRI on the phagocyte surface

Less avid binding to microbes may occur via lectins, e.g. mannose, molecules recognized by the macrophage's scavenger receptor or by a coating of fibronectin, fibrinogen or C-reactive protein (CRP)

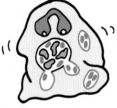

(b)   Phagosome forms

(b) Engulfing foreign material:
Once the receptor is triggered the cytoskeleton alters shape and the membrane invaginates and reseals, forming a phagosome

(c) Killing:
Phagosome fuses with lysosomes packed with pre-formed destructive enzymes, e.g. lysozyme, acid hydrolases, lactoferrin, major basic protein

Macrophages and polymorphs generate reactive oxygen species and superoxide anions by activating NADPH oxidase in the phagolysosome membrane

Polymorphs form highly toxic HOCL using myeloperoxidase and halide ions; macrophages generate nitric oxide to form nitrogen dioxide

(c)   Lysosome fuses to phagosome to form a phagolysosome

(d) Damage to surrounding tissues:
Occurs if enzymes leak before the surface membrane has fused (regurgitation during feeding)

Intentional secretion of cytotoxic agents occurs if microbe too large to be engulfed, e.g. a parasite, or antibody is attached to a fixed substrate, e.g. antigens trapped in glomerular or alveolar basement membrane

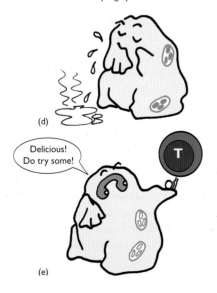

(d)

(e)

(e) Antigen presentation:
Macrophages which have phagocytosed foreign material usually select whether to become killers or antigen-presenting cells (APC) – this is to remind you that the latter present processed antigen to Th cells via MHC type II antigens

cell cytoplasm encircles the particle so that it becomes wrapped in what was originally cell surface membrane. This new intracytoplasmic membrane-bound sac is termed a phagosome. Another such sac, normally present in the cell and packed with destructive enzymes, is the lysosome. A lysosome fuses with the phagosome producing a phagolysosome. This allows the enzymes to have access to the engulfed particle and it is within this vesicle that the killing takes place. If some proteolytic enzymes leak out of the phagolysosome, as may occur if the lysosome fuses with the phagosome while the phagosome is still open to the cell surface, they may damage adjacent tissue; a phenomenon described, rather poetically, as 'regurgitation during feeding'. Fusion of a lysosome with the cell membrane and, hence, local release of toxic metabolites can be deliberate and is important for attacking large organisms, such as worms, that are too large to be ingested. The system can backfire, as happens if antibody–antigen complexes lodge in capillaries (e.g. farmer's lung, a type III hypersensitivity reaction, or glomerulonephritis in which the glomerular basement membrane is damaged because ab–ag complexes lodged within it stimulate the release of lysosomal contents). The lysosomal membrane may be traumatized by phagocytosed agents such as silica or urate crystals, causing the release of its contents into the tissues.

MECHANISMS FOR BACTERIAL KILLING

There are essentially two mechanisms for bacterial killing: oxygen-dependent and oxygen-independent.

The oxygen-dependent system involves toxic oxygen radicals that have an unpaired electron (indicated by a dot). These include superoxide (O_2^-), singlet oxygen ($O^{\cdot}$) and the hydroxyl radical ($OH^-{}^{\cdot}$). These molecules are produced by the respiratory burst that occurs during the process of phagocytosis. Oxygen is reduced to superoxide ion which is then converted to hydrogen peroxide (H_2O_2). A brilliant mechanism protects the neutrophil from being damaged by these products: they are not produced until the cell has been activated. To achieve this, some of the chemical components are moved from the cytoplasm to the membrane of the lysosome, where they combine to form NADPH oxidase. This converts oxygen within the lysosome to hydrogen peroxide and the toxic oxygen radicals. Iron

is required as a cofactor. This is not, however, the most powerful bactericidal chemical. Neutrophils contain an enzyme, myeloperoxidase, which converts H_2O_2 to HOCl (hypochlorous acid, or hypochlorite) in the presence of halide ions (e.g. chloride) and nitric oxide, produced by macrophages, reacts with superoxide anion to form the strong oxidant, nitrogen dioxide. These are powerful oxidants active against bacteria, fungi, viruses, protozoa and helminths. This system is of clinical importance as its absence produces 'chronic granulomatous disease of childhood', an inherited disease in which the neutrophils are able to ingest bacteria but unable to kill them. This is because the child lacks the enzyme NADPH oxidase, which leads to a failure of production of superoxide anion (O_2^-) and hydrogen peroxide.

There are a number of oxygen-independent mechanisms that are useful in microbial killing. These include

- lysozyme, an enzyme which attacks the cell wall of some bacteria (especially Gram-positive cocci)
- lactoferrin, an iron-binding protein that inhibits growth of bacteria
- major basic protein (MBP), which is a cationic protein found in eosinophils and is active principally against parasites
- bactericidal permeability increasing protein (BPI), which as the name implies, causes changes in the permeability of the membranes of the microorganisms.

Also the low pH found in the phagolysosomes, besides being bactericidal itself, enhances the conversion of hydrogen peroxide to superoxide. Unfortunately, the leucocyte is not successful in killing all organisms and some bacteria, such as the mycobacterium which causes tuberculosis, can survive inside phagocytes, happily protected from antibacterial drugs and host defence mechanisms.

This takes us on to consider the chemical mediators involved in inflammation.

CHEMICAL MEDIATORS

Since Sir Thomas Lewis demonstrated the role of histamine, an enormous number of possible mediators have been put forward and some remain putative rather than having an established role. Some inflammatory mediators are derived from cells in the blood or tissues, whereas others are circulating proteins, most of which are manufactured in the liver.

Cell-derived mediators

Lysosomal contents

Since we have just been discussing the role of phago-cytes such as neutrophils and macrophages in the acute inflammatory response, we will now talk about the destructive power of their lysosomal contents. Lysosomal enzymes and accessory substances are present in neu-trophils and monocytes, packaged in membrane- bound vesicles ('granules') to prevent them from damaging their own cell.

In the neutrophil there are two types of granules, the smaller *specific* and the larger *azurophilic*. These contain substances which increase vascular permeability and are chemotactic. The myeloperoxidase which gives the azurophilic granules their name causes the greenish-yellow colour seen in pus, which is an accumulation of dead and dying neutrophils plus liquefied tissues and (often) microbes. The lysosomes contain phospholipase A2 and plasminogen activator (see below).

Monocytes and macrophages also contain lysosomes with a powerful array of hydrolytic and pro-teolytic enzymes, phospholipase A2 and plasminogen activator.

The lysosomal enzymes destroy many extracellular components including collagen, fibrin, elastin, cartilage and basement membrane and can activate complement; as well as producing intracellular killing in the phagolysosome as already described.

If these processes were unopposed, there would be massive tissue destruction. So there are anti-proteases within the serum and tissue fluids to neutralize these enzymes and therefore regulate the extent of tissue damage. Does this seem a far-fetched idea, distant from clinical practice? Well not so!

A deficiency of one such anti-protease, alpha-1-antitrypsin, leads to unopposed action of elastase and hence destruction of elastic tissue, especially in the lungs and liver. Clinically, a patient with alpha-1-antit-rypsin deficiency may suffer from emphysema of the lungs and liver cirrhosis (Fig. 4.11).

Arachidonic acid derivatives

These are the prostaglandins and the leukotrienes. Just like the clotting and fibrinolytic system, they play a part in thrombosis as well as inflammation. They are best thought of as local hormones. They have a short range of action, are produced rapidly and degenerate sponta-neously or are degraded by enzymes. Arachidonic acid,

Key facts

Mediators of acute inflammation

Cell-derived

- Arachidonic acid derivatives (thrombin, prostaglandins and leukotrienes)
- Cytokines (interleukins, colony-stimulating factors, interferons, chemokines, growth factors such as EGF, PDGF, FGF and TGF)
- Platelet activating factor
- Vasoactive amines (histamine and serotonin)
- Lysosomal contents
- Nitric oxide

Plasma-derived

- Kinins
- Clotting and fibrinolytic systems
- Complement

the parent molecule, is a 20-carbon polyunsaturated fatty acid that is derived either from the diet or from essential fatty acids. It is not found in a free state but is present esterified in the cell membrane phospholipid. The two main pathways of arachidonic acid metabo-lism, involving the cyclo-oxygenase (COX) and lipoxy-genase pathways, and their products are shown in Fig. 4.12 which also depicts some of the roles of the prod-ucts in inflammation. Drugs such as corticosteroids, aspirin and indomethacin act to reduce inflammation by inhibiting the production of prostaglandins. Unfortunately the stomach relies on the production of prostaglandins for the generation of a protective bicar-bonate layer, thus suppression of the COX pathway by aspirin and other NSAIDs can cause gastric erosion and peptic ulceration. A therapeutic breakthrough was expected when it was discovered that a subtype of COX enzymes, COX-2, was only expressed during inflam-mation whereas COX-1 is expressed as part of normal cell metabolism. Drugs were developed which selec-tively inhibited COX-2. This prevented the gastro-intestinal tract side effects but unexpectedly led to an increase in cardiovascular diseases like stroke and myocardial infarction in susceptible individuals, the reasons for which are currently being unravelled.

Figure 4.11 Alpha-1-antitrypsin (A-1-AT) is a 394-amino-acid glycoprotein secreted by the liver that is produced during the acute inflammatory response. It inhibits serine proteases, especially neutrophil elastase, which can cleave a wide variety of extracellular matrix components, including elastin. Elastin is what gives tissues such as lung their elastic recoil. Inflammatory episodes are more severe and prolonged than normal, with more tissue damage leading to scarring. The severity of A-1-AT deficiency varies because the disease can be caused by several different mutations

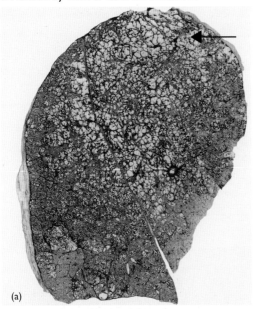

(a)

Lung with emphysema: the 'holes' (arrowed) are hugely distended, coalescent, alveolar spaces. If blood A-1-AT levels are less than 75% of normal, patients are at severe risk of developing emphysema. Any inflammatory stimulus exacerbates the risk – this patient was a coal miner.

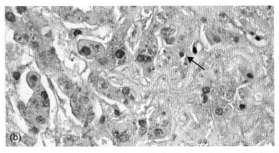

(b)

Mutations in the genes encoding A-1-AT lead to abnormally folded protein, which cannot be secreted into the blood by the liver. Instead, it accumulates within endoplasmic reticulum, shown here (arrows). These patients are at increased risk of cirrhosis. Drinking alcohol stimulates an acute inflammatory response in the liver and increases the risk of this complication.

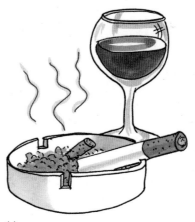

(c)

Cytokines, e.g. lymphokines and monokines, and chemokines

A large array of these polypeptides are being identified Most cytokines are produced by macrophages and activated lymphocytes, and can be termed monokines or lymphokines respectively, but some are made by endothelial and epithelial cells and some cells in the connective tissue. They act principally to regulate immune and haemopoetic cell proliferation and activity (Table 4.3). In addition they have effects in the inflammatory response. The two most important are interleukin-1

(IL-1) and tumour necrosis factor (TNF). They have a variety of important effects as shown in Fig. 4.13, amongst which are the release of chemokines.

Cytokines can be grouped broadly as:

- interleukins
- colony stimulating factors
- interferons
- growth factors.

Chemokines Interleukins are secreted by leucocytes, and predominantly act on other leucocytes. There are

Figure 4.12 Arachidonic acid derivatives

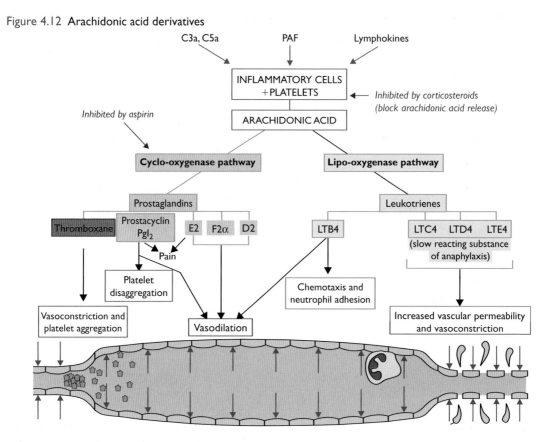

many interleukins of which IL-1, IL-6 and IL-8 are most important in acute inflammation.

Colony stimulating factors (CSFs) act on the bone marrow to stimulate the production of various haemopoeitic cell lines, e.g. neutrophil production is greatly increased during the acute inflammatory response.

Interferons are secreted by many cell types, particularly activated macrophages. Various forms exist, of which IFN-α, β and γ are the most well-characterized.

Growth factors have a role in chemotaxis as well as inducing healing and repair of tissues and playing a part in the development of malignant tumours.

The principal growth factors are:

- epidermal growth factor (EGF)
- platelet-derived growth factor (PDGF)
- fibroblast growth factor (FGF)
- vascular endothelial growth factor (VEGF)
- transforming growth factor (TGF).

Most of these can be produced by macrophages, which are numerous in areas of chronic inflammation.

Chemokines are responsible for attracting inflammatory cells from the circulation to the site where they are needed. There are numerous chemokines, which are mainly produced by activated macrophages or endothelial cells. They attract specific types of inflammatory cell; for instance IL-8 attracts neutrophils rather than macrophages or eosinophils, whereas MCP-1 (monocyte chemoattractant protein-1), macrophage inflammatory protein-1 (MIP-1) and RANTES (regulated and normal T-cell expressed and secreted) attract monocytes, eosinophils, basophils and lymphocytes rather than neutrophils.

Platelet activating factor (PAF)

This is derived from the phospholipid membrane of activated antigen-stimulated IgE-sensitized basophils as well as neutrophils, macrophages and endothelial cells. In addition to activating platelets and causing them to aggregate, it can cause bronchoconstriction and vasoconstriction changes (though at low levels it causes vasodilatation plus a marked increase in venular endothelial

Figure 4.13 The sources and effects of the major cytokines involved in inflammation

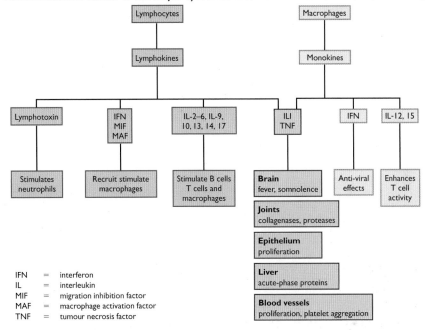

IFN	=	interferon
IL	=	interleukin
MIF	=	migration inhibition factor
MAF	=	macrophage activation factor
TNF	=	tumour necrosis factor

permeability), leucocyte adhesion and chemotaxis. It can also stimulate the production of other mediators, in particular the arachidonic acid metabolites, and stimulate the 'respiratory burst' to produce oxygen-dependent inflammatory metabolites in the lysosomes of neutrophils and macrophages. PAF activity is inhibited by specific PAF aceteylhydrolase enzymes (Fig. 4.14).

Vasoactive amines (histamine and serotonin)

Histamine (5-hydroxytryptamine) is stored in and released from mast cells, basophils and platelets. Mast cells are found in the tissues lying close to blood vessels, where the effects of histamine and other vasoactive mediators are most evident. Mast cells degranulate (release their granule contents by fusing the lysosomal membranes of the granule with the plasma membrane) in response to many types of stimulus.

These stimuli include physical trauma such as injury by force, cold or heat, antibody-binding, complement fragments C3a and C5a, releasing factors produced by neutrophils, monocytes and platelets and interleukin-1, neuropeptides such as substance P and some cytokines, such as IL-1 or -8.

Serotonin (5-hydroxytryptamine or 5-HT) is present in platelets and enterochromaffin cells in humans (and mast cells in some other animals).

When platelets are activated by contact with collagen, histamine and 5-HT are released.

By contrast, when mast cells are activated by the cross-linking of bound IgE, they release platelet activating factor (PAF), causing platelet aggregation and release of platelet granule contents.

The release of histamine causes bronchoconstriction, vasodilatation of arterioles (but constriction of arteries) and increases the permeability of venules. The action of histamine on vessels is mediated via H1 receptors on endothelial cells, while some of its other actions (e.g. bronchoconstriction) are effected via H2 receptors.

Mast cells and platelets (these are cytoplasmic fragments of megakaryocytes, rather than true cells) are the first to be involved in the acute inflammatory response (along with the tissue macrophage and NK cells). The role of these amines is thought to be in the early phase of inflammation as it has been shown that antihistamines blocking H1 receptors have no effect on the permeability that is present after 60 minutes.

Nitric oxide

Nitric oxide (NO) is produced by endothelial cells, macrophages and specific neurons in the brain and has roles in smooth muscle relaxation, reduction of platelet

Table 4.3 The main actions of some of the most important cytokines

Cytokine	Origin	Action
IL-1	Secreted by macrophages, antigen presenting cells and B cells	Activates T cells and NK cells, causes liver to produce acute-phase proteins, elevates core temperature (fever)
IL-2	Secreted by Th cells	Stimulates proliferation of activated T and B cells and NK cells
IL-3	Secreted by Th cells and NK cells	Stimulates haemopoeisis by activation of stem cells, stimulates mast cells to proliferate and release histamine
IL-4, -5, -6	Secreted by Th cells	Stimulate proliferation and differentiation of B cells and antibody secretion by plasma cells
IL-5	Secreted by Th cells	Stimulates bone marrow production of eosinophils, e.g. parasitic infection, induces IgE class switch in B cells
IL-6	Secreted by Th cells, macrophages, stromal cells	Elevates core temperature (fever), release of acute-phase proteins, induces stem cell differentiation
IL-7	Produced by stroma of marrow and thymus	Induces lymphoid stem cells to form B and T cell precursors
IL-8	Made by macrophages and endothelial cells	Important for neutrophil chemotaxis
IL-10	Made by Th cells	Stimulates B cell activation and macrophages to secrete cytokines
IL-12	Made by macrophages and B cells	Activates NK cells and acts synergistically with IL-2 to induce Ts/c cells to differentiate into cytotoxic T lymphocytes
Interferons (IFN-α, β, γ)	IFN-α is produced by most white cells, IFN-β is produced by fibroblasts, and IFN-γ is produced by Th, Tc and NK cells	All act to induce MHC expression and increase viral replication in a variety of cells. IFN-γ has more extensive effects on T and B cells and macrophages and induces class switch to IgG
Tumour necrosis factor (TNF)	Can induce the death of tumour cells. Receptors for the TNF family include Fas	When this is bound by Fas-ligand on Tc cells, apoptosis is induced. CD40 on activated B cells belongs to this group
TNF-α	Secreted by macrophages, mast cells and NK cells	Acts on macrophages to increase cytokine production and cell surface receptor molecule expression, induces class switch to IgA
TNF-β	Secreted by Th and Tc cells	Stimulate phagocytosis by macrophages and polymorphs and NO production by endothelial cells

aggregation and adhesion, and acts as a toxic radical to certain microbes and tumour cells. NO can also decrease leucocyte adhesion to endothelium and thus can diminish the inflammatory response (under-production by endothelial cells in diabetics or vessels with atherosclerosis may contribute to the vascular damage common in these diseases). It has a half-life of seconds, so acts only on immediately adjacent cells.

Macrophage nitric oxide production only occurs when induced by cytokines, such as gamma interferon, whereas endothelial and neural nitrous oxide is produced constitutively. Uncontrolled production by

Figure 4.14 Activation and actions of platelet-activating factor (PAF)

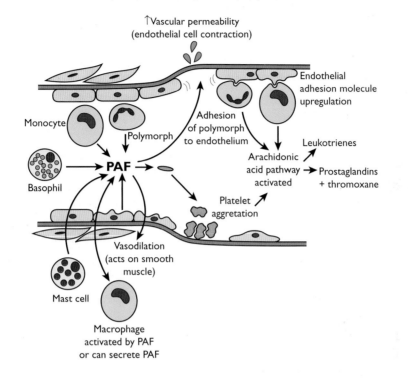

macrophages can lead to massive peripheral vasodilatation and shock.

Plasma-derived mediators

Kinin system

Bradykinin is the major active product of this system. It is a polypeptide which is one of the most powerful vasodilators known to man, increases vascular permeability and also induces pain when injected into the skin. The kinin cascade is activated by Hageman factor (clotting factor XII), which activates prekallikrein to form kallikrein. Kallikrein in turn activates high molecular weight kininogen (HMWK) to form bradykinin. The relationship to the coagulation system is shown in Fig. 4.15. As with other cascades, this contains an amplification step because kallikrein itself acts to stimulate production of Hageman factor. Kallikrein is a highly active substance which is a chemotaxin in its own right, but can also cleave complement component 5 to make C5a (a highly potent chemotaxin) and it also converts plasminogen to plasmin, which dissolves fibrin (the end-product of the coagulation cascade).

The clotting and fibrinolytic systems

This system is not only important in inflammation but is also central to blood clotting, see also chapter 7 (Fig. 7.3, page 173). The end-product, fibrinopeptides, act as chemical mediators in inflammation. They increase vascular permeability and are chemotactic for neutrophils. As in the kinin system, the cascade is activated by Hageman factor – this is activated by contact with collagen and basement membrane, exposed when vascular endothelial damage occurs, or by HMWK and kallikrein from the kinin cascade – and includes an amplification loop so that plasmin stimulates Hageman factor.

Plasmin is a multifunctional protease which also lyses fibrin clots to produce fibrin degradation products, which themselves induce permeability changes and also trigger the complement system by cleaving C3.

The complement system

The system comprises nine liver-derived plasma proteins (C1–9) which are split into about 20 cleavage products; these are involved in increasing vascular

Figure 4.15 The coagulation cascade and fibrinolytic pathways and their interactions with the kinin and complement systems. Pink arrows (→) denote activation of other systems. Inhibition pathways are not shown.

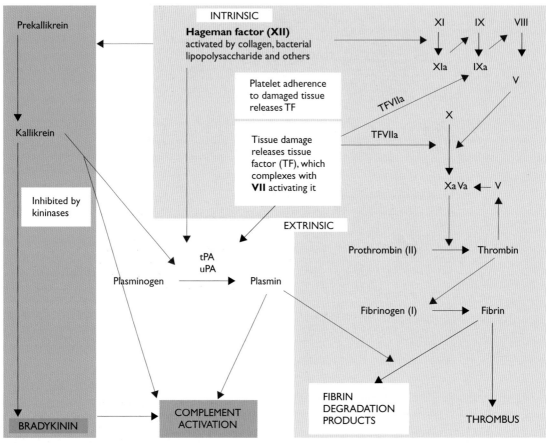

permeability, chemotaxis, opsonization and direct lysis of organisms (Fig. 4.16). The most important components concerned with the inflammatory reaction are:

- C3a and C5a, which increase vascular permeability and are chemotactic for neutrophils and macrophages (particularly C5a)
- C3b and C3bi, which opsonize microbes for phagocytosis
- C5b–9, which form the membrane attack complex (MAC), which causes cell lysis by assembling a port-hole in the microbial membrane which causes unregulated movement of ions and fluids and cell death.

There are three main pathways by which complement can be activated. The classical pathway is rapidly initiated by antigen–antibody complexes; IgM is the best at activating C1, because its pentameric structure clusters many antigens together in one place.

Activation through the alternative pathway is slower because its initiation requires a little bit of luck.

C3 is abundant in the blood, and there is some in tissue fluid as well. C3 spontaneously breaks into its active sub-parts, C3b and C3a all the time. C3b is inactivated by binding to water in less than a second, but if a microbe lies nearby it attaches to amino or hydroxyl groups in its wall and this stabilizes C3b. The bound C3b binds another complement protein, B; this becomes cleaved by protein D to make complex C3bBb. Together this complex can cleave more C3 (preventing the need for spontaneous events) and can also

Figure 4.16 The complement system

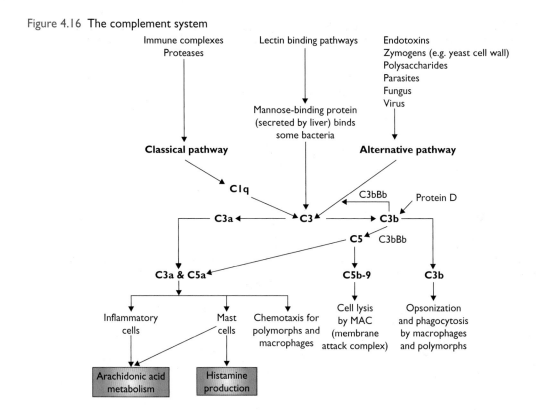

cleave protein C5 into C5a and b. The actions are summarized in Fig. 4.16.

The third pathway is the mannose or lectin binding pathway. Mannose is a carbohydrate constituent of many bacterial cell walls, especially Gram-positive bacteria, and also some important fungi such as *Candida albicans* ('thrush') and some viruses and parasites. Lectins are proteins which bind carbohydrates. Mannose-binding lectin (or protein) is present in the blood in a protected state, bound to another protein. When the lectin binds mannose on the surface of a microbe, the other protein functions with it to become a C3 convertase. Thus C3b is formed and the pathway continues.

Protection of human cells from the actions of complement C3b include the secretion by all our cells of defensive proteins, such as decay accelerating factor, which speeds the breakdown of the C3bBb complex by other blood constituents. CD59 on the cell surface of human cells prevents the MAC complex from forming and penetrating the cell wall.

THE SYSTEMIC EFFECTS OF INFLAMMATION

Having considered acute inflammation, we have an idea of the *local* effects involved. We have alluded to the fact that, at the same time, there are many *systemic* effects which may take place, such as the stimulation of leucocyte production by the bone marrow, fever, rigors, tachycardia, drop in blood pressure, loss of appetite, vomiting, skeletal weakness and aching. These are known collectively as acute-phase reactions.

Fever is a regular accompaniment of inflammatory responses and occurs due to the 'resetting' of the thermo-regulatory centre in the anterior hypothalamus (Fig. 4.17). The hypothalamus reacts to the new setting by causing a rise in the body's core temperature by constricting vessels in the skin, so reducing blood flow and limiting heat loss, and by promoting heat production in muscles by shivering. Biological substances that induce fever are called pyrogens. Many bacteria and viruses produce molecules that act as pyrogens and these are

Figure 4.17 Normal control of body temperature and the mechanism of fever

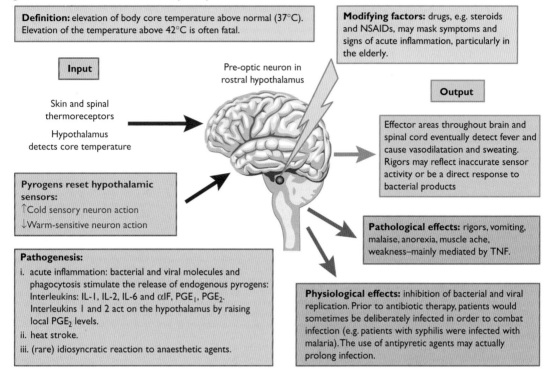

Definition: elevation of body core temperature above normal (37°C). Elevation of the temperature above 42°C is often fatal.

Modifying factors: drugs, e.g. steroids and NSAIDs, may mask symptoms and signs of acute inflammation, particularly in the elderly.

Input

Pre-optic neuron in rostral hypothalamus

Output

Skin and spinal thermoreceptors

Hypothalamus detects core temperature

Pyrogens reset hypothalamic sensors:
↑Cold sensory neuron action
↓Warm-sensitive neuron action

Effector areas throughout brain and spinal cord eventually detect fever and cause vasodilatation and sweating. Rigors may reflect inaccurate sensor activity or be a direct response to bacterial products

Pathological effects: rigors, vomiting, malaise, anorexia, muscle ache, weakness—mainly mediated by TNF.

Pathogenesis:
i. acute inflammation: bacterial and viral molecules and phagocytosis stimulate the release of endogenous pyrogens: Interleukins: IL-1, IL-2, IL-6 and αIF, PGE$_1$, PGE$_2$. Interleukins 1 and 2 act on the hypothalamus by raising local PGE$_2$ levels.
ii. heat stroke.
iii. (rare) idiosyncratic reaction to anaesthetic agents.

Physiological effects: inhibition of bacterial and viral replication. Prior to antibiotic therapy, patients would sometimes be deliberately infected in order to combat infection (e.g. patients with syphilis were infected with malaria). The use of antipyretic agents may actually prolong infection.

called exogenous pyrogens. Endogenous pyrogens are produced by the body and are listed below. It is thought that exogenous pyrogens stimulate leucocytes to release the endogenous pyrogen IL-1 or IL-6, which act on the hypothalamus by raising local prostaglandin E2 levels. Aspirin is useful for lowering the temperature because it interferes with PGE2 production. Paracetamol reduces temperature by directly acting on the temperature centre.

THE ACUTE-PHASE PROTEINS

Localized inflammatory responses lead to changes in plasma proteins due to alterations in liver metabolism. These proteins are called acute-phase proteins and this change is thought to be mediated by IL-1, IL-6 and TNF. There is increased production of clotting factors and complement which is of importance because they are consumed during the inflammatory process.

Transport proteins, such as haptoglobins, may be important in regulating the amount of amines and oxygen free radicals. Iron is an important constituent of lactoferrin and a cofactor in the respiratory burst, which probably explains the increase in plasma transferrin in inflammation. Ferrous iron is also an essential factor in the cross-linking of collagen which occurs during wound healing.

Many other acute-phase proteins, such as C-reactive protein (CRP) and serum amyloid A, are produced but their role is not entirely clear. We know that CRP can coat invading organisms and stimulate complement activation or phagocytosis. The acute-phase reaction varies depending on the cause of inflammation. Viral infection is a poor inducer of acute-phase proteins whereas bacterial infections produce a major response, probably by bacterial endotoxins acting indirectly through raised TNF-α levels. When investigating a patient, CRP is the most useful acute-phase reactant to measure because it rises soon after an inflammatory stimulus is encountered and has a short half-life. If symptoms are equivocal, it may help to establish that there is organic disease rather than psychosomatic disease. In those patients with chronic diseases, a rise

Figure 4.18 C-reactive protein (CRP) fluctuations are an accurate reflection of inflammatory disease activity. CRP levels rise within 4–6 hours and have a half-life of 12 hours. This graph, from a patient with bronchopneumonia, shows the parallel between the patient's temperature, CRP levels and treatment with a first line antibiotic, followed by a second antibiotic, given once microbiological culture and sensitivity results were known (Courtesy of Dr Jo Sheldon, St George's Hospital)

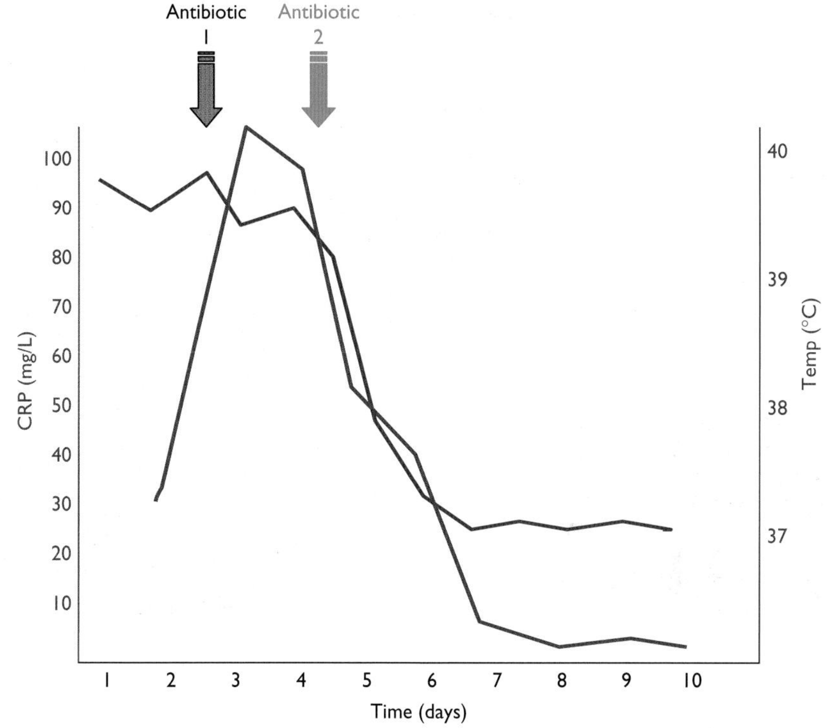

in the level may be an indication of an acute exacerbation or of intercurrent infection (Fig. 4.18).

The number of leucocytes in the peripheral blood increases in many forms of inflammation so that they are available to fight infection. Cytokines act through colony stimulating factors to increase the production and release of cells from the marrow. Again there are differences depending on the type of infection and this may be helpful in making a diagnosis. Bacterial infection provokes an increase in neutrophils, viral infections cause a rise in lymphocyte numbers, and allergic reactions or parasitic infections result in more eosinophils.

Trauma or stress of any kind also affects the hypothalamus–pituitary–adrenal axis resulting in the production of growth hormone, prolactin, ADH, ACTH and adrenaline. These hormones are responsible for the breakdown of glycogen, changes in fatty acid metabolism and sodium–potassium transport. It is these metabolic changes that are responsible for the malaise, weakness, loss of appetite and other varied systemic effects observed during injury.

Although it is now rarely seen clinically because antibiotic treatment halts the usual course of the disease, lobar pneumonia is often used to illustrate the process of acute inflammation (Figs 4.19–4.22). This is because it exemplifies the process of resolution; complete restoration of normality after a period of intense inflammation.

It is so named because the lung parenchyma is involved in continuity so that the process affects a whole lobe or contiguous lobes. *Streptococcus pneumoniae*, a Gram-positive diplococcus bacterium, is the commonest cause of lobar pneumonia.

The first the body may know of this is when the organism invades the lung, or is encountered by a macrophage lining the alveolar space, leading to changes in the microvasculature. These result in a massive outpouring of fluid into the alveolar spaces resulting in congestion (a). This fluid is rich in fibrin and red blood cells.

Figure 4.19 The stages of lobar pneumonia

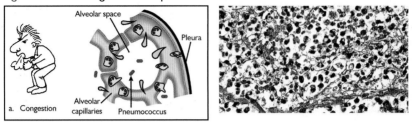

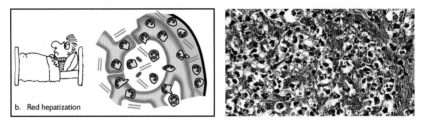

Acute congestion: Bacteria invade alveolar spaces of lung. Acute inflammatory response characterized first by increased vascular permeability, with the formation of a fibrin-rich exudate

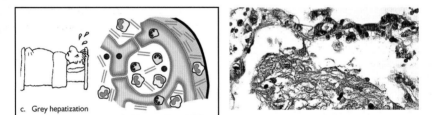

Red hepatization: Neutrophils are quickly attracted to the site, accompanied by red blood cells. The fluid spreads between alveolar spaces via pores of Kohn and soon the entire lung lobe is consolidated (solidified) due to a mixture of fibrin, red and white blood cells. Neutrophils phagocytose the bacteria. The texture and colour of the lobe resembles fresh liver

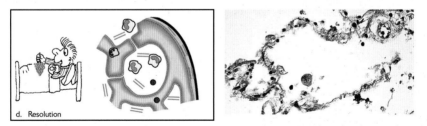

Grey hepatization: Macrophages are attracted to the site, also lymphocytes. Further phagocytosis occurs. Bacteria and dead red and white cells are removed and the fibrin mesh starts to be digested. The grey/white colour of the lobe is due to the high fibrin and white cell content; the texture resembles cooked liver (ugh!)

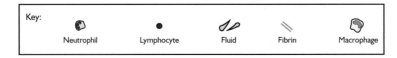

Resolution: The last few fibrin strands and white cells are removed, together with any remaining bacterial corpses and the lung returns to normal. This is possible because the basic skeleton of the lung (formed by reticulin, a type of collagen) is not damaged, unlike bronchopneumonia, in which the inflammatory process is centred on infected bronchioles and is characterized by destruction of the adjacent lung framework (this is usually followed by scarring of lung tissue)

Key:

Neutrophil   Lymphocyte   Fluid   Fibrin   Macrophage

Soon afterwards, neutrophils follow and the fibrin-rich fluid and cells spread from alveolus to alveolus via the pores of Kohn. The neutrophils attack the organisms and phagocytose them, leading to the death of many organisms and neutrophils. Not surprisingly, the alveoli are now airless and the lung is firm and red, with the texture of liver; the stage is termed 'red hepatization' (b).

As this process progresses, the macrophage is recruited not only to phagocytose dead neutrophils and bacteria but also to digest the fibrin mesh. The lung is still firm but the large inflammatory cell infiltrate and reduction in vasodilatation give it a grey colour and, hence, the term 'grey hepatization' (c).

The final outcome will depend on the competence of this system and whether the basic framework of the lung tissue is intact. Ideally, the degenerate cells and dead organisms in the alveolar spaces will be cleared and re-aerated and resolution (d) will take place.

If the alveolar framework has been destroyed or the exudate has not been cleared, organization will occur, leading to scar formation. The infection may persist, destroying lung tissue, but become localized so that an abscess is formed. This is a collection of pus walled off by fibrous tissue. Alternatively it may spread to the rest of the lung, involve the pleura, cause an empyema, or disseminate via the blood stream to other areas of the body and can lead to death due to septicaemia or respiratory failure.

Figure 4.20 Left lung with consolidation (grey hepatization) of the lower lobe

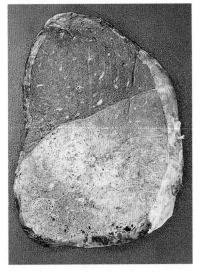

Figure 4.21 Chest X-ray showing consolidation in the right upper lobe (blue arrow) and an enlarged right hilum due to lymphadenopathy (red arrow)

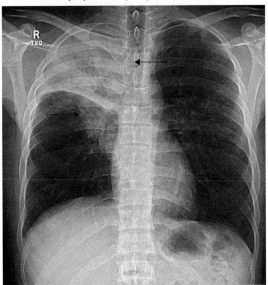

Figure 4.22 Photomicrograph of lung alveoli filled with inflammatory exudate and fibrin passing through the pores of Kohn

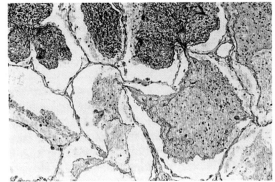

Clinicopathological case study   lobar pneumonia

A 60-year-old man presented to the casualty department complaining of a productive cough, fever, rigors and general malaise. The onset of symptoms was sudden and he had been perfectly well two days previously. He had no past medical history of note and he was not on any medication.

Systemic enquiry
Respiratory system – he was coughing up rusty coloured sputum and also complained of chest pain on inspiration.
Allergies: Nil known

Examination
Temperature 39.4°C (normal 37°C)

Pulse 90/min, regular (normal, approx 70/min)

Respiratory rate 30/min (normal, approx 14/min)

Examination also revealed a dull percussion note in the right lower zone and auscultation confirmed decreased air entry and bronchial breathing. There was also a pleural rub over the affected area.

Investigations
Full blood count: White cell count 18×10^9/L (95 per cent neutrophils) (normal $4-11 \times 10^9$/L with approx 65 per cent neutrophils)

Chest X-ray: Opaque right lower lobe

Sputum culture: Streptococcus pneumoniae

Diagnosis
A diagnosis of lobar pneumonia was made and he was started on a course of penicillin. He did not have a history of allergy to this drug.

The **symptoms** are due to local respiratory irritation from the inflammatory process and the fever is secondary to the production of pyrogens.

Inflammation causes vasodilatation, followed by margination and emigration of cells. Together with increased permeability, this leads to a purulent exudate within alveoli which is coughed up as sputum. The chest pain is due to friction between two inflamed pleural surfaces which are roughened and adherent due to the inflammatory exudate. This is also responsible for the pleural rub heard on auscultation.

Pyrogens cause a rise in body temperature by resetting the thermoregulatory centre in the hypothalamus. A rise in temperature will also increase the metabolic rate and therefore an increase in cardiac output. Decreased gas transfer plus the rise in temperature will lead to an increase in the respiratory rate. The decreased air entry due to the inflammatory exudate within alveoli is responsible for the dull percussion note and the findings on auscultation.

Cytokines cause bone marrow stimulation and hence a leukocytosis. Airless alveoli full of exudate appear white on X-ray. *S. pneumoniae* is the most common organism causing lobar pneumonia.

With **effective treatment,** there will be complete reversal of all the clinical and radiological signs as the exudate is cleared away from the alveoli. This ideal process may not occur and healing may take place by scarring. Lobar pneumonia differs from the more common bronchopneumonia in that the latter tends to be patchy and caused by a variety of organisms, e.g. *H. influenzae.*

CHAPTER 5

CHRONIC AND GRANULOMATOUS INFLAMMATION, HEALING AND REPAIR

CHRONIC INFLAMMATION

Chronic inflammatory disorders are some of the most common, fascinating, devastating and mysterious diseases to affect mankind. They include tuberculosis, sarcoidosis, syphilis, leprosy, Crohn's disease, rheumatoid arthritis, systemic lupus erythematosus and the pneumoconioses. Despite the availability of treatment and some information on prevention, tuberculosis remains a significant worldwide problem. For this reason, (and because it turns up in exams with frightening regularity!), we shall discuss tuberculosis in a moment.

First we had better consider what chronic inflammation is; the definition is not as clear-cut as one might like. You might expect that acute and chronic inflammation are the ends of a spectrum and that after a certain length of time has elapsed, an inflammatory process is considered to be chronic. To some extent this is true.

Acute inflammation peaks at about 3 days and resolves within 5 days; if the stimulus persists, chronic inflammatory cells (lymphocytes, plasma cells and macrophages) begin to accumulate at the site, and this is now a chronic inflammatory process. Thus we are defining chronic inflammation by the type of cell present as well as by the length of time involved. Sometimes the acute phase is so transitory that the disease is not usually detected during this phase and is thought of as a chronic inflammatory process; examples are *Helicobacter* gastritis and tuberculosis.

Viral hepatitis is a special case, because even the acute event is characterized by an infiltrate of lymphocytes. Viral hepatitis is considered chronic after it has persisted for more than 6 months.

Curiously, there are instances in which acute inflammatory cells persist, for example when neutrophils become walled off by fibrous tissue to form abscesses. Some of you will have experienced a dental abscess, in which bacteria enter the jaw through a cracked or carious tooth and thrive in the oxygen-poor environment of the dental root and surrounding bone. This is an example of chronic suppurative inflammation. Microscopical examination of the abscess would show pus and acute inflammation in the centre of the abscess, with many surrounding chronic inflammatory cells, and fibrous tissue.

Osteomyelitis is a fascinating example of what the body does when it cannot rid itself of a focus of infection which causes persistent acute inflammation. In this case, infectious organisms such as *Staphylococcus aureus* from skin or wound infections, or *Salmonella typhi* (which causes typhoid and may persist in bile in the gallbladder for months or years) can spread to bone via the blood. You would think that this would be the worst place for a bug to survive, given that bone marrow is where the inflammatory cells are made! A suppurative focus in the bone becomes walled off by new bone formation (the 'involucrum') and multiple sinuses may form between the purulent focus and the skin. Because numerous anastomosing canals full of pus form within the bone and these are poorly vascularized, it can be very difficult to cure with antibiotics and in extreme circumstances the area may need to be excised. A focus of infection within the body always carries the potential to break into the bloodstream and cause septicaemia or the formation of multiple abscesses in far-flung parts of the body, such as the heart valves or other organs. However, much of the time we find that chronic inflammatory diseases appear to have either a negligible or no acute component and that the disease is typified by a chronic inflammatory cell infiltrate from the start. Rheumatoid arthritis is a good example of a *de novo* chronic inflammatory condition, in which abundant plasma cells and lymphocytes expand the synovium of joints, which becomes greatly thickened and covered in a thick membrane, or 'pannus' of fibrin and chronic inflammatory cells. The pathogenesis of rheumatoid arthritis is not entirely understood, but about 70 per cent of patients have circulating IgM antibodies directed against the Fc component of IgG. Why these patients form antibodies against their own body constituents ('autoimmune disease') and why joints and connective tissues are the major targets are some of the puzzles which are still to be wholly resolved (see page 155). The inflammatory process destroys bone, leading to severe joint deformities, typically in the knee, wrists and the small bones of the hands.

We will discuss other autoimmune diseases, such as SLE, a little later when antibodies have been explained in more detail.

GRANULOMATOUS INFLAMMATION

Granulomatous inflammation is a special type of chronic inflammation, characterized by the presence of granulomata. A granuloma is a collection of

macrophages and is frequently surrounded by a rim of lymphocytes. The macrophages are usually modified to become larger with more abundant pink cytoplasm and are referred to as 'epithelioid' cells.

Typical situations in which granulomatous chronic inflammation occurs are summarized in Fig 5.1. Two main scenarios are encountered: a response to the phagocytosis of inert foreign material and an immune-driven response.

In the former, an inert substance such as a splinter of glass, which cannot be destroyed by the lysosomal contents, causes multiple macrophages to fuse during the attempt to phagocytose and destroy the substance.

Immune-mediated granuloma formation occurs when an antigenic substance, usually microbial, is ingested. Selected components from the microbe are processed by the macrophage and presented via its type II MHC molecules to helper T cells. These become activated and secrete IFN-γ, which activates the

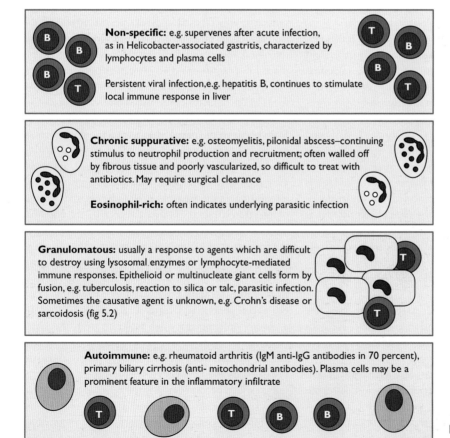

Non-specific: e.g. supervenes after acute infection, as in Helicobacter-associated gastritis, characterized by lymphocytes and plasma cells

Persistent viral infection,e.g. hepatitis B, continues to stimulate local immune response in liver

Chronic suppurative: e.g. osteomyelitis, pilonidal abscess—continuing stimulus to neutrophil production and recruitment; often walled off by fibrous tissue and poorly vascularized, so difficult to treat with antibiotics. May require surgical clearance

Eosinophil-rich: often indicates underlying parasitic infection

Granulomatous: usually a response to agents which are difficult to destroy using lysosomal enzymes or lymphocyte-mediated immune responses. Epithelioid or multinucleate giant cells form by fusion, e.g. tuberculosis, reaction to silica or talc, parasitic infection. Sometimes the causative agent is unknown, e.g. Crohn's disease or sarcoidosis (fig 5.2)

Autoimmune: e.g. rheumatoid arthritis (IgM anti-IgG antibodies in 70 percent), primary biliary cirrhosis (anti- mitochondrial antibodies). Plasma cells may be a prominent feature in the inflammatory infiltrate

Figure 5.1 **Main types of chronic inflammation**

Figure 5.2 (a) Non-caseating granuloma from a patient with sarcoidosis. (b) Components of a non-caseating granuloma

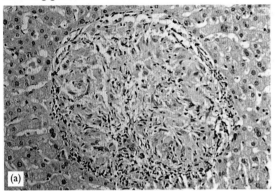

(a)

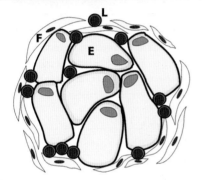

(b)

Group of epithelioid cell (E), with variable numbers of lymphocytes (L) and fibroblasts (F)

macrophage and stimulates it to transform into an epithelioid giant cell, or multinucleate giant cell.

The factors influencing granuloma formation are largely unknown but a variety of cytokines appears to be involved. Animal experiments suggest that IL-1 is important in the initiation of granuloma formation and that TNF is responsible for their maintenance. IL-2 has been shown to increase their size and IL-5 can attract eosinophils to the granulomata, as seen in parasitic disease. IL-6 is believed to have an important role in tuberculous granulomata. We will discuss tuberculosis (TB) as an example of a chronic granulomatous inflammatory disease.

TUBERCULOSIS

Tuberculosis is a worldwide problem and it is caused by *Mycobacterium tuberculosis*. Two strains infect humans; these are *M. tuberculosis hominis* and *M. tuberculosis bovis*. Bovine tuberculosis is passed from cattle to humans in

Key facts

Koch's postulates

It was clear to Koch that in order to implicate a particular organism as the cause of a disease, he must:

- demonstrate the organism in the lesions in all cases of that disease
- be able to isolate the organism and cultivate it in pure culture outside the host
- produce the same disease by injecting the pure culture into a healthy subject.

These three criteria are known as **Koch's postulates.**

milk so that it enters through the gastrointestinal tract to produce abdominal tuberculosis. It is uncommon in developed countries now that dairy herds are generally free of mycobacteria and milk is pasteurized. Infection with *Mycobacterium tuberculosis hominis* is the common form and it produces pulmonary tuberculosis.

Patients with tuberculosis may present with a cough producing bloodstained sputum, or more subtly, with night sweats, weight loss and vague symptoms of ill-health.

Having dipped in the early part of the twentieth century, tuberculosis has increased in incidence: in 2005 there were 2 million deaths from tuberculosis.

The WHO estimates that around 14 million people had TB in 2005. However, the good news is that the number of new cases appears to have peaked in 2004–5. Tuberculosis is more common in the young and the very old and there are definite racial and ethnic differences in incidence. The incidence is highest in Asians, black Africans, Native Americans, the Irish and Inuit (incidence ranges from 100/100 000 to 200/100 000 population).

TB is seen in only 5/100 000 in the UK white ethnic group and is generally seen as reactivation of tuberculosis in migrants to the UK, born in countries with a high prevalence of tuberculosis. The disease also flourishes in socially deprived areas and poverty and malnutrition appear to be important predisposing factors. There is a higher incidence in men and in people suffering from alcoholism, chronic lung diseases and conditions causing immunosuppression, e.g. cancer and AIDS.

About 12 per cent of deaths from TB are in patients who are also infected with HIV. Tuberculosis is the major cause of death in patients with HIV/AIDS. The risk of contracting tuberculosis is much higher in HIV/AIDs patients because the organisms act synergistically: both infect and proliferate in macrophages and HIV also infects helper T cells (Th cells). Tuberculosis assists HIV by stimulating a T-cell mediated immune response; when the Th cells proliferate, so does HIV virus and this leads to Th-cell death. HIV infection depresses immune system function by causing the death of T-helper cells, which makes it difficult for the body to generated a T-cell mediated immune response against tuberculosis. Th cells are at the heart of all immune responses (see Fig. 6.8).

Mycobacterium tuberculosis is a slender, rod-shaped organism, approximately 4 μm in length. It is not visible on haematoxylin and eosin stained sections but is stained using the Ziehl–Neelsen method (Fig. 5.3). This reaction relies on the fact that, once stained, the organisms are resistant to decolouration with acid and alcohol (hence 'acid and alcohol fast bacilli', AAFB). Mycobacteria grow very slowly in culture and may not be apparent for 6 weeks. Observing the bacilli in excised tissues will allow faster diagnosis and treatment, but they will not be seen in sections unless there are approximately one million bacteria per millilitre of tissue. Using a polymerase chain reaction (see page 69) to detect mycobacterial nucleic acid is both reasonably fast and more sensitive but technically more difficult and not generally available.

Mycobacterium tuberculosis does not possess any toxins with which to harm its host, although a number of cell

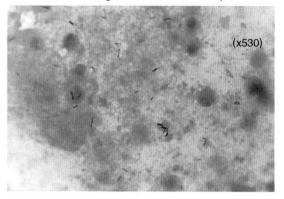

Figure 5.3 ZN stain showing presence of acid-fast (red) bacilli (reproduced with permission from Lydyard, P. *et al.* 2000: *Pathology Integrated: An A–Z of Disease and its Pathogenesis.* London: Arnold)

(x530)

membrane glycolipids and proteins, including bacterial stress proteins, act to provoke a hypersensitivity reaction. It is the hypersensitivity reaction that causes the tissue destruction that is so characteristic of this disease.

PRIMARY TUBERCULOSIS

This occurs in individuals who have never been infected with *Mycobacterium tuberculosis*.

Inhalation of the organism produces a small lesion (approximately 1 cm in diameter), usually in the subpleural region in the lower part of the upper lobe or the upper part of the lower lobe of lung. This is referred to as the Ghon focus. Lesions occur in these sites because the bacterium is a strict aerobe and prefers these well-oxygenated regions. When the tissue is first invaded by the mycobacteria, there is no hypersensitivity reaction, but an initial transient acute, non-specific, inflammatory response with neutrophils predominating. This is followed rapidly by an influx of macrophages, which ingest the bacilli and present their antigens to T lymphocytes, leading to the proliferation of a clone of T cells and the emergence of specific hypersensitivity. The lymphocytes release lymphokines, which attract more macrophages. These accumulate to form the characteristic granuloma, containing a mixture of macrophages, including epithelioid cells and Langhan-type giant cells. Tissue destruction leads to necrosis in the centre of the granuloma called caseous necrosis (Fig. 5.4) because, macroscopically, the necrotic area resembles cheesy material! Tubercle bacilli, either free or contained in macrophages, may drain to the regional lymph nodes and set up granulomatous inflammation,

Figure 5.4 **Photomicrograph showing lymph node with caseous necrosis (arrow)**

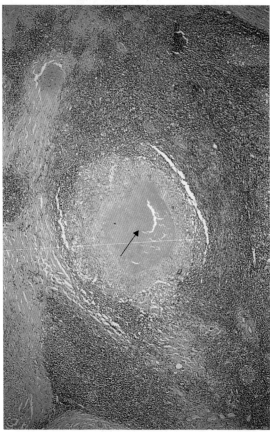

causing massive lymph node enlargement. The combination of the Ghon focus and the regional nodes is called the primary complex (Fig. 5.5).

Thus, the development of hypersensitivity results in tissue destruction but also improves the body's resistance to the mycobacterium by promoting phagocytosis and reducing intracellular replication of bacilli. It is not known why the granulomatous response to mycobacteria produces caseation whereas most other granulomatous reactions do not. Another puzzle is why the attraction of macrophages in most inflammatory responses produces a dispersed infiltrate while in granulomatous reactions they form well-demarcated collections: granulomata.

To return to our patient with TB, as stated above, in about 90 per cent of otherwise healthy people, the primary Ghon complex (Ghon focus plus enlarged hilar lymph nodes) will heal. There will be replacement of the caseous necrosis by a small fibrous scar and the lesion will be walled off. Calcification may also occur in these lesions. Despite this, the mycobacterial organisms may survive and lead to reactivation infection at a later date, especially if the host defences become lowered, as can occur with cancer or steroid treatment for diseases such as rheumatoid arthritis.

There are, however, alternative outcomes. If the hypersensitivity reaction is severe, it will lead to a florid inflammatory response and the patient may present with a systemic illness. If the caseous necrosis is extensive, the tissue destruction may erode major bronchi and allow airborne spread of organisms to produce satellite lesions in either lung. Alternatively, tubercle bacilli may enter the bloodstream. If they enter a small pulmonary arteriole, then the bacilli will lodge in lung tissue. However, if they enter a pulmonary vein the bacilli may disseminate throughout the systemic circulation. If this occurs, numerous small granulomas may be encountered in almost any organ including meninges, kidneys and adrenals. This type of disease is called miliary tuberculosis (Fig. 5.6a), so-called because the lesions look like millet seeds! This is a disastrous complication, associated with a high risk of death. Fortunately, systemic spread is not a common event in primary disease.

SECONDARY TUBERCULOSIS

Secondary, or post-primary, tuberculosis refers to infection occurring in a patient previously sensitized to the mycobacteria. Most of these cases are due to reactivation of latent mycobacteria following an asymptomatic primary infection (Fig. 5.6b). The latency period can vary tremendously and reactivation may not occur for many decades. Reactivation of latent tuberculosis tends to occur if the immune system becomes compromised, as happens in patients treated with steroids or immunosuppressives (e.g. transplant recipients, patients with autoimmune disease, sarcoidosis or chronic inflammatory bowel disease). A particular risk group is patients with HIV/AIDS. Some immune modulation drugs which depress T-cell function have been linked with the reactivation of tuberculosis. (Occasionally there is reinfection from an exogenous source.)

Secondary infection tends to affect the subapical region of the upper lobe. Although the reasons for this are far from clear, it is believed that at the time of primary infection, some tubercle bacilli spread to other parts of the lung and the body via the bloodstream. Most die off as a result of the immune response but a few may survive. Recent studies suggest that the bacillus can survive within macrophages in several ways.

Figure 5.5 Typical sites involved by primary, secondary and miliary tuberculosis

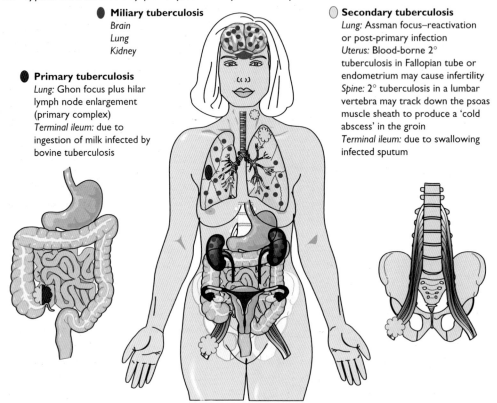

● Miliary tuberculosis
  Brain
  Lung
  Kidney

● Primary tuberculosis
  Lung: Ghon focus plus hilar
  lymph node enlargement
  (primary complex)
  Terminal ileum: due to
  ingestion of milk infected by
  bovine tuberculosis

○ Secondary tuberculosis
  Lung: Assman focus–reactivation
  or post-primary infection
  Uterus: Blood-borne 2°
  tuberculosis in Fallopian tube or
  endometrium may cause infertility
  Spine: 2° tuberculosis in a lumbar
  vertebra may track down the psoas
  muscle sheath to produce a 'cold
  abscess' in the groin
  Terminal ileum: due to swallowing
  infected sputum

Figure 5.6 (a) Chest X-ray showing fine nodules throughout both lungs (nodules you would have to pick with a tweezer) in a patient with miliary TB. (b) Coronal CT showing a cavitating lesion at the right lung apex; secondary reactivation of TB (arrow)

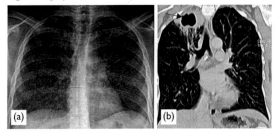

(a)   (b)

First, it may interfere with the fusion of the phagosome with the lysosome. This appears to happen if the tubercle bacillus can form protein kinase G (PknG).

Second, it may become dormant in response to low oxygen states. Low levels of secretion of nitric oxide (NO) by macrophage cell-signalling pathways appears to induce tubercle bacillus dormancy genes (high levels cause the organism to be stressed).

The favoured site for reactivation is the upper lobe of a lung, which is thought to be due to the higher oxygen concentration in this part. (If you remember, tubercle bacilli are obligate aerobes.) Macrophages and other inflammatory cells are programmed to work in inflamed, often poorly oxygenated, tissues and perform less well if the oxygen concentration is higher than normal. This focus of reactivation in the upper lobe is called the Assman focus.

There are three possible outcomes of secondary tuberculous infection: healing, cavitation or spread. Since there has been previous infection, the host will have some degree of immunity. If this is sufficient, the reactivated infection will heal with scarring and subsequent calcification. Intervention with anti-tuberculous drugs will also enhance and modify the healing process. If, on the other hand, the host's degree of hypersensitivity is high and/or the organisms are particularly virulent, there may be considerable lung tissue destruction and caseous necrosis (Fig. 5.7), which can lead to the formation of a cavity. The infected caseous material may spread through destroyed tissue or via bronchi to adjacent

Figure 5.7 Cut surface of the lung showing white areas of caseation due to reactivation of tuberculosis in the upper and lower lobes

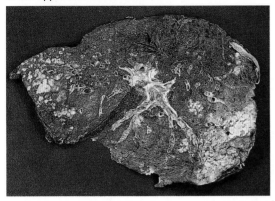

Figure 5.8 Raised skin lesion in sarcoidosis. Microscopy would show epitheloid granulomata

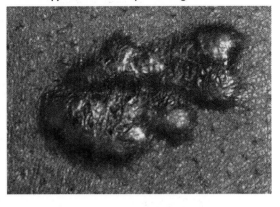

parts of the lung and extend the local disease. Patients with cavitation and bronchial erosion are usually highly infectious, since they can cough up large numbers of organisms. (In survivors, the cavity may be colonized by fungi such as *Aspergillus*, which may later invade the lung and disseminate via the blood.) The pleura may become involved, with the production of an effusion, which can contain caseous and necrotic material, a tuberculous empyema. Infected sputum may be swallowed, spreading the disease to the gastrointestinal tract. Systemic spread to produce miliary tuberculosis is more common in post-primary tuberculosis because tissue destruction is greater and there is more likelihood of venous disruption and dissemination of organisms.

The natural history of the disease will depend on the host's immunity, hypersensitivity and factors such as nutritional status, associated disease and intervention with (preventative) BCG vaccination or treatment of active disease with anti-tuberculous drugs. Tuberculosis is a treatable disease, yet despite this, it remains a major problem in under-developed countries and there is a worrying trend towards the development of antibiotic-resistant strains in the developed countries. Inoculation with the BCG vaccine has greatly reduced the incidence of tuberculosis meningitis in children with primary infection, and also the risk of developing post-primary tuberculosis, though it has had less effect on reactivation tuberculosis. BCG does not prevent the organism from causing an initial infection. Its function is to simulate a primary infection, thus priming the immune system for a rapid response within days of encountering the organism, unlike the 3–4 weeks required to generate *de novo* cell-mediated immunity.

It is important that those people with active tuberculosis are isolated until they have been treated, since it has been estimated that untreated individuals spread the disease to an average of 12 other people.

Traditional tuberculous therapy requires the use of multiple drugs for 6 months to 1 year. Many patients fail to complete the course, partly because it is so long and also some drugs have side effects such as loss of colour vision and tinnitus (buzzing and ringing in the ears). A worrying feature has been the emergence of drug-resistant and multi-drug resistant strains of tuberculosis; the latter is defined as TB which is resistant to the two most important anti-tuberculous drugs, rifampicin and isoniazid. Multi-drug resistance is a particular problem in Russia.

The WHO launched a drive (the 'Stop TB strategy') to eradicate tuberculosis in 2006 and recommended treatment using 'directly observed therapy, short-course' (DOTS). This has been found to be highly effective with an average success rate of around 75–84 per cent.

SARCOIDOSIS

Sarcoidosis is a baffling systemic disease of unknown aetiology and is characterized by the presence of granulomas which, unlike tuberculosis, do not exhibit caseous necrosis and so are termed 'non-caseating granulomas' (Fig. 5.8).

It is a systemic disorder of variable severity, hence it can present in numerous ways. Many patients are asymptomatic and in some the diagnosis is only made at post mortem. Almost every organ in the body may be affected, the commonest being lung, liver, spleen, skin and salivary glands with the heart, kidneys and central nervous system slightly less commonly affected. Most patients present with respiratory symptoms (shortness of breath, haemoptysis and chest pain) but some have a more rapid course with fever, erythema nodosum and polyarthritis. Patients may also present with signs and symptoms of hypercalcaemia, and lytic bone lesions, especially in the phalanges, are strong supportive evidence for the disease.

OTHER TYPES OF CHRONIC GRANULOMATOUS DISEASE

Some other causes of granulomatous inflammation are listed below. Many are due to infections (if eosinophils are also present, parasitic disease is most likely), some are of autoimmune aetiology and sometimes we do not know the cause, as in the cases of sarcoid and Crohn's disease. A tissue biopsy can help when trying to establish the cause of granulomatous disease. The only way to be certain of the cause of granulomatous disease is either to see it under the microscope, as for instance with fungal hyphae or acid- and alcohol-fast bacilli, or to culture the organism. However, some macrophage variants are more common in specific conditions and the type seen may offer a clue as to the underlying cause. We will discuss the origin and activity of this remarkable cell in the following section, but for now will

Key facts

Some causes of granulomatous inflammation

Bacterial	tuberculosis
	leprosy
	syphilis
Fungal	cryptococcus
	coccidioides
Protozoal	toxoplasmosis
	pneumocystis
Parasitic	schistosomiasis
Inorganic material	silicosis
	berylliosis
	foreign material
Autoimmune	rheumatoid arthritis
	primary biliary cirrhosis
Unknown	sarcoidosis
	Crohn's disease

consider briefly the ways in which macrophages may adapt to fight particular diseases, becoming morphologically distinctive in the process.

Having read about acute inflammation, chronic inflammation and a little about the immune system, you will appreciate the complex interplay which exists between cells and mediators. It is a veritable orchestra! The helper T cell is probably the conductor, but a key player (the first violin, to continue the analogy) is undoubtedly the macrophage and it is useful to summarize inflammation and repair by reviewing macrophage function.

MACROPHAGES

Macrophages are involved in all inflammatory processes with their ability to phagocytose particles, process and present antigens and secrete an array of mediators. Macrophages are derived from the same stem cells in the bone marrow that give rise to polymorphonuclear leucocyte precursors. These marrow cells produce monocytes which circulate in the blood for a day or two before migrating into the tissues where they are called macrophages or (a more old-fashioned term) histiocytes. Macrophages can continue to proliferate, slowly, within the tissues. Their role is a mixture of simple scavenger, litter collecting and generally keeping the extracellular tissues tidy, and they scout for trouble in the form of invading pathogenic organisms.

Apart from the 'free-range' tissue macrophages there are also populations of relatively fixed macrophages in the epithelium and lining the endothelial aspects of vessels in the liver (Kupffer cells), spleen, bone marrow and lymph nodes; the so-called reticulo-endothelial system (RES). Other macrophages of the RES line part of the central nervous system (microglial cells).

Particularly in the spleen, sinusoidal macrophages remove from circulation those red blood cells which have either passed their sell-by date (the life span of a normal red cell is 120 days) or become battered and worn. This can happen in inherited diseases of the red cell membrane (e.g. hereditary spherocytosis, in which the red cells are round and incompressible, or sickle cell anaemia in which a point mutation alters the shape of the red cell under conditions of poor oxygenation, and causes sludging of the sickled cells within blood vessels) or autoimmune diseases, in which antibodies are produced against the body's own red cells. The sinusoidal macrophages also phagocytose bacteria which have been opsonized with antibody. A common misconception is that the spleen is redundant and can be removed with impunity: splenectomy patients are particularly susceptible to severe infection by encapsulated bacteria, such as *Haemophilus influenzae* or *Streptococcus pneumoniae*. Splenectomized patients must receive lifelong antibiotic therapy if it has not been possible to vaccinate them prior to the removal of the spleen.

A crucially important function is a macrophage's ability to scavenge and phagocytose; it does this in its resting state and also in areas of tissue damage. Macrophages possess scavenger receptor molecules, which are important in self-/non-self-discrimination and appear able to bind to a wide range of modified molecules. Most important of these is modified LDL (low density lipoprotein), but modified albumin and probably other molecules can also be bound and phagocytosed. Unlike LDL receptors on other tissue cells, these surface receptors are not downregulated as the LDL content of the cytoplasm increases. This means that macrophages keep taking up lipid, etc. and become foamy macrophages, seen in areas of tissue damage and atheromatous plaques (see page 196).

Just like the neutrophils in acute inflammation, macrophages emigrate and become activated under the influence of chemotactic factors, adhesion molecules, cytokines and microbial components. An activated macrophage increases its size and its lysosomal enzyme content and speeds up its metabolism and ability to phagocytose and kill microbes. When macrophages become hyperactivated they start to secrete tumour necrosis factor (TNF), which is a multifunctional cytokine that can activate other immune cells or cause viral-infected or tumour cells to die by apoptosis.

Hyperactivation is a red-alert status which is usually achieved when microbial molecules such as lipopolysaccharide (LPS), found in Gram-negative bacteria, or mannose, found in many Gram-positive bacteria, and other organisms are encountered.

Macrophages are also important because they synthesize and secrete factors which promote granulation tissue formation and enhance healing and repair. For example, macrophage derived growth factors such as PDGF, FGF and TGF-β stimulate cell growth, angiogenic factors stimulate new vessel formation and fibrogenic stimuli and collagenases permit the remodelling and laying down of scar tissue. This, together with factors released from other cells, results in new vessel formation, and fibroblasts for collagen and extracellular matrix production.

After acute, transient insults, macrophages will assist in healing and repair and then depart, continuing their nomadic, scavenging lifestyle. However, in chronic inflammation, macrophages produce a variety of substances that maintain the inflammatory process and attract and stimulate other inflammatory cells, contributing to local tissue injury and fibrosis. This is potentially harmful to the body. Their continued presence is due principally to continued emigration from the blood, a reduction in movement out of the tissues and some local proliferation, all of which is in response to cytokines, inflammatory mediators or microbial products. They are naturally longer lived cells than the neutrophils; they can live for weeks or months in the tissues.

Key facts

The role of the macrophage in chronic inflammation

- Antigen presentation to T cells and B cells leading to clonal expansion
- Scavenging abnormal cells, particles, large molecules, immune complexes, etc.
- Chemotactic factors for other leucocytes
- Stimulate endothelium for adhesion molecule activation and granulation tissue formation
- Fusion with other macrophages to form giant cells
- Phagocytosis and killing of some organisms
- Harbouring of some organisms
- Exocytosis for attacking parasites or damaging tissues

Key facts

Macrophage products involved in tissue injury

- Toxic oxygen metabolites
- Nitric oxide
- Proteases
- Eicosanoids
- Coagulation factors
- Neutrophil chemotactic factors

MACROPHAGES IN SPECIFIC DISEASES

Epithelioid cells occur in all types of granulomatous disease. They have some resemblance to epithelial cells as they possess abundant pink cytoplasm, packed with endoplasmic reticulum, Golgi apparatus and vesicles. Thus the cells are well adapted to synthesize macrophage products, such as arachidonic acid metabolites, complement, coagulation factors and cytokines. However, they are less mobile and less proficient at phagocytosis than ordinary macrophages. The multinucleate giant macrophages principally form by fusion of epithelioid cells. Each may have 50 nuclei or more and it is the arrangement of these nuclei which distinguishes the types. The Langhan giant cell is typical of (though not exclusive to) tuberculosis or sarcoidosis and has its nuclei arranged as a horseshoe at the periphery. The foreign-body giant cell, predictably, often contains identifiable foreign material (for instance suture material or shards of glass) in its cytoplasm. Its nuclei are randomly arranged throughout the cell. Foreign body giant cells are also seen often in parasitic infections, such as schistosomiasis ('bilharzia').

These are the most important macrophage variants but, for completeness, we will mention two others (Fig. 5.9). These are the Warthin–Finkeldey cell, pathognomonic of measles and characterized by the presence of eosinophilic nuclear and cytoplasmic inclusions, and Touton giant cells, which have a central cluster of nuclei surrounded by foamy lipid-laden cytoplasm. Touton cells occur in xanthomas, which are benign tumorous collections of lipid-laden macrophages in the skin.

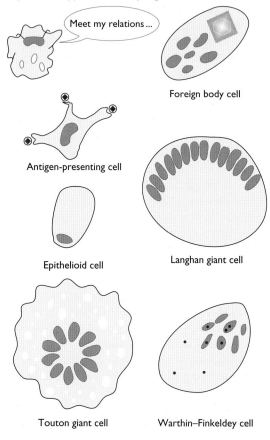

Figure 5.9 **Types of macrophage**

Meet my relations...

Foreign body cell

Antigen-presenting cell

Epithelioid cell

Langhan giant cell

Touton giant cell

Warthin–Finkeldey cell

WOUND HEALING AND REPAIR

CLINICAL CASE: ACUTE TRAUMA

Edward, a 19-year-old student, is rushed to the Accident and Emergency department. He has been rescued from the wreck of a small car, entangled with a juggernaut, the result of a miscalculated overtaking manoeuvre on a rainy night. He is unconscious on admission, but he almost immediately regains consciousness and appears lucid and in pain. He has obviously broken his left thigh, which is swollen and shows early bruising. A grating sensation is palpable when the thigh is gently pressed. He has a gaping wound on his right thigh, about 6 cm diameter and 1 cm deep, through which the underlying fatty tissue can be seen, along with much oozing and crusted blood.

His blood pressure is low, at 95/40 mmHg, and his pulse rate is 120 beats per minute: these features are signs of shock and indicate that he is probably bleeding internally (page 227). He may have lost a litre of blood or so into the tissues surrounding his broken femur. The presence of tenderness and guarding over his upper left abdomen raise the possibility of a ruptured spleen.

Whilst his blood is being cross-matched for transfusion, fluids and plasma expanders are infused to maintain his circulation. An emergency scan indicates that he does indeed have a ruptured spleen.

Edward undergoes an emergency splenectomy. His fractured femur is set at the same time, and the gaping wound in his right thigh is debrided (the injured tissue is scraped away) and the site is packed with gauze impregnated with iodine (a disinfectant). By the time his parents have been tracked down and retrieved from a party by the police, Edward is settled in intensive care, in traction, and is beginning to regain consciousness after the anaesthetic.

Once his parents have recovered from the shock of the events they begin to fire questions at the consultant orthopaedic surgeon. Edward was unconscious on arrival – will he suffer any permanent brain damage? He is a keen rugby player – when, if ever, will he be able to play again? And what about the loss of his spleen – isn't it important? How long will his operation scar take to heal? He supplements his student grant by stacking supermarket shelves late at night, a job that involves lifting heavy boxes and crates. When will he be able to return to work?

The surgeon tackles the questions when he can get a word in. It is too early to tell whether Edward has any lasting brain injury, but the speed of his return to consciousness bodes well.

The spleen *is* an important organ, with a particular role in removing certain bacteria from the blood (page 123). Without going into too much detail, he tells them that Edward must be inoculated against pneumococci and will have to take lifelong antibiotic prophylaxis against other bacterial infection, but should otherwise manage very well.

Edward will not be fit for shelf stacking for at least 3 months, not just because of the fractured femur but also because his abdominal wound will take that long to regain sufficient strength. His fracture is uncomplicated and should heal well. As long as all goes according to plan, he should be walking on crutches in 6 weeks and be ready for rugby after several months of rehabilitation.

Edward's parents are content with this, but let us examine the surgeon's statements about wound and bone fracture healing in a little more detail.

We know already that any tissue injury will initiate acute inflammation (see chapter 4) and neutrophil polymorphs will soon arrive at the scene of the damage, along with macrophages, to start phagocytosing the debris. If any microorganisms have penetrated the skin wounds, they will be immobilized and phagocytosed, opsonized by a combination of circulating antibody and complement. But what happens next?

CELL CAPACITY FOR REGENERATION

What happens when injury causes loss of normal tissue and leaves a defect, for example a cut in the skin? In this situation the end result depends on the size of the defect and the capacity of the tissue to regenerate. Not all tissues of the body have the same capacity to regenerate

Figure 5.10 **Types of fracture**

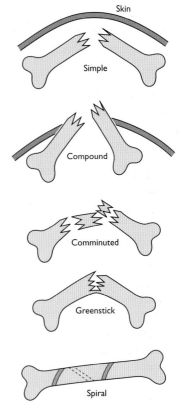

and cells can be divided into three major types: labile, stable and permanent (Fig. 5.11).

The labile cells include epithelial and blood cells; these divide and proliferate throughout life and the cells have a set lifespan. Stable cells normally divide extremely slowly but can proliferate rapidly if required. If you remove half the liver, the cells will regenerate and return it to its original size! Other examples of stable cells are fibroblasts, vascular endothelial cells, smooth muscle cells, osteoblasts and renal tubular epithelial cells. Permanent cells cannot divide but may be capable of some individual cell repair if the nucleus and synthetic apparatus are intact. Examples include neurones and cardiac muscle cells. If a permanent cell is damaged but not destroyed, as in injury to a nerve axon, there may be regrowth of the damaged portion. However, if the whole cell is destroyed, it will be replaced by a small scar because its neighbouring cells are incapable of proliferating to replace it.

When injury takes place and the processes of inflammation are set in motion, the elements of repair and

Key facts

Fracture types and general treatment (see Fig. 5.10)

Simple: no communication between bone and skin surface

Compound: bone fragments breach skin, thus has potential for infection

Comminuted: multiple bone fragments due to more than one breakage site

Greenstick (typical in young children): incomplete fracture, with part of a fractured long bone remaining intact

Stress: the result of abnormal stresses applied to bone (similar to metal fatigue)

Pathological: the bone is abnormal and fractures easily: 4 types: congenital disease, such as osteogenesis imperfecta; inflammatory disease, such as osteomyelitis; neoplastic disease, such as primary or metastatic tumour in bone; metabolic disease, such as osteoporosis.

Fracture management

Reduction: to restore bony alignment

Immobilization: to maintain the alignment until union has occurred; if this cannot be achieved by external fixation in a plaster cast, internal fixation with pins, screws or plates may be required

Rehabilitation: to restore normal function if possible, or cope with residual disability

---

healing are also activated. Briefly, the processes that take place during and after the injury are:

- removal of dead and foreign material
- regeneration of injured tissue from cells of the same type
- replacement of damaged tissue by new connective tissue.

Wound healing requires

- haemostasis
- inflammation
- cell proliferation and repair
- adequate nutrition.

Ideally, adequate tissue repair will occur within 3 weeks. This process of restoring the tissue to pristine condition is called resolution. Resolution requires that the inflammatory process deals quickly with the insult, the tissue has not lost its basic scaffolding and any damaged specialized cells are capable of regeneration. The size of the defect is very important, as any destruction of the tissue scaffold will result in scarring.

Although the basic mechanisms involved in wound healing are the same, by convention, the healing of cleanly incised wounds, where the edges are in close apposition, is considered separately from those in which there is extensive loss of epithelium, a large subepithelial tissue defect which has to be filled in by scar tissue and where the edges cannot be brought together with sutures. These two circumstances are described as 'healing by primary intention' or 'healing by secondary intention'. These terms first appeared in a surgical treatise published in 1543, although Thomson (1813) in *Lectures on Inflammation*, gives Galen the credit for introducing these terms.

HEALING BY PRIMARY AND SECONDARY INTENTION

HEALING BY PRIMARY INTENTION

Let us return to Edward and consider his abdominal surgical incision, made at the time of splenectomy. This is about the cleanest type of wound you can get, in both senses. Not only is surgery performed using aseptic technique, but also a sharp knife makes the wound, with the minimum of tissue trauma. The healing in this type of instance, in which the two sides need merely to be pushed back together and held still (by sutures) in order to heal, is known as 'healing by primary intention' (Fig. 5.12).

The skill of the surgeon has a role to play in the outcome of course, not least in the selection of an incision

Figure 5.11 The capacity for cell regeneration after damage depends on the type of tissue involved

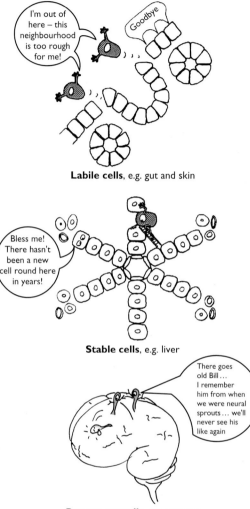

Labile cells, e.g. gut and skin

Stable cells, e.g. liver

Permanent cells, e.g. neurons

Figure 5.12 Healing by primary intention

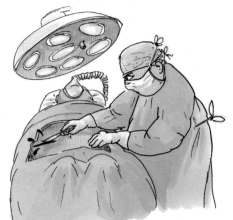

Primary intention
'Clean' wounds e.g. incisions.
which heal with little scarring

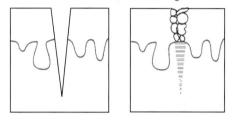

site that will not come under undue tension, which will tend to pull the wound sides apart as soon as the sutures have been removed.

HEALING BY SECONDARY INTENTION

What about the large gash on Ed's thigh? You will recall that this was not sutured, but left open, packed with gauze. How will this wound heal? And why not suture the sides together, so that the skin can form a barrier to infection from marauding bacteria?

This was a very large wound – almost the size of the palm of Edward's hand – it would have been impossible to appose the sides without generating unbearable

tension on the tissues. Also, there was severely damaged tissue at the wound base, not the clean edges of a surgical excision. Dead tissue may form a nidus for infection, and it is quite possible that microorganisms had already entered the wound site by the time Ed arrived at the A&E department. The surgeon has cleared away the obviously dead tissue. By allowing this wound to granulate up, i.e. heal by what is called 'secondary intention', the patient will stand a good chance of an uncomplicated repair, though at the expense of an unsightly scar.

The processes involved in healing by secondary intention are the same as those for primary intention, but the amount of scar tissue generated is greater. One feature that helps to speed up the healing process and which is not seen in relation to healing of incised wounds is wound contraction. Interestingly, wound contraction, which diminishes the size of the wound bed, begins at about 1–2 days. This is before collagen deposition has been fully established. Myofibroblasts within the dermis at the wound edges, possibly controlled by sympathetic nerves, contract and draw the wound edges closer. Wound contraction continues at just under 1 mm per day. It peaks at 5 days but continues for up to 15 days.

Figure 5.13 Healing by secondary intention: repair of a large tissue defect generates scar tissue

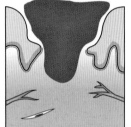

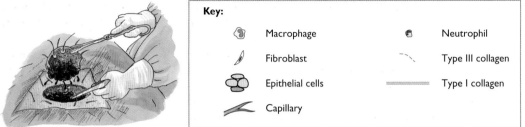

Key:

Macrophage		Neutrophil	
Fibroblast		Type III collagen	
Epithelial cells		Type I collagen	
Capillary			

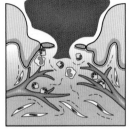

Wound gap

a. Fibrin clot

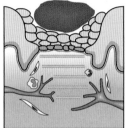

Wound gap

b. Day 1–2: cellular infiltrate, temporary matrix, wound contraction, epithelial migration, clot dissolution

c. Day 3–4: surface intact, new basement membrane, definitive matrix

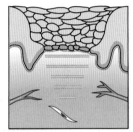

d. Day 5: scar

Because scar contraction is so effective, even a 6 cm gash like Edward's will reduce to about half the diameter or less once it has scarred. Whilst not a problem on his thigh, in a wound at a more strategic site — over a joint, for instance — scarring of this degree could interfere with function and an alternative approach, such as skin grafting, may have to be employed.

Wounds of this size can alternatively be closed in a two-stage operation. First, the wound is cleaned by washing and debridement, and left to granulate for 5–7 days. When it is clear that it is healing well, the surgeon will then scrape the wound base and sides until there is pinpoint bleeding, indicating good vascularity, and the edges, now under less tension due to diminished tissue oedema, can be apposed and sutured together. (This will still result in healing by secondary intention, with the production of moderate amount of scar tissue, since there has been appreciable tissue loss.)

Most wounds, whether of skin or internal organs, will heal in this way but an interesting exception is bone. This breaks the rules and does not heal with a fibrous scar. Even if the 'scaffold' is completely distorted, as with a traumatic fracture, it will remodel to resemble the original structure and function. If it didn't the bone would remain flexible at the breakpoint.

WHAT DOES WOUND HEALING LOOK LIKE AT THE TISSUE LEVEL?

There are several phases to wound healing: initially there is inflammation and the removal of dead or damaged tissues, then there is a cellular phase of proliferation of epithelial cells, fibroblasts and new blood vessels, and finally a healing phase with tissue maturation and regression of any excess inflammatory cells and vessels.

The simplest form of healing occurs with an incisional wound, with clean edges in which the sides can be easily pushed together, as in Ed's surgical incision. This is known as healing by primary intention. Healing by secondary intention is when a large defect is involved and the tissue has to heal from the base upwards, because the sides of the wound are too far apart to be closed by suturing (Fig. 5.13).

Since healing by primary and secondary intention involves the same processes, they will be discussed together.

Removal phase and acute inflammation

A skin wound causes injury to epidermal and connective tissue cells, sparking off the first steps in the acute inflammatory response.

First there is bleeding (haemorrhage), due to damage to the small blood vessels of the skin. This exposes clotting factors and platelets to collagen in the basement membrane and the extravascular tissues, which stimulates the formation of a blood clot. This is achieved by the activation of Hageman factor (factor XII) in the intrinsic pathway and tissue factor (factor III) in the extrinsic pathway, found in extravascular cells, which becomes activated in the presence of factors III and Va. Fibronectin and von Willibrand factor (vWF) bind extracellular tissues and are molecules to which platelets can bind (see Figs 7.2 and 7.3).

Fibrin and fibrinogen formed by the coagulation cascade help to 'glue' the wound edges together and provides the protective dry surface scab. We have already discussed how the combination of tissue damage and the activation of the coagulation cascade can kick off acute inflammation and the way that activation of Hageman factor also activates the kinin system and more indirectly leads to complement activation (Fig. 4.15).

Reflex vasoconstriction for the first 5–10 minutes after injury (mediated by serotonin, prostaglandins, adrenaline, noradrenaline and thromboxane released by tissue cells such as mast cells and macrophages and also by platelets) slows the blood flow and thus makes it easier for platelets to aggregate and form a primary haemostatic plug. Activated platelets release many agents, including thrombospondin, serotonin, platelet-derived growth factor (PDGF), proteases and other growth factors. (Haemostasis is discussed further in chapter 7.)

After 5–10 minutes of vasoconstriction there is vasodilatation, due to the actions of histamine (mast cells), other prostaglandins, leukotrienes (inflammatory and endothelial cells and platelets) and kinins (plasma). This leads to an increase in vascular permeability, allowing the exudation of protein-containing fluid from the plasma into the tissues, carrying supplies of plasma proteins such as fibrinogen and complement. Swelling occurs.

The upregulation of endothelial cell selectins and ICAM-1 attracts neutrophils to the vessel walls. The neutrophils marginate and then migrate from the vessels to the damaged area, following a chemotactic pathway of cytokines and complement fragments (see Figs 4.8 and 4.9).

Neutrophils are very important if pathogenic microorganisms have been introduced at the time of the injury, but otherwise have a relatively minor role in wound healing, confined to their phagocytic activity (removal of microbes and debris) and the production of inflammatory mediators. They are short-lived and disappear after about 2 days unless an inflammatory stimulus persists.

There are fewer monocytes in the blood than there are neutrophils, but these are recruited in a similar fashion and begin to move to the damaged tissues. Don't forget that the macrophages already present in the tissues will migrate to the site of damage and immediately begin work. Macrophages can also proliferate locally. Their roles are the phagocytosis of debris, the destruction of microbial pathogens which have breached the tissue defences, and the secretion of inflammatory cytokines such as PDGF, vascular endothelial growth factor (VEGF) and proteases.

Later on, at about 3 days, a few T lymphocytes are attracted to the wound site. They may participate in wound healing by interacting with macrophages, other antigen presenting cells, B cells and other T cells and, if required, begin the processes involved in the generation of a specific immune response to particular microbial pathogens.

The regenerative phase

Meanwhile epidermal cells begin to re-cover the surface. Within a few hours of the injury, a single layer of epidermal cells starts to migrate from the wound edges to form a delicate covering over the raw area exposed by the loss of epidermis. Normal keratinocytes are nonmotile but can alter their phenotype to produce contractile actin microfilaments in response to growth factors to re-epithelialize a surface defect.

The distance the cells need to cover is reduced by an early phase of wound contraction. Epidermal cell movement can provide an initial covering for very small wounds (such as sutured incisional wounds), but in most instances new cells are derived from the stem-cell compartment in the basal layer of the epidermis, stimulated by growth factors secreted by platelets and damaged endothelial cells (and the absence of inhibition of growth by neighbouring epithelial cells).

From about 12 hours after wounding, new epidermal cells begin to proliferate and they grow under the protective fibrin/fibronectin clot. Epithelial cells secure their grip by attaching to fibronectin in the matrix which has formed at the wound site. They secrete collagenases and plasminogen activator, dissolving the clot and the matrix.

They also grow for a little distance down the gap between the cut edges to form a small 'spur' of epithelium which afterwards regresses. If the wound has been sutured, a similar downgrowth of new epidermis occurs in relation to the suture tracks and, on occasion, these may form the basis of keratin-forming cysts within the dermis, the so-called 'implantation dermoid cysts'. (This ability of epidermal cells to grow along tracks created by sutures or other foreign material is of course the basis for piercing ears for earrings.)

Once re-epithelialization is complete, basement membrane proteins will reappear and the epithelial cells revert to their normal non-migratory phenotype and attach to each other and to the basement membrane. Covering a wound keeps it from drying out and this enhances epithelial cell migration.

Thus a switch to a migratory epithelial cell phenotype, with a capacity to dissolve surrounding tissues and interact with connective tissue matrix proteins, is a normal response to wound healing. (One can begin to understand how cancer cells, which can express inappropriate or mutated genes, can invade and migrate through the tissues with such ease.)

The replacement phase: granulation tissue formation and repair

Meanwhile, there is an influx of macrophages, proliferation of fibroblasts and production of collagen within a connective tissue matrix gel and ingrowth of many fine capillaries (granulation tissue). This combination of a richly vascularized gel in which both inflammatory cells and collagen-producing fibroblasts are present is known as granulation tissue. The term is derived from the observation that the raw surface of a wound shows a granular appearance rather like that seen on the surface of a strawberry. Each of these 'granules' contains a loop of capillaries and hence bleeds easily if traumatized.

Granulation tissue production is a fascinating process common to all forms of repair.

Macrophages and fibroblasts are key cells in wound healing and are responsible for the demolition and removal of tissue debris and inflammatory exudate and for restoring the tensile strength of the subepithelial connective tissue.

Macrophages secrete chemoattractants which recruit fibroblasts to the wound site. Macrophages also expand the existing small fibroblast population by stimulating them to proliferate. Several agents do this, including fibroblast growth factor (FGF), transforming growth factor-α (TGF-α), PDGF and C5a. Some of these may come from sources other than the macrophage, for instance platelets and endothelial cells. As with the proliferating epithelial cells, migrating fibroblasts attach to fibronectin in the connective tissue matrix to facilitate movement.

Fibroblasts are very important cells, as they synthesize and secrete the collagen and elastins required for tissue repair. They also secrete fibronectin and matrix components. Fibroblasts secrete procollagen, which is split to form tropocollagen which aggregates to form collagen fibrils. These fibrils align to form collagen fibres. Collagen deposition requires a framework of fibronectin to be present. Surplus collagen is removed by collagenases secreted by several cell types, including fibroblasts and macrophages.

The ingrowth of new small blood vessels (angiogenesis) into the area undergoing repair is initiated by macrophages, which secrete angiogenic factors in response to a low oxygen tension and the accumulation of lactic acid in the tissues. Angiogenesis involves the budding of new endothelial cells from small intact blood vessels at the edges of the wound, and chemoattraction of these new endothelial cells into the fibrin/fibronectin gel within the wounded area.

Growth factors such as FGF and VEGF can stimulate the endothelial cells of capillaries and post-capillary venules to secrete proteases that digest the surrounding basement membrane. The endothelial cells then proliferate to produce a bud of cells protruding through the gap in the wall towards the source of the stimulus and into the matrix gel in the wound area. At first the bud of endothelial cells is solid but eventually it canalizes to allow the flow of blood, although quite how the circulatory loop is completed is not known.

Anti-angiogenic factors exist to control and limit the extent of new vessel formation. As the inflammatory process subsides, those new vessels which are no longer useful regress by undergoing apoptosis. In diabetic retinopathy and cataract formation these mechanisms fail to prevent the ingrowth of new vessels into the retina and lens, respectively. Angiogenesis is an important aspect of tumour growth and some successful new treatments for cancer involve the use of anti-angiogenic drugs such as thalidomide.

The late repair phase: scar tissue formation and remodelling

We talk about repair because the healed site is rarely as good as new (this is called resolution). Usually, the repair site is marked by a collagen scar. An exception is when damage is done to a fetus (e.g. by intra-uterine surgery), when complete resolution is usual, and in lobar pneumonia, where there is little or no tissue destruction. Much interesting research is being directed towards trying to find a way of achieving this in adults, possibly by switching on dormant embryological genes.

At this stage, around day 3, there is a temporary matrix of type III collagen. Epithelial migration over the wound surface halts by contact inhibition and a definitive matrix with type I collagen is laid down. The vessels and inflammatory cells reduce in number. Usually by day 5, bundles of collagen have been laid down across the damaged tissue to form a scar and the epidermis has returned to normal thickness.

Continuing collagen production may occur for two or more weeks.

Remodelling of the collagen starts at about 3 weeks, when fibronectin is reduced, the matrix proteins have altered in favour of proteoglycans, the proportions of type I and other collagens are roughly normal and much of the excess fluid has been reabsorbed so that the collagen fibres lie closer together. Collagenases are secreted in tandem with new collagen fibres.

Replacement and remodelling of the collagen formed early in wound healing is an important part of the healing process. Initially the scar is red, because of the increase in small vessels, but it will pale over the next few weeks as the vessels regress and the collagen thickens.

If the cut is fine and there is good wound apposition, the scar tissue is limited and the cosmetic result good, but how strong is the repair? Immediately after surgery, the sutured wound has around 70 per cent of the strength of normal skin, but this is principally conferred by the sutures. When these are removed, after 7 to 10 days, the wound strength drops to 10 per cent of normal; a point to emphasize to patients. Strength then

increases rapidly over the next month to reach a maximum at around 2 to 3 months, when a well-healed scar will have 70–80 per cent of the tensile strength of uninjured skin.

The strength of a scar does not correlate with the amount of collagen but may be related to the type, with type I being stronger than the type III deposited early in the repair process. The ultimate development of tensile strength in a wound depends on the production of adequate amounts of cross-linked collagen and on the final orientation of that collagen. Type I collagen must be cross-linked by hydroxylation of proline or lysine residues; this requires adequate supplies of oxygen, vitamin C and ferrous iron. Tensile strength is also referred to, somewhat alarmingly, as 'wound-bursting strength'!

BONE HEALING

We have not forgotten Ed's fractured femur. The femur is a tubular bone, which means that it is formed of a hollow sheath of lamellar bone, which is filled with fat, bone marrow and a delicate meshwork of bony trabeculae. The tubular shaft imparts the strength of the bone, and the lamellae (or layers) indicate the direction in which the bone has been laid down, in line with the direction of stress. The direct trauma imparted on the femur by the car crash caused it to fracture transversely across its shaft. About a litre of blood will have oozed from vessels damaged at the site, causing a localized haematoma. Early bruising and swelling of the thigh was evident by the time he reached hospital, since extracting him from the car crash took well over an hour. The two free fracture ends grated together when the leg was moved, which caused Edward great pain and produced the sensation of crepitus at the fracture site, as noted in the A&E department.

The fracture was reduced, i.e. pulled back into alignment, and maintained in this position by traction. The site was immobilized in a plaster cast to allow optimal conditions for healing. Inside the leg, the body is beavering away at much the same thing. At the fracture site a kind of internal splint is formed by the haematoma, formed from clotted blood, and also the localized tissue swelling, secondary to the release of inflammatory mediators (Fig. 5.14). Polymorphs and macrophages from the blood and surrounding tissues appear within hours and increase in number over the

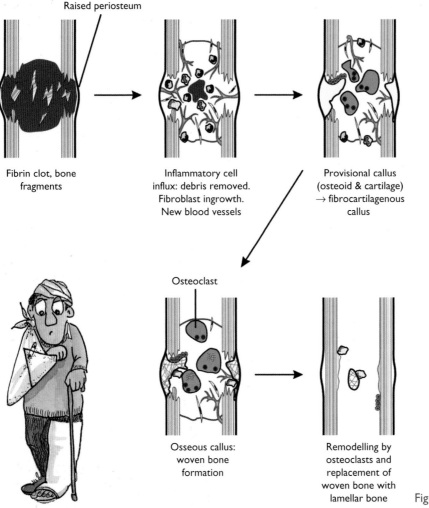

Raised periosteum

Fibrin clot, bone fragments

Inflammatory cell influx: debris removed. Fibroblast ingrowth. New blood vessels

Provisional callus (osteoid & cartilage) → fibrocartilagenous callus

Osteoclast

Osseous callus: woven bone formation

Remodelling by osteoclasts and replacement of woven bone with lamellar bone

Figure 5.14 **Bone healing**

next 2 days. They phagocytose the debris: bony fragments, blood clot and damaged connective tissue. Under the influence of inflammatory mediators, fibroblasts invade the wound site and the ingrowth of new capillaries is stimulated, carrying nutrients to the site. If pressed, the site is still slightly mobile at this stage, but is 'sticky,' and is still tender. As the healing process progresses, fibrous tissue and cartilage is laid down, and this ossifies to form woven bone. In Ed's case, this takes 6 weeks.

At this point the fracture is considered to be united, and is no longer tender or mobile under pressure, although it remains swollen. Radiologically, there is a clear difference between the original tubular lamellar bone, still obviously sundered but linked by a cuff of

woven bone around the wound site, which appears as a loose bony meshwork on X-ray. Several factors influence the rate at which fractures heal, particularly the type and site of the fracture (upper limb heals quicker than lower, oblique or spiral fractures more quickly than transverse) and the age and nutritional state of the patient. For instance a child with a simple spiral fracture of the humerus may heal in 3 weeks whereas an elderly patient, an adult with a comminuted fracture, or any patient with a fracture at a poor-healing site, such as the lower leg, may take 24 weeks to achieve union.

It will take several weeks/months more for the woven bone to be remodelled by osteoclasts within the bone, and for osteoblasts to lay down lamellar bone along the lines of stress, and the patient must be gently mobilized as soon as possible to assist this process. Once union has occurred and the patient is bearing weight, the lumpy new cortical bone gradually becomes resorbed and smoothed out and the excess medullary new bone is removed, restoring a normal medullary cavity. Woven bone, which is quite rapidly formed and which is much less efficient at weight bearing, is resorbed completely and is replaced by lamellar bone. This restoration to normality may take up to a year.

Fortunately, Edward is young and well nourished, and heals quickly. He is back on the rugby pitch 9 months later. He returns to his supermarket job rather more quickly than is sensible, and develops a small incisional hernia in his abdominal scar. It is causing him no problem at present and he has decided to put up with it.

HEALING IN OTHER SPECIALIZED TISSUES

Central nervous system

Cerebral infarction is a typical example of neuronal loss. Neurons are a 'permanent' tissue and it has always been thought that once lost, they are gone forever. Encouragingly, there is now some evidence to suggest that a limited degree of regeneration can take place in the hypothalamic–neurohypophyseal system. Scarring is not a major feature following necrosis within the central nervous system – dead brain tissue liquefies and is gradually cleared, leaving empty spaces often called 'lacunar infarcts'. The process stimulates the proliferation of glial cells which, together with the ingrowths of capillaries, may form a physical barrier to the regeneration of new neuronal fibres. There is encouraging new work in this field, particularly involving the use of stem cells.

Peripheral nervous system

Severed axons can regenerate. New fibrils sprout from the proximal end of the severed axon, each invaginating the surrounding Schwann cells as they grow, at a rate of about 1 mm per day. If a fibril grows down an existing endoneurial sheath, its function may be recovered. If the sprouts grow away from the correct pathway, substances secreted by stromal cells in the connective tissue bind to the tips and prevent them growing further. Often, this does not happen and instead the regenerative efforts result in a tangle of fibres embedded in fibrous scar, a 'traumatic neuroma'.

History   Friedrich Schwann (1810–1882)

Friedrich Schwann was a German anatomical professor who made two major contributions: he showed that fermentation was associated with living organisms and he developed the cell theory with Schleiden and Müller. He submitted his manuscript describing how cells with their nucleus and protoplasm are the building blocks of all animal and plant tissues to a Catholic bishop for approval before publication.

He discovered the axon sheath cells that bear his name, the striped muscle in the upper part of the oesophagus, the importance of bile for digestion and the enzyme, pepsin. He also studied muscle contraction and demonstrated that the tension of a contracting muscle varies with its length.

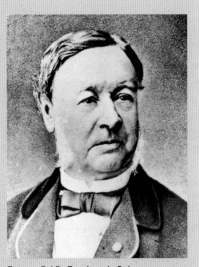

Figure 5.15 Frederick Schwann (1810–82) (Reproduced with permission from Wellcome Trust)

Liver

The liver is an amazing organ, capable of regenerating from half to two thirds of its volume after an acute insult. In fact it is so good at regeneration that it is possible for a live donor to supply a liver transplant by division of his own liver, and survive the event. Possible, but not particularly recommended!

The liver can regenerate in three ways. In day-to-day insults, in which a single hepatocyte might die, the adjacent cell will divide and take its place. In a more elaborate injury, stem cells which lie in the liver tissue next to the portal tracts ('oval cells') proliferate to form new liver; sometimes they are confused and make new bile ducts as well – they can form either. A really major insult, such as a paracetamol overdose, may overwhelm the system and stem cells from the bone marrow may migrate to the site to assist.

The new liver produced is indistinguishable from the original, except that it contains less age-related pigment (lipofuscin).

WHAT CAN GO WRONG WITH THE HEALING PROCESSES?

When it comes to wound healing, it is not any one thing but rather a complex and dynamic interplay between many factors within an intricate network that determines the final outcome. Failure to heal satisfactorily can be the result of either systemic or local factors.

SYSTEMIC FACTORS

Nutrition

Deficient protein intake may inhibit collagen formation and so inhibit the regaining of tensile strength. Sulfur-containing amino acids such as methionine seem to be particularly important. Lack of vitamin C has been found to inhibit the secretion of collagen fibres by fibroblasts and adversely affect the deposition of chondroitin sulphate in the extracellular matrix of granulation tissue. Vitamin A has important functions in relation to epithelial proliferation and epithelial differentiation, important in wound healing. A role for zinc in wound healing was discovered more or less by accident. In the course of a study on the effects of certain amino acids on wound healing, a phenylalanine analogue which had been expected to impair healing instead accelerated it. Careful study of this analogue revealed that the sample used had been contaminated by zinc. Zinc deficiency,

such as is found in patients who have been on parenteral nutrition for long periods and in patients with severe burns, is associated with poor healing.

Steroid treatment, chemotherapy and radiotherapy

It is well known that steroids damp down the inflammatory response and are of great use in diseases where the inflammatory response is causing more harm than good. The effect on healing may be a secondary phenomenon related to this effect on inflammation. This is probably due to a reduction in macrophages entering the wound and, hence, a reduction in macrophage-derived factors important in healing. There may also be a direct effect on fibroblasts to reduce collagen production. Steroids are therefore administered in situations where inappropriate scarring is taking place, such as in interstitial fibrosis in the lung.

Chemotherapy and radiotherapy also reduce the number of circulating monocytes and so probably cause a reduction in wound macrophages.

LOCAL FACTORS

Foreign material and/or infection

The presence of infection or of a foreign body will increase the intensity and prolong the duration of the inflammatory response to injury. It is worth remembering that fragments of dead tissue, such as bone, and other elements of the patient's own tissues which have become misplaced, such as hair or keratin, act as foreign bodies.

Poor immobilization of wound edges

Excess mobility in any tissue will impair healing and prolong the time to full recovery. Anything which leads to undue tension or excess movement at the wound site, such as poor siting of an incision, may interfere with healing.

In bones, movement at the fracture site may cause non-union or the development of pseudarthrosis.

Vascular supply

If the arterial perfusion of the wound site is compromised by stenosis or occlusion, as for instance in atherosclerosis, healing may be delayed or completely inhibited. Adequate venous drainage is also important, and impairment of this may play a part in the genesis of chronic ulcers, which often occur on the anterior surface of the legs in elderly patients (Fig. 5.16). Poor oxygenation of adequately perfused tissue, for instance in severe anaemia, will also impair healing.

Abnormal scar formation

The scar may remain well vascularized and contain an exuberant excess of collagen. A hypertrophic scar bulges from the original wound site, develops immediately and often regresses over time, whereas a keloid scar gradually protrudes out of and then beyond the original site, starting to develop up to a year after the wound has healed. Keloids do not regress.

Both hypertrophic scars and keloids tend to occur in dark-skinned people and particular sites are involved, typically the ear lobes, shoulders and over the sternum, or at a site which is under tension, such as the natural facial creases. The exact mechanisms are not known but there is an immature, hypervascularized collagen matrix present and it may be that there is abnormal expression of regulatory genes controlling interactions between epithelial and mesenchymal cells. Genetic factors may be important.

Scar contractures

This is usually a complication of severe burns or injuries in which a large amount of tissue has been lost. Marked contraction may cause deformities of joints because of involvement of the underlying tendons.

Cirrhosis of the liver

Although the liver is amazingly good at regenerating after its cells have been killed by one-off insults, e.g. hepatitis A infection or paracetamol overdose, if the insult continues over many months and years eventually haphazard bands of fibrous scar tissue are laid down. The delicate irrigation system required for normal blood flow and normal liver function is interrupted.

Back-pressure leads to linkages forming between the portal blood supply to the liver and the systemic veins which drain the rest of the body, sometimes with catastrophic consequences, such as when engorged veins in the oesophagus (oesophageal varices) rupture and can cause death due to massive haematemesis.

> **Dictionary**
>
> Haematemesis: vomiting blood

PROBLEMS SPECIFIC TO BONE HEALING

Non-union is often a result of excess movement in the fracture ends; the gap is bridged by fibrous scar tissue

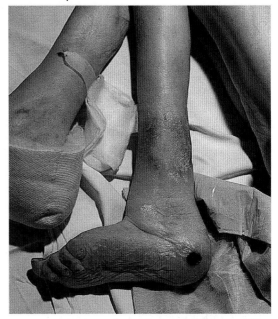

Figure 5.16 Poor blood supply, oedema of the lower limbs, poor nutrition and infection may all contribute to the failure to heal of a pressure sore in a bed-ridden patient

instead of the usual bone-forming process. This can result in a useless bone, which cannot resist the pull of attached muscles. If the fibrous segment is extremely short, a good union may be achieved, at the cost of bone strength.

Pseudarthrosis is analagous to non-union, but here a joint develops, sometimes with a synovial space and cartilagenous lining. Obviously this creates a useless bone.

In mal-union the bony ends are poorly apposed, and may overlap. Mal-union may result in a shortened, deformed bone with a degree of normal function. In other forms of mal-union, adhesions may form between adjacent muscle and the bone, as a result of scarring following inflammation.

In osteomyelitis a focus of infection may persist following a compound fracture. However, osteomyelitis more commonly results from blood-borne spread of bacteria.

IMPROVING WOUND HEALING

The discussion of factors modifying wound healing emphasises that a clean, uninfected, immobile wound with the sides closely apposed in a healthy patient is most likely to heal quickly and neatly. There are several

Figure 5.17 Male alcohol-related death rates by age group, United Kingdom, 1991–2006. (Data source: National Statistics website: www.statistics.gov.uk. Crown copyright material is reproduced with the permission of the Controller Office of Public Sector Information (OPSI))

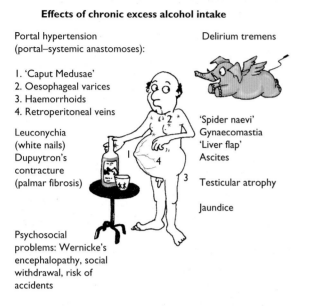

Effects of chronic excess alcohol intake

Portal hypertension
(portal–systemic anastomoses):

1. 'Caput Medusae'
2. Oesophageal varices
3. Haemorrhoids
4. Retroperitoneal veins

Leuconychia
(white nails)
Dupuytron's
contracture
(palmar fibrosis)

Psychosocial
problems: Wernicke's
encephalopathy, social
withdrawal, risk of
accidents

Delirium tremens

'Spider naevi'
Gynaecomastia
'Liver flap'
Ascites

Testicular atrophy

Jaundice

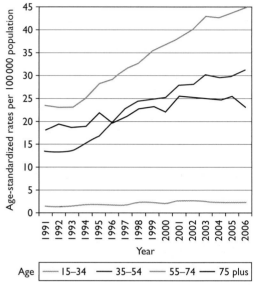

Age 15–34 35–54 55–74 75 plus

Figure 5.18 Coronal CT in a patient with alcoholic liver disease, showing a shrunken, cirrhotic liver (white arrow), splenomegaly (blue arrow) from portal venous hypertension, and ascites (red arrows)

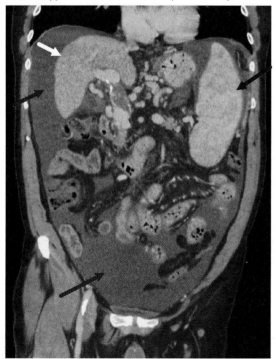

new approaches to wound healing which are under investigation.

Wound healing may be improved by the local use of ultrasound or laser therapy, which are thought to increase vascular permeability.

Synthetic growth factors, applied topically, may stimulate the healing of chronically ulcerated sites and there has been particular interest in the topical application of keratinocyte growth factor and transforming growth factor beta.

Stubborn bone fractures may be persuaded to unite by the passage of electrical currents through the bone, and skin wounds may also benefit.

Figure 5.19 Cirrhosis of liver The irregular nodular pattern is visible to the naked eye

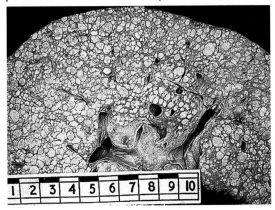

Figure 5.20 Photomicrograph of liver with cirrhosis showing nodules of hepatocytes (H) separated by fibrous bands (F). The hepatocytes are distended with fat, which together with inflammation was the injurious stimulus

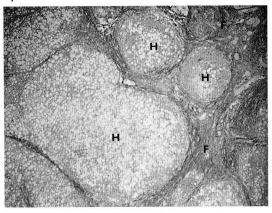

Clinicopathological case study   alcoholic liver disease

Clinical

A 60-year-old man with long-standing history of alcohol abuse presented with a 3-week history of general malaise, weight loss, loss of appetite and productive cough.

Examination

He was noted to be short of breath with an increased respiratory rate and was jaundiced. He had a fever and tachycardia of 110 beats/min. He also had supraclavicular lymphadenopathy and a mildly enlarged and tender liver. Auscultation of his chest revealed coarse crackles over both his lung fields.

Investigations

The liver function tests were abnormal with a raised bilirubin of 45 μmol/L and a raised γ-GT of 90 IU/L. His chest X-ray showed bilateral consolidation with a small right pleural effusion. A lymph node and liver biopsy were carried out.

The lymph node showed numerous caseating granulomata with calcification. The Ziehl–Neelson stain showed abundant acid-fast mycobacteria. The liver biopsy showed an acute alcoholic hepatitis with marked fatty change and liver fibrosis, but without cirrhosis.

Pathological

He had a long history of alcohol abuse and this predisposes to many illnesses. Alcoholics tend to be malnourished as they derive most of their calories from alcohol and are therefore deficient in many vitamins, especially the B group. They damage the liver by episodes of hepatitis which heals with scarring, producing fibrosis and eventually cirrhosis. They are also predisposed to infections because of depression of the immune system caused by the alcohol, and, in this man, clinical examination revealed signs of a chest infection. Tuberculosis is a particular problem in alcoholics.

The liver function tests were in keeping with alcoholic damage with raised bilirubin and liver cell enzymes. The chest X-ray confirmed a pneumonic process involving both lungs.

Caseous necrosis with granuloma formation is a classical picture of tuberculosis and special stains revealed mycobacteria. Immune suppression due to alcohol abuse is responsible for the reactivation of secondary tuberculosis. In areas of necrosis, calcification is common and this type is called dystrophic calcification. The serum calcium levels are normal as opposed to metastatic calcification in which serum calcium levels are raised.

Clinicopathological case study   alcoholic liver disease

His liver showed the classical fatty change common in alcohol abuse with some hepatitis, i.e. inflammation of the hepatocytes with liver cell necrosis. The result is healing by scarring with resultant fibrosis. He did not have cirrhosis which is irreversible, unlike fatty change which is.

Management and progress:

He was started on anti-tuberculous therapy and was counselled for his alcohol abuse.

While in hospital, he had a bout of abdominal pain and diarrhoea. Endoscopy showed gastritis but sigmoidoscopy was unremarkable. The rectal biopsy revealed the presence of amyloid in the mucosa. He was discharged on anti-tuberculous therapy and sent for rehabilitation for his alcohol abuse but he defaulted from his appointments and was lost to follow-up.

Alcoholics are predisposed to gastritis, i.e. inflammation of the gastric mucosa. They may also have gastric ulcers. Other complications include oesophageal varices if portal hypertension has developed due to cirrhosis. Patients with long-standing chronic inflammatory diseases such as rheumatoid arthritis and tuberculosis are prone to reactive amyloidosis (AA). Rectal biopsy is a good way of diagnosing amyloid. The amyloid may have been responsible for the diarrhoea but infective causes should be excluded.

Lack of compliance is a common problem with alcoholics.

CHAPTER 6

THE IMMUNE DEFENCE AGAINST INFECTION

Students can become confused when pathologists talk about acute and chronic inflammation whereas immunologists speak of innate and adaptive (or acquired) immunity.

As we have already seen in chapter 4, acute inflammation is an immediate response to injury or to invasion by pathogens and particularly involves neutrophils, macrophages, mast cells and platelets, plus numerous inflammatory mediators. When immunologists refer to an innate response they are considering the body's standard response to invasion by microbial pathogens.

Innate immunity is a bit like setting a minefield just in case someone tries to invade your country: if a mine is stepped on, an immense explosion takes place, usually killing whatever set off the mine and causing a considerable amount of local damage in the process (Fig. 6.1).

The adaptive immune response is a precisely targeted response to a pathogen, the body having been alerted by sentries or scouts on duty at the border. A photograph of the invader is circulated to a highly trained sniper, who recognizes and assassinates the target cleanly, with little 'collateral damage'.

THE LYMPHATIC SYSTEM IN INFLAMMATION

Before we go on to discuss the acquired immune response, we must consider the role of the lymphatic system in inflammation.

The lymphatic system comprises several collections of organized lymphoid tissue and their interconnecting network of vessels, the lymphatics. Lymphocytes are produced and mature in the bone marrow and thymus. They migrate in the blood to populate and proliferate in the lymph nodes, the spleen and the lining of the gut and respiratory tract, the so-called mucosa-associated lymphoid tissue or MALT. The lymphatic vessels comprise a one-way circulatory system linked to, but separate from, the blood circulation. Once the lymphocytes have been returned to the bloodstream via the thoracic duct, the cycle is repeated. The recirculation of lymphoid cells is important, as it allows information about invading organisms in one part of the body to be shared with other areas of lymphoid cell production. A lymphocyte which has come from a specific area,

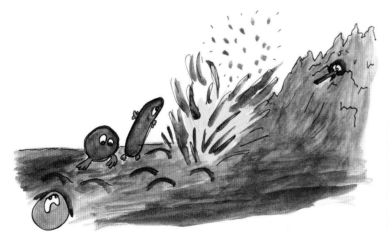

Figure 6.1 The innate immune response relies on non-specialized defence systems at strategic sites whereas the acquired immune reponse is a targetted response to a specific threat. These immune responses largely translate to acute and chronic inflammation

such as the gut, recognizes particular surface molecules on the endothelial cells of that area (addressins) that allow it to 'home' back to the same tissue.

Lymphatic channels begin as blind-ended sacs, with ultra-thin walls. They consist of little more than endothelial lining cells supported by delicate collagen fibres initially, but as these vessels drain into larger ones they start to resemble veins, eventually developing a muscularized wall. The lymph is all eventually channelled into one large vessel, the thoracic duct, which empties into the venous system at the junction of the left subclavian and internal jugular veins. Like the venous system, lymphatic channels have valves and rely on the pumping action of adjacent muscles to create flow. A distinctive feature of the lymphatic system is the presence of a chain of lymph nodes, stationed at strategic points within the body; these form check points at which the contents are filtered and screened for miscreants. Unlike the venous system, the lymphatics form a branching network which does not follow a uniform course back to the heart, but may allow lymph to meander through quite disparate sites. We know this because of studies in melanoma patients, whose skin is injected with radioactive material and special dye in an attempt to find the immediately draining lymph node. One of our patients, with a skin lesion on the back of the right shoulder, was found to have a 'sentinel node' in the right groin! This was an extreme example, but shows that lymph nodes are not necessarily anatomically adjacent to the tissues they drain.

What is lymph? When we considered fluid flow across vessels (see Figs 4.6 and 4.7) it became clear that more fluid moves out of tissue capillaries due to the pump pressure within the system (hydrostatic pressure) than is returned to the bloodstream due to the pull of plasma proteins (plasma oncotic pressure). This is increased if there is nearby inflammatory activity, when plasma proteins also leak out of the excessively permeable vascular endothelium. The tissue fluid is termed lymph and it drains into the lymphatic channels which are present in all tissues. In addition to the fluid, lymph also contains a variety of inflammatory cells, particularly lymphocytes and cells of monocyte/macrophage lineage. The actual number of cells is very variable and increases if the tissue is inflamed. Foreign antigens and particles can also enter the lymph, sometimes loose but often within specialized cells of the monocyte/macrophage lineage.

Let us consider the case of a 10-year-old boy complaining of a severe sore throat which is making it

Figure 6.2 An immune response to infection such as *Streptococcus* causes a sore throat because antigen presenting cells present first to the mucosa-associated lymphoid tissue in the oropharynx. Persistent infection causes enlargement and tenderness of the lymph nodes which drain this region

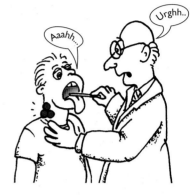

painful to swallow. Examination of his pharynx shows red, swollen tonsils with a purulent exudate on the surface. He also complains of painful lumps in his neck; these are the lymph nodes on either side of the sternomastoid muscle which have enlarged in response to the throat infection (Fig. 6.2).

A swab taken from the tonsil grows *Streptococcus pyogenes*. Lancefield group A streptococci, along with other Gram-positive bacteria, have mannose, a carbohydrate moeity in their outer wall, which stimulates the inflammatory response and is the cause of the boy's throat symptoms and the enlargement of the local lymphoid defences in the pharynx. But why are the lymph nodes swollen too? If, for the sake of illustration, one of the nodes were to be excised for microscopical examination, it would show a number of changes (Fig. 6.3).

The changes arise because lymph fluid, with cellular and particulate matter containing foreign bacterial antigens and complement fragment C3b, drains into the lymph nodes of the neck. This initiates a specific adaptive immune response which causes proliferation and differentiation of T and B cells (these are the same as T and B lymphocytes, but use less printing ink).

The response of T cells and B cells requires help from other cells as they are incapable (T cells) or inefficient (B cells) in recognizing native foreign antigens such as bacterial products.

These helper cells are called accessory cells and fall into two broad categories.

Figure 6.3 (a) Photomicrograph of a lymph node. (b) Diagram of a lymph node

- Lymph carries antigens, antigen-presenting cells (APC) and complement fragments. It enters the node via afferent lymphatics, trickles through the B zone (cortex), T zone (paracortex) and medulla and exits via the efferent lymphatic.
- Lymph passes through a chain of lymph nodes before returning to the venous system via the thoracic duct.

- Lymphocytes circulating in the blood move into the lymph node through 'high endothelial venules' which express lymphocyte adhesion molecules.
- Lymphocytes exit the node in lymph fluid and are carried through other nodes in the chain before being returned to the blood.

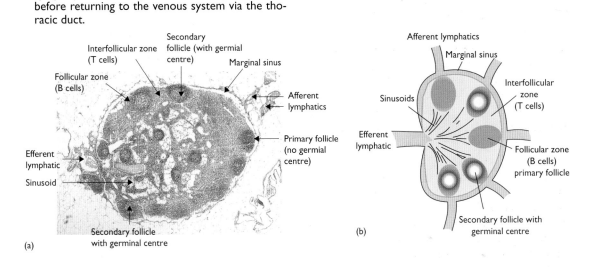

(a)
Secondary follicle (with germial centre)
Interfollicular zone (T cells)
Marginal sinus
Follicular zone (B cells)
Efferent lymphatic
Sinusoid
Secondary follicle with germinal centre
Afferent lymphatics
Primary follicle (no germial centre)

(b)
Afferent lymphatics
Marginal sinus
Sinusoids
Efferent lymphatic
Interfollicular zone (T cells)
Follicular zone (B cells) primary follicle
Secondary follicle with germinal centre

The first group belongs to the macrophage/monocyte lineage. These cells are widely distributed in the skin and the mucosa and are originally formed in the bone marrow, from where they migrate to their stations in the body's perimeter defence system. They can take up antigen in a variety of ways, including via immunoglobulin (Fc) or complement (C3b) receptors. Many of these accessory cells have processes to increase their cell surface contact area and are called dendritic cells (Fig. 6.4). Dendritic cells live within the epithelium or in the immediately adjacent connective tissue at most portals of entry to the body, so they are well placed to encounter any invading pathogens. The foreign antigen is sampled by these cells at the site of entry (the tonsils in this case) and is carried to the lymph node where an army of T cells and B cells resides.

The dendritic cells are also called the antigen-presenting cells (APC) as after sampling the antigen, they can break it to smaller fragments (epitopes) and present the antigen to T cells in a suitable form on type II MHC receptors. APC express high levels of co-stimulatory molecules on their surfaces. In order for T-cell activation to take place, both antigen presentation and engagement of co-stimulatory molecules must occur.

Figure 6.4 Langerhans cells (stained here for S100 protein) are dendritic antigen-presenting cells (APC) found in skin and other squamous epithelium, such as that found in the oropharynx

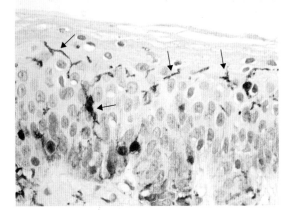

Although dendritic APCs are the most efficient cells for the presentation of antigen to T cells, there are other cells which could perform this function. These include B cells, macrophages, epithelial and endothelial cells.

The dendritic APCs should not be confused with follicular dendritic cells (FDCs), the second type of accessory

Figure 6.5 Diagram of a secondary follicle and adjacent paracortex to illustrate the anatomical relationship between B cells and FDCs, and T cells and APCs

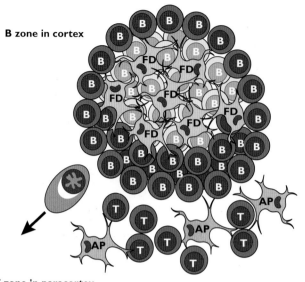

B zone in cortex

T zone in paracortex

The follicle dendritic cells in the B zones (follicles) and the antigen-presenting cells in the T zones form a mesh resembling a sieve. They catch and present antigen to B and T lymphocytes

A highly specific immune response is generated. B cells produce antibody and T cells produce helper and suppressor/cytotoxic cells

B and T memory cells are generated and guard against another infection by the same agent

cell. The FDCs are confined to the lymphoid follicles, and can be found in lymph nodes during embryonal development. They are possibly not of macrophage/monocyte lineage but nevertheless express Fc and complement receptors. FDCs cannot phagocytose or process antigen, but can trap and display it on their surfaces as whole molecules and they are potent stimulators of B-cell differentiation.

The APCs carrying the antigen reach the lymph node through afferent lymphatics and filter through the paracortex where they meet an army of T cells ready to respond. The T cells recognize the antigenic epitopes presented by APC, proliferate and differentiate into helper T cells which co-ordinate key aspects of the immune response (page 143) and initiate the B-cell response. FDCs stimulate B cells to produce antibodies tailored to fit a particular antigen (page 144). These changes lead to enlargement of the lymph node which can be palpated in the neck as in this case.

As we discussed, APCs can trap organisms (in this case, streptococci) to prevent their dissemination into the blood; they do this by grabbing attached portions of immunoglobulin (Fc component) or complement (C3b). These, of course, are opsonins (see chapter 4). The opsonins are fixed to the surface of the bug itself or to any soluble antigenic fragments which it may have

released. You already know that bacterial wall fragments can directly stimulate the complement cascade to produce C3b (see Fig. 4.16), but as the adaptive immune response has not yet been stimulated at this initial stage and antibody production is a function of the immune response, how can there be any immunoglobulin for the phagocyte to adhere to?

Like any good general anticipating a possible attack, the body prepares itself during the early months of a baby's life. At this time the bone marrow generates millions of different B-cell clones, each capable of secreting an antibody likely to be of use in combating infection, and these cells patrol the body. If an antibody is a reasonable 'fit' with an antigen, it can stick to it well enough to opsonize the particle.

The type of microbial agent which initiates an inflammatory reaction determines the most appropriate host immune response.

The lymph node is organized into zones to optimize the immune response: B lymphocytes, which can develop into plasma cells that produce antibodies, are gathered into aggregates called follicles. These are situated in the cortex of the lymph node. T lymphocytes reside outside the follicles in the inter-follicular zone (Fig. 6.5). Bacterial infections, such as the streptococcal infection suffered by our patient, are characterized by

Figure 6.6 Lymphoid stem cells differentiating to form B and T lymphocytes, which circulate to the lymph nodes and spleen

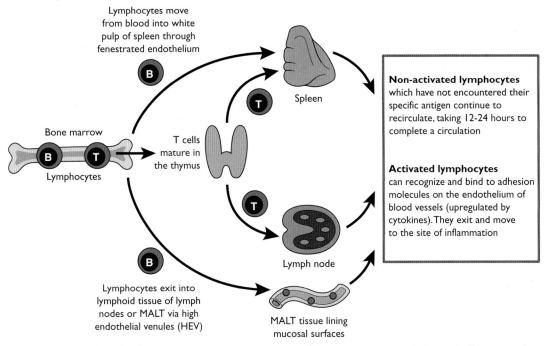

Lymphocytes move from blood into white pulp of spleen through fenestrated endothelium

Spleen

Bone marrow

Lymphocytes

T cells mature in the thymus

T

Lymph node

Lymphocytes exit into lymphoid tissue of lymph nodes or MALT via high endothelial venules (HEV)

MALT tissue lining mucosal surfaces

Non-activated lymphocytes which have not encountered their specific antigen continue to recirculate, taking 12-24 hours to complete a circulation

Activated lymphocytes can recognize and bind to adhesion molecules on the endothelium of blood vessels (upregulated by cytokines). They exit and move to the site of inflammation

the enlargement of the B cell areas (follicular hyperplasia). If a virus had caused the sore throat, as is usually the case, then the T-cell response would be more important than antibody production and there would be paracortical hyperplasia.

With any luck, the defence systems activated in our 10-year-old patient's lymph nodes will stop the infection from spreading to the rest of the body. If the systems fail, the streptococcal infection may reach the blood. Infection of the blood (septicaemia) can also occur if tissue organisms directly enter blood vessels instead of lymphatics.

A septicaemic patient is gravely ill with fevers, shivering attacks (rigors) and a dangerous lowering of the blood pressure ('shock', see page 212). The spleen is all-important here; its structure and functions are analogous to those of the lymph node. It has sinusoids lined by macrophages and specific B- and T-cell areas, but the fluid percolating through is blood rather than lymph. It exists to trap organisms, debris and particulate matter and to promote immune cell proliferation. The most serious risk of infection is from capsulated bacteria, such as the pneumococcus (*Streptococcus pneumonia*) and *Haemophilus influenzae*, which are better at evading the body's innate defences than other bacteria.

THE ADAPTIVE IMMUNE RESPONSE

The adaptive immune response can be split into humoral immunity and cell-mediated immunity.

Humoral immunity is due to antibody production by B cells which transform to plasma cells and produce immunoglobulin (antibodies).

Cell-mediated immunity is mediated by T cells. There are several subsets of T cells, but the two most important are the T suppressor/cytotoxic cells, capable of direct attack and lymphokine production, and the T helper-cells, which act to regulate the immune response and interact widely with other immune-reactive cells. A third important type of lymphocyte, probably a T subtype, is the NK cell (page 155).

We start life with an army of B and T cells, raw recruits perhaps, but willing to go into action at the press of a button. Both originate from stem cells in the bone marrow, but early on the T cells are lured away to the thymus; the mechanisms governing how they get there are still not clear (Fig. 6.6).

The 'action' buttons, or cell surface receptors, on the B and T cells have been prepared by an intelligence service which has attempted to anticipate every eventuality.

Each cell has a unique receptor for antigen on its surface, generated after the B cells have undergone a series of rearrangements in their heavy chain genes whilst in the bone marrow the T cells have similarly rearranged their T-cell receptor genes during their maturation process in the thymus.

HUMORAL IMMUNITY

How does a B cell produce the correct antibody for a new antigen?

Surprisingly, it is the antigen which chooses the B cell best equipped to fight it, rather than the other way round! The B cell has no choice in the matter. Mother Nature equips the body with an enormous number of B cells, each armed with a receptor for a unique antigen.

Imagine the B cells, lined up around the wall of a dance hall, waiting for the right antigen to ask them to dance! Each B cell has the genetic code for a single antibody and it displays this antibody on its own cell surface. This 'B cell receptor complex' (BCR) consists of an immunoglobulin molecule which is stuck to the membrane and binds antigen (Fig. 6.7). Like antibody, the BCR has both heavy and light chain components. The Fc end (see Fig. 6.10) of the antibody is anchored to the surface of the B cell by a transmembrane component. Other than this, the BCR is identical to the antibody it will produce when the BCR binds antigen.

The BCR is unique to that B cell. The BCR is complexed with other proteins which traverse the cell membrane. This protein anchors the BCR in the membrane and is essential for signal transduction after antigen binding. Only B cells with a BCR that binds the antigen will be stimulated to proliferate and secrete antibody with an identical structure to the BCR, only lacking the transmembrane component. The type of immunoglobulin molecule in the BCR is usually an IgM monomer or sometimes IgD.

Figure 6.7 Each B lymphocyte bears a unique B-cell receptor (BCR) which is tethered to the membrane but is otherwise identical to the antibody it will secrete. Antibody secretion occurs when B cells are activated by antigen, either by cross-linkage of BCRs on the surface or by Th cells, with which they interact via MHC II and co-stimulatory molecules

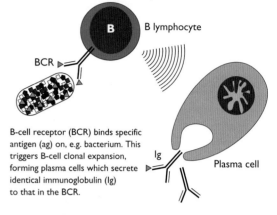

B-cell receptor (BCR) binds specific antigen (ag) on, e.g. bacterium. This triggers B-cell clonal expansion, forming plasma cells which secrete identical immunoglobulin (Ig) to that in the BCR.

Of course, it requires an enormous number of B cells with different genetic codes (and thus BCRs) to ensure that the body has a B cell equipped to fight any new foreign antigen. Several B cells may have receptors which can bind to different parts of the antigen (epitopes); only those which fit closely are used. (There are at least 10^8 different immunoglobulin molecules in the serum.) Nature discovered a brilliant way of producing this variety of codes, which we shall describe below, and then used a similar approach for T-cell receptor molecules (TCR) (Fig. 6.8).

While we are discussing the receptors displayed on the surface of a B cell, we should mention CD40, which binds to the CD40 ligand present on helper T cells (Fig. 6.6). Without this, B cells cannot mature to form plasma cells or 'class switch' (page 146) to secrete IgG, IgA or IgE antibodies. B cells also express a number of other 'co-stimulatory' cell surface molecules, such as CD80 and CD86 which interact with CD28 on T cells and are critical in the development of the T-cell–B-cell interaction.

B cells, like macrophages, express MHC class II molecules and carry receptors for complement (CD21) and the Fc component of immunoglobulin molecules, although they do not phagocytose. In order for a B cell to be activated, there must be multiple binding of the BCR to antigenic sites. B cells can recognize complement which is bound to the surface of a microbe (and complement only binds to foreign cells) and the BCR is much

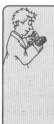

Dictionary

Transduction: the translation of a signal into an action, usually involving messengers which refer the signal to the nucleus. Here particular genes are switched on and translated into proteins with actions appropriate to the initial stimulus.

Figure 6.8 Interactions between antigen-presenting cells and T and B lymphocytes; arrows indicate direction of stimulation

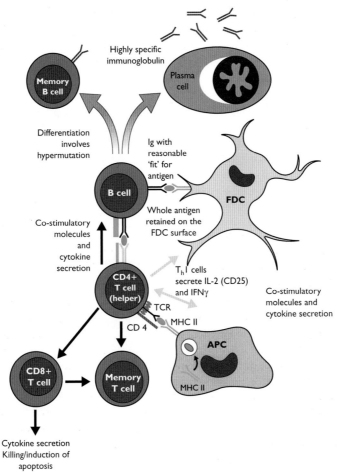

Follicle dendritic cells (FDC) trap bound antigen in the lymph using complement or Fc receptors. The antigen is not processed, but is presented to the B cell and is a potent stimulator for B cell maturation, including hypermutation of the immunoglobulin antigen recognition site to create high-affinity antibodies

Antigen-presenting cells (APC) process phagocytosed antigen and combine it with MHC II, which moves to the cell surface and interacts with T (helper) cells in conjunction with CD4 and the T-cell receptor complex (TCR)

Helper T-cells are of two types:

- T_h1 cells secrete IL-2 and interferon gamma. IL-2/IL-2 receptor interaction is the target of much current interest, since if it can be 'mopped up' by administration of antibody, the stimulus for cell proliferation may be reduced or removed, with implications for inflammation-driven disease

- T_h2 cells stimulate antibody production and activate eosinophils and mast cells

more easily activated if the B cell also binds to complement. The FDC cells in the lymph node's germinal centre can bind complement and use it to gather complement-bound antigen for presentation to the B cell.

You will probably have come across glandular fever (infectious mononucleosis), caused by Epstein–Barr virus (EBV). The virus infects B cells with ease since its antigen is the same as the complement receptor (CD21), so it has a key to the door. EBV can be a nuisance. (See later under autoimmune disease and neoplasia.)

At the first encounter between a B cell and an appropriate antigen, there is a proliferation of immunologically identical B cells, called a clone, together with memory cells. However the 'fit' between the antibody and the antigen can be improved considerably by a bit of adjustment, the difference you might say between an off-the-peg and a tailored garment. The tailoring is achieved through interactions between B cells and antigen presented by follicle dendritic cells. The follicle dendritic cell (see Fig. 6.5) is a potent inducer of hypermutation in the hypervariable region of the antibody.

A large population of daughter B cells is produced through cloning and these differentiate to form plasma cells; a population of circulating memory B cells is also generated.

Plasma cells secrete huge quantities of antibody into the bloodstream and tissues, deluging the antigen. Initially, the antibody is of IgM type and later the B-cell clone switches to produce IgG. This 'heavy chain switch' is useful clinically; the presence of IgM antibody in the blood of a patient indicates a recent infection, of no more than a few weeks' duration.

Finding IgG antibody is less useful, as it can indicate that the patient has been exposed to the antigen at almost any time in the past, from weeks to years. If the particular antigen is encountered again, the memory cells will quickly undergo clonal proliferation and swamp it with specific antibody. They require far less stimulation and co-stimulation than an unprimed B cell.

It is worth stating that a B-cell inflammatory reaction will lead to the generation of numerous different antibodies, all directed at different antigenic sites (epitopes). Imagine a class of students, all asked to give a one-line answer to the question 'How are antibodies generated?' We would see as many different variants on a theme as there are students. However, if one student was asked to write an answer, no matter how many times he was asked, his answer would be the same.

In a similar way, different B cells, with different BCRs and therefore antibody properties, stimulated by the same antigen, will produce a variety of different antibodies. This is a 'polyclonal' response, i.e. several different B-cell clones are stimulated and each will produce its own particular antibody.

This is very different from what happens in multiple myeloma, a malignant disease of plasma cells. All malignancies originate from a single mutated cell, so it

Figure 6.9 Myeloma: M band (arrowed), compared with normal plasma electrophoresis (Courtesy of Dr Jo Sheldon, St George's Hospital, London)

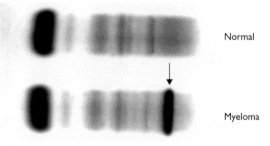

Normal

Myeloma

An extra band is present in an electrophoretic strip from a patient with myeloma, due to very large quantities of a single type of immunoglobulin secreted by a malignant clone of plasma cells. The control strip shows no significant bands in the gamma region

follows that all the antibodies secreted by a malignant proliferation of plasma cells will be identical. Compare the electrophoretic strips shown in Fig. 6.9.

This is an important concept since certain cancers which affect the lymphoid system may be difficult to differentiate from an inflammatory condition. Multiple myeloma is a tumour of bone marrow caused by a malignant proliferation of plasma cells. Malignant lymphomas representing cells at earlier stages in the path from B cell to plasma cell may secrete antibodies. The finding that all the antibodies are the same is of diagnostic value.

This is probably a good moment to think about antibodies! What do they look like and exactly how do they bind to antigen? Why are there antibody subtypes? We have come across IgM and IgG so far. And how can such a large number of diverse antibodies have been generated from cells with a common ancestor?

What are antibodies and how do they work?

Immunoglobulins are collectively known as 'gamma globulins' because of their motility on electrophoresis although this is an historical term you may still hear it used. For instance an immunodeficient patient is likely to be treated with 'pooled gammaglobulin', i.e. concentrated immunoglobulins derived from blood from a number of different donors.

Each immunoglobulin molecule is formed from two identical heavy chains and two identical light chains joined by interchain disulfide links. There are two types of light chain (kappa and lambda) and five types

Figure 6.10 The immunoglobulin molecule is active at both ends! The antigen-binding site is a three-dimensional structure, with three key sites at which bonds are made. Through a process of hypermutation, low-affinity binding sites can mutate to show high affinity for antigen

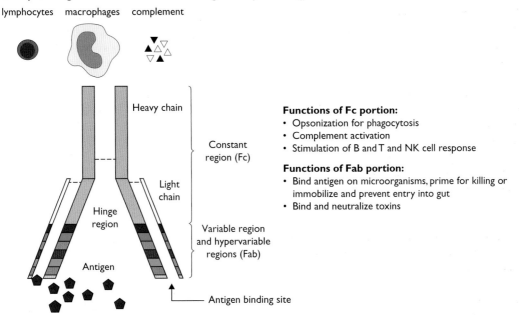

Functions of Fc portion:
• Opsonization for phagocytosis
• Complement activation
• Stimulation of B and T and NK cell response

Functions of Fab portion:
• Bind antigen on microorganisms, prime for killing or immobilize and prevent entry into gut
• Bind and neutralize toxins

of heavy chain (G, A, M, D, E). The light chains can combine with any type of heavy chain and do not influence biological function whereas each heavy chain type supports different biological functions (Fig. 6.10 and Table 6.1).

IgM is the largest: five monomeric units are joined by a J-chain to make a massive pentamer. By clustering antigen together in one spot (10 antigen molecules can be bound by one IgM pentamer), it is good at mopping up large quantities of invading pathogens at the start of an infection. IgM can also activate the C1 fragment of the complement pathway. A key feature of this molecule is that it is too large to cross the placenta (see Fig. 2.17, rhesus incompatibility).

IgG is the most prevalent antibody in the blood and exhibits the most basic immunoglobulin structure, referred to as a monomer. There are several subtypes, whose constant regions are slightly different. IgG$_3$, for instance, is best at fixing complement, whereas IgG$_1$ is the best at opsonizing for phagocytosis, since phagocytes such as macrophages and neutrophils bear specific receptors for FcIgG1. In general, IgG is the best antibody for attacking bacterial pathogens. IgG can cross the placenta, carrying passive immunity from mother to fetus to 'tide it over' until the newborn child can produce its own antibody about 3 months later.

In the blood, IgA exists in a monomeric form, but IgA is most important as a mucosal protector, in gut secretions, for instance. At these sites it exists as a dimer, linked by a J-chain and a 'secretory component' derived from the gut epithelial cell. Its constant (Fc) region ends are linked by a chain, which prevents mucosal enzymes from digesting and destroying the antibody. Also, the dumbbell-shaped dimer can bind antigen at either end, clumping bugs together and making it easier for them to be caught up in mucin and carried out of the body. In the gut-associated lymphoid tissue (such as the Peyer's patches in the terminal ileum) there are 20–30 times more IgA-producing than IgG-producing cells. This means that IgA is the most plentiful antibody in the body but most of it is on the mucosal surfaces, not in the blood. Look out for trick questions in exams! IgA defends both the luminal and subepithelial zones. About 1/600 people are IgA deficient. They may be asymptomatic or present with recurrent ear or sinus infections. An interesting finding is that patients with coeliac disease (page 50) are 10–15 times more likely to be IgA deficient (2–3 per cent of coeliac patients). In a clever extension of mucosal immunity, intestinal B lymphocytes can be stimulated by antigens and then migrate via the lymphatics and blood to localize in other areas, such as breast or salivary glands, so that specific IgA defends these sites also.

IgE binds mast cells and has a major role in the defence against parasites. When IgE is made, its Fc end is bound by mast cells, which are long-lived cells in the tissues. Here the antibody is ideally placed to recognize pathogens such as worms or flukes which invade the tissues. When two IgE molecules bound to the same mast cell are cross-linked, by binding to epitopes on a marauding parasite, they stimulate the immediate release of toxic granules from the mast cell onto the parasite. This is clever, but backfires when IgE recognizes repeated epitopes on an allergen such as a bee sting and mast cell degranulation sets off an allergic or anaphylactic (body-wide allergic) response.

IgD is a slightly mysterious monomeric immunoglobulin: it is found in mucosa-associated lymphoid tissue, particularly in the wall of the gut, but its precise role is not clear. It is present on the surface of B cells, where it seems to be very important in the primary activation of a naive B cell; that is, a B cell which has never before encountered its unique antigen. Such 'virgin' B cells have more surface IgD (sIgD) than sIgM on their surfaces, whereas those which are 'experienced' bear more sIgM. Whether they have sIgD or sIgM on their surfaces, the first immunoglobulin produced and secreted into the blood is almost always IgM. There is very little IgD in the circulating blood.

Most importantly, immunoglobulin *recognizes antigen* through the variable regions on the molecule. After that, the constant regions *initiate the biological functions*, such as complement fixation and opsonization, appropriate for the immunoglobulin class. Although diagrams generally depict antibody molecules as simple bent dinner forks (see Fig. 6.10) they actually have a complex three-dimensional structure with many 'folds' (Fig. 6.11).

Antigen binds to the variable end of the antibody molecule (Fab), in which there are three hypervariable regions forming a potential 'pocket' for antigen attachment. The shape of the pocket is dependent on the outer electron clouds of its atoms, which of course determines the antigen *shape* that it recognizes. The important point is that this interaction depends on the antigen and antibody having complementary profiles; no covalent bonding is involved, so the chemical composition is not crucial. The shapes don't have to be a perfect fit but a close fit gives the strongest binding. As mentioned

above, fine-tuning can be undertaken by a B cell in conjunction with follicle dendritic cells (FDCs) in the germinal centre and Th cells in the paracortex of the lymph node. The genetic make-up governing the three hypervariable regions in each pocket can be adjusted for a better antigen fit before the clonal expansion of the B cell is undertaken. This requires new instructions from the cell's genome and the alterations within the genome to generate better-fitting BCR proteins produce the phenomenon of hypermutation. The B cell is the only cell in the body in which it is normal for the body to play about with its genetic make-up! This generates a population of antibodies with excellent binding properties.

In hypermutating B cells, spontaneous mutation is encouraged in order to generate a hypervariable region which more closely fits the antigen. Of course, mutation generates daughter B cells with new hypervariable regions in their BCR, each slightly different from that of the first cell which bound the antigen presented to it by the FDCs.

In the germinal centre, those B cells with new BCRs are tested to see if they fit the antigen more snugly than the original. It is a bit like the story of Cinderella! The failures (the ugly sisters) die by apoptosis. The best fitting are rescued by binding with CD40 ligand on Th cells (Prince Charming) and the debris from the dead B cells is hoovered up by macrophages; their clear cytoplasm, speckled with debris, makes the germinal centre appear rather like a 'starry sky'.

Binding of antigen to antibody can lead to a variety of effects. Cross-linking of antigenic particles or cells will produce precipitation or agglutination while binding of antibody to an active site on a virus or toxin can result in neutralization. Other components of the immune response can become involved as when antibody fixes complement to produce lysis or enhanced phagocytosis. Antibody can also promote cell-mediated cytotoxicity involving NK cells, so-called antibody-dependent cell-mediated cytotoxicity (ADCC).

Nature has found this approach so useful that a common structure, the immunoglobulin homology unit, is the basic building block for a range of molecules involved in cell–cell recognition, the so-called immunoglobulin gene superfamily (Fig. 6.11). Its members include the MHC I and II receptors, CD4 and CD8, amongst others: CD4, expressed on helper T cells, binds to MHC II, and CD8, on suppressor/cytotoxic T cells, binds to MHC I.

These interactions are essential; in fact T-cell activation requires there to be both antigen binding by the

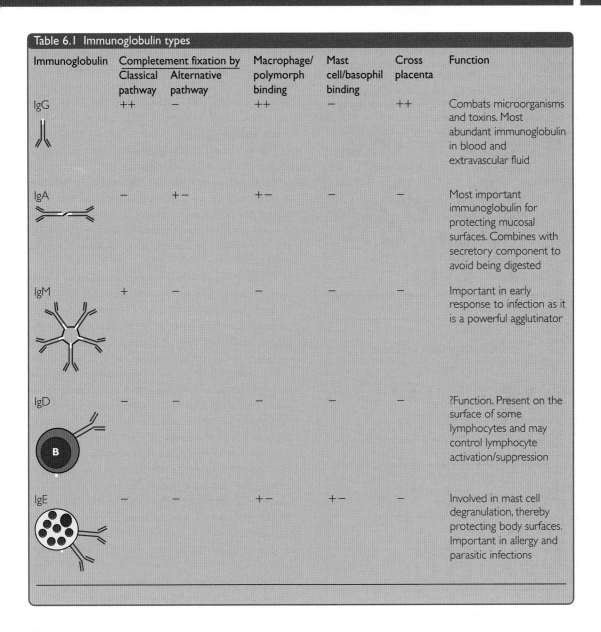

Table 6.1 Immunoglobulin types

Immunoglobulin	Completement fixation by		Macrophage/ polymorph binding	Mast cell/basophil binding	Cross placenta	Function
	Classical pathway	Alternative pathway				
IgG	++	−	++	−	++	Combats microorganisms and toxins. Most abundant immunoglobulin in blood and extravascular fluid
IgA	−	+ −	+ −	−	−	Most important immunoglobulin for protecting mucosal surfaces. Combines with secretory component to avoid being digested
IgM	+	−	−	−	−	Important in early response to infection as it is a powerful agglutinator
IgD	−	−	−	−	−	?Function. Present on the surface of some lymphocytes and may control lymphocyte activation/suppression
IgE	−	−	+ −	+ −	−	Involved in mast cell degranulation, thereby protecting body surfaces. Important in allergy and parasitic infections

TCR *and* T-cell stimulation by the binding of either CD4 or CD8 to their respective MHC receptors. There also are several co-stimulatory molecules which are very important in cell–cell interactions.

THE MHC SYSTEM

The human major histocompatibility complex (MHC) system is also called the HLA (human leucocyte antigen) system and is coded for on chromosome 6 where there are six loci, three for class I antigens (A, B and C) and three for class II antigens (DP, DQ and DR). Class I molecules are expressed on virtually all nucleated cells while class II molecules are restricted to antigen-presenting cells (APC), other macrophages and B cells, but can be expressed on many other cell types, if they are stimulated with γ-interferon.

Figure 6.11 The immunoglobulin homology unit is the basic building block for a range of molecules involved in cell–cell recognition, the 'immunoglobulin gene superfamily'. These often interact with other Ig superfamily members, e.g. the T-cell receptor complex/CD4 or 8 and MHC molecules. Several other molecules play an important role in immune reactions, such as intercellular adhesion molecules (e.g. ICAM-1) and lymphocyte function antigen (e.g. LFA-3)

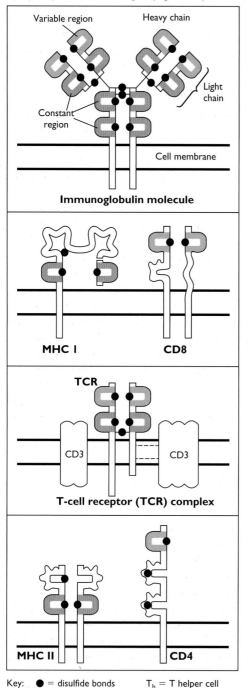

Key: ● = disulfide bonds T_h = T helper cell

Each person has an (almost) unique set of MHC molecules which are present on most cells and are inherited: three class I MHC and three class II MHC from each parent The A, B and C HLA proteins encoded by the class I MHC loci are paired with their other halves and linked to α2-microglobulin to make up the whole class I MHC molecule.

This is relevant to transplantation where it is essential to have a good 'match' between the donor and the recipient to minimize the risk of rejection. An identical twin will provide an excellent match. Some siblings are a good match but other people's organs carry MHC antigens which will be identified by the recipient's immune system as foreign and the tissue will be rejected.

The MHC molecules are important because T cells cannot react with free, native antigens (that is a job for the immunoglobulin molecules). T cells can only bind to antigens which have been processed by special antigen-presenting cells or macrophages and are then displayed on the cell surface *alongside* MHC molecules.

The class I molecules on all nucleated cells present antigens on the cell surfaces which reflect the protein content within the cell. Intracellular protein is processed through an organelle called a proteasome, cut into small polypeptide chunks and placed in a lysosome along with an MHC I molecule. The polypeptide molecule fits into a groove on the MHC I molecule and is transported to the cell surface for display. This mechanism is brilliant for declaring to the world that a virus has infected the cell, and attracting T cells or NK cells to come and kill the cell by inducing it to undergo apoptosis. Class I MHC antigens bind CD8+ T cells (suppressor/cytotoxic); see Fig. 6.13.

Class II molecules are very different. For a start they appear normally on antigen-presenting cells and their job is to reflect what is happening in the world around them. They engulf microbial particles, digest them into small fragments and place these small peptides in lysosomes, which fuse with lysosomes containing class II MHC molecules. The class II molecule has a 'clip' mechanism which protects it from binding intracellularly derived protein. The clip is only released by a special protein, allowing the binding of MHC II with extracellularly derived protein. This is then moved to the APC surface for presentation to CD4+ T cells (helper), and the generation of an immune response.

Thus class I antigens show what is happening within the cell and class II antigens show what is happening in the tissues outside the cell. APC are mobile and can travel to lymph nodes to stimulate Th cells.

GENERATION OF DIVERSITY IN THE IMMUNE SYSTEM

If you have forgotten what genes are made of and how they can be translated to form proteins, refer to Fig. 2.34.

You will be aware that much of our DNA appears to code for nothing, and that the important sections which encode genes are called exons and the in-between stuff consists of introns.

A similar mechanism exists for the generation of multiple unique antigen recognition sites in T cells and B cells, for the chains which make up the T-cell receptor and those which make up the immunoglobulin molecule, respectively. For the sake of simplicity we will consider, in a small amount of detail, only the processes involved in generating diversity in the B-cell heavy chains (Fig. 6.12).

The immunoglobulin heavy chain is constructed from four building blocks, the variable (V), diversity (D), joining (J) and constant (C) regions. These are four groups of exons separated by introns and, in lymphoid cells during maturation, one gene from each of three of the groups is rearranged by creating loops of DNA, so that they lie adjacent to each other. The genes coding for each chain are not a continuous structure in non-lymphoid cells but are groups of exons separated by long non-coding introns.

There is great diversity within the V, D and J groups but the constant region genes are limited in number with only a single gene for each subclass of molecule; thus, for immunoglobulin heavy chains these are $C\mu$, $C\gamma$, $C\alpha$, $C\delta$ and $C\epsilon$, which will code for Ig's M, G, A, D and E, respectively.

Once the chosen V, D and J regions have been aligned satisfactorily the intervening DNA is snipped away and the contiguous segments are joined (excising and splicing). The process is rather like cutting and pasting using a computer. Immunoglobulin heavy chain gene rearrangement is a two-stage process. Having rearranged the V, D and J regions satisfactorily, within the nucleus, the cell must make its choice of heavy chain. V, D and J are separated from the five C genes by a long intron. Just as the mRNA is formed, the constant region selection is made, the intron is excised and the mRNA leaves the nucleus for the cytoplasm, to be translated into protein by the ribosomes.

Why is the C region treated differently? Probably because a lymphocyte that has recognized an antigen with the variable region on its surface molecule may need to produce molecules with different constant regions. Each immunoglobulin molecule has slightly different functions. For example IgG is better at opsonizing bacteria for phagocytosis or NK cell killing, whereas IgM is best at activating the complement complex, IgE is best at eliminating parasites and IgA is designed to neutralize microbes in the mucosal surfaces. The switch of constant region occurs during the germinal centre reaction before differentiation to plasma cells. The antigen recognition site and the variable region remain the same; only the constant region has changed.

It is easy to see how an enormous variety of molecules can be produced in this way. For example, the mouse immunoglobulin heavy chain molecule genome is produced from a choice of 500 V gene segments, 15 D gene segments and 4 J gene segments. This gives a possible repertoire of $500 \times 15 \times 4$ combinations for the heavy chain. That chain will be combined into an immunoglobulin molecule and, in humans, approximately 108 different immunoglobulins are produced in this way.

Although exactly the same type of process is undertaken for the generation of diversity in the T cell receptor and other similar molecules, it must be emphasized that the V, D, J and C groups of genes are different for each type of molecule (i.e. heavy chain, light chain, TCRα, TCRβ etc.). Also, the genes for each chain are rearranged independently. Only the genes on one of a

Figure 6.12 **Gene rearrangement in the B-cell heavy chain.** This example shows two different heavy chains being produced in each cell

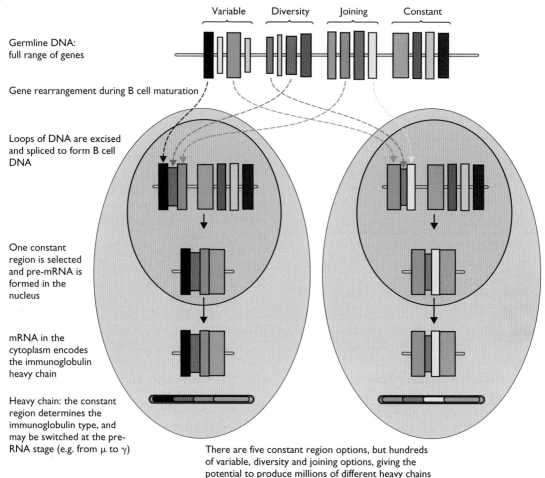

Germline DNA: full range of genes

Gene rearrangement during B cell maturation

Loops of DNA are excised and spliced to form B cell DNA

One constant region is selected and pre-mRNA is formed in the nucleus

mRNA in the cytoplasm encodes the immunoglobulin heavy chain

Heavy chain: the constant region determines the immunoglobulin type, and may be switched at the pre-RNA stage (e.g. from μ to γ)

There are five constant region options, but hundreds of variable, diversity and joining options, giving the potential to produce millions of different heavy chains

pair of chromosomes is rearranged, the locus on the paired chromosome is inhibited (allelic exclusion). Unlike B cells, T cells do not undergo hypermaturation with alteration of the binding site.

CELL-MEDIATED IMMUNITY

Cell-mediated immunity is achieved by T cells. There are several types of T cell, which differ in their biological roles (Table 6.2). Some act as helper cells, some as cytotoxic cells, some as killer cells and some as suppressor cells. A population of null lymphocytes, which is neither T nor B, is called the natural killer (NK) cell. The NK cell is a strange cell – technically a lymphocyte,

but with actions akin to the innate immune system (see page 154). It is particularly important in killing tumour cells.

T cells bear a variety of surface molecules, some of which are common to many T cell types (e.g. CD3) while others are individual to the various subtypes (e.g. CD4, CD8). These molecules are involved in antigen recognition by combining with the T-cell receptor.

How is antigen recognized by T cells?

We have mentioned already that T-cell recognition of antigen is similar to that of B cells, though it is a bit more complicated. The T-cell receptor (TCR) on the

Table 6.2 T-lymphocyte subsets

Mode of action	CD4+			CD8+	
	Suppressor / inducer	Helper / Th1	Inducer Th2	Suppressor cells	Cytotoxic cells
Genetic restriction (MHC)	II	II	II	I	I
Suppressor activity	++ (provide help)	–	–	++	–
Cytotoxic activity	–	+	–	–	++
Help for immunoglobulin	–	+	+++	–	–

MHC, major histocompatibility complex.
T cells are important against infections, in graft rejection, in graft-versus-host disease, in some hypersensitivity reactions and in tumour immunity. Th1 cells assist macrophages in stimulating cell-mediated immunity. Th2 cells assist B cells by stimulating immunoglobulin production and regulating immunoglobulin class.

Small print

Cluster designations

CD (cluster designation) numbers indicate that a particular cell has a surface antigen that can be detected with a specific antibody. This has proved very useful for identifying leucocytes.

Some CD antigens useful in leucocyte identification

Antigen	Principally expressed on
2	Most T cells
3	Mature T cells
4	'Helper/inducer' T cells
8	'Suppressor/cytotoxic' T cells
15	Monocytes and granulocytes
16 and 56	Natural killer cells
20	Most B cells
79a	Most B cells, including plasma cells
68	Monocytes/macrophages

Antigen binds to a receptor site on the TCR. The TCR is linked to a cluster of polypeptide chains, collectively named the CD3 molecules; together, TCR and CD3 make up the T-cell receptor complex. We have already said that the TCR and immunoglobulin molecule belong to the same family. In fact, the similarities between the TCR and immunoglobulin structure go even deeper, as the genetic mechanisms for producing the necessary enormous diversity are almost identical. As in the immunoglobulin molecule, rearrangement of germline DNA during the T-cell maturation process (in the thymus, rather than the bone marrow, where B cells mature) generates a series of somatic mutations such that every T cell has a unique receptor.

As with B cells, self-reacting cells are deleted at an early stage.

Like the immunoglobulin molecule, the T-cell antigen receptor site depends on a three-dimensional fit to form non-covalent bonds with antigen. However, the hypermutation mechanism so important in generation of high-affinity immunoglobulin molecules does not affect the T-cell receptor genes.

What is the difference between helper (Th) and suppressor/cytotoxic (Ts/c) T cells and NK cells?

Helper cells, which have the molecule CD4 included in the T-cell receptor complex, make up about 60 per cent of the body's mature T cells (Fig. 6.13). They will only recognize processed antigen if the CD4 receptor combines with class II MHC molecules. By a combination of releasing interferon, interleukins and binding co-stimulatory molecules, helper T cells stimulate other T cells, NK cells, macrophages and B cells.

surface of the majority (about 95 per cent) of T cells is composed of an alpha chain and a beta chain with constant and variable regions analogous to those of immunoglobulins. The remaining minority of T cells have a receptor made up of gamma and delta chains. These T cells tend to migrate to epithelial surfaces, such as the gut or respiratory epithelial lining cells, and are thought to act independently of antigen-presenting cells (APCs).

In AIDS the immune system is devastated because the human immunodeficiency virus (HIV) has a receptor for CD4, and thus enters and destroys the function of the cell most centrally placed in co-ordinating cell-mediated immunity and much of humoral (antibody-mediated) immunity. Macrophages and dendritic antigen-presenting cells express low levels of CD4 on their surfaces and are also target cells for HIV infection.

Cytotoxic or suppressor T cells, with CD8 included in the TCR complex, make up about 30 per cent of mature T cells (Fig. 6.14). They bind to processed antigen

associated with class I molecules (pages 150–151). In fact, they cannot recognize any antigen which is not presented in conjuction with MHC class I molecules, which are expressed by every nucleated cell in the body.

One of their most important roles is that of recognizing viral-infected cells. When viruses replicate within cells, viral antigen is expressed on the cell surface. When this viral antigen is presented, together with MHC I, to a cytotoxic T cell, it springs into action, and lyses the cell membrane, destroying the infected cell. CD8 + T cells are also thought to be pivotal in the generation of peripheral tolerance (see later) and in tumour cells; both the cytotoxic cells which can lyse other cells, and the suppressor cells, which just induce anergy, are important in this process.

Natural killer (NK) cells are neither T nor B cells and make up 10–15 per cent of the circulating blood lymphocytes (Fig. 6.15). They contain cytoplasmic granules and have three important membrane receptors: one for the Fc component of IgG, one antigen receptor and a non-CD8 type receptor for MHC I receptor (present on all normal nucleated cells). Cells coated with antibody will be recognized via the Fc receptor and lysed by NK cells (this process is known as antibody-dependent cell-mediated cytotoxicity or ADCC). The lysis is achieved by molecules such as perforin and granzyme contained within the cytoplasmic granules. Other cells whose antigens bind with the NK cell antigen receptor are saved from death by possession of their MHC I molecule, which represses NK cell lysis. If the NK cell cannot 'see' the MHC I receptor due to its alteration (for

Figure 6.13 T helper (Th) cells recognize processed antigen presented to their unique T-cell receptor (TCR) by MHC II molecules on the surface of antigen-presenting cells (APC). CD4 is the co-stimulatory molecule. Their role is to activate Ts/c and B cells and stimulate them to proliferate and form circulating memory cells. Without T-cell help, class-switching of antibody and the formation of memory B cells does not occur

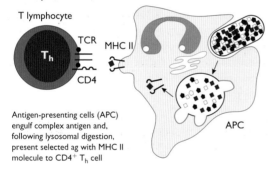

T lymphocyte

Antigen-presenting cells (APC) engulf complex antigen and, following lysosomal digestion, present selected ag with MHC II molecule to CD4+ T$_h$ cell

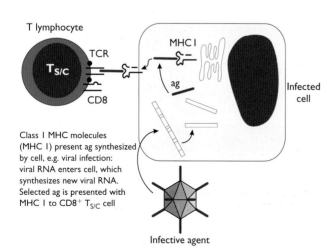

Class I MHC molecules (MHC I) present ag synthesized by cell, e.g. viral infection: viral RNA enters cell, which synthesizes new viral RNA. Selected ag is presented with MHC I to CD8+ T$_{S/C}$ cell

Figure 6.14 T suppressor/cytotoxic (Ts/c) cells recognize processed antigen presented to the unique TCR by MHC I molecules on the surfaces of infected host cells and cause the cells to undergo apoptosis. CD8 is the co-stimulatory molecule

instance by tumour, viral infection, or drug binding) the target will be lysed.

TOLERANCE

This ability of the body to mount an immune response against foreign antigens raises a very important question. How does the immune system distinguish between an antigen that is foreign and one that is normally present on the cells in the body?

This process, known as tolerance, can be acquired at two stages. The first occurs during lymphopoiesis (lymphoid cell maturation) and is known as central tolerance. The second occurs once the mature B and T cells have been released into the peripheral tissues and is referred to as peripheral tolerance. Tolerance is achieved by a mixture of cell deletion or the generation of anergy in self-reacting cells (Fig. 6.16). These mechanisms induce tolerance such that antigens that are exposed to the immune system during fetal life are not capable of eliciting a response in later life.

So, nature has devised a neat system of differentiating self from non-self. Or has it?

AUTOIMMUNE DISEASE

As the heading suggests, the body can on occasion turn on itself and begin to react with self-antigens, to destructive purpose. Autoimmune diseases are estimated to affect up to 7 per cent of the population. Mostly this is due to a breakdown in tolerance, but occasionally new antigens are generated which cross-react with the body's cells. For reasons that are, as yet, unknown, middle-aged women seem to be the most likely to develop autoimmune disease.

It is thought that this loss of tolerance can occur in several ways: exposure of the immune system to sequestered (hidden) antigens is the most easily explained. Parts of the body that are not exposed to the immune system during fetal life can produce a response later on; lens protein and spermatozoa are just two examples. A person who has suffered severe trauma to one eye, with the release of lens protein into the blood, runs the risk of forming antibodies to the protein. A few weeks later, the other eye may be severely damaged by an antibody-mediated inflammatory reaction (a condition known as sympathetic opthalmitis). Mumps may give rise to inflammation of the testis (orchitis) which causes sperm antigens to be released into the

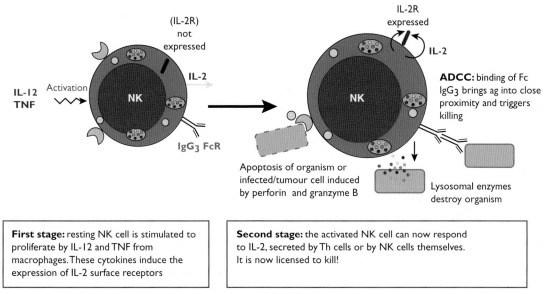

Figure 6.15 NK cells act independently of MHC molecules and may directly cause apoptosis of cells displaying stress antigens or indirectly induce apoptosis when stimulated by binding antibody attached to antigens on a cell surface. They are particularly useful in defence against intracellular particles such as viruses, or altered host cells, e.g. tumour cells

First stage: resting NK cell is stimulated to proliferate by IL-12 and TNF from macrophages. These cytokines induce the expression of IL-2 surface receptors

Second stage: the activated NK cell can now respond to IL-2, secreted by Th cells or by NK cells themselves. It is now licensed to kill!

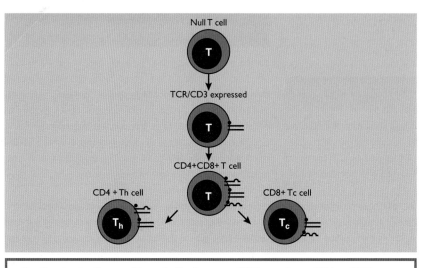

- T cells enter the thymus without the T-cell receptor/CD3 complex or CD4 or CD8. To prevent these T-cells from encountering any antigen too early in their development, macrophages phagocytose any loose antigenic material, such as apoptotic debris.

- They mature and proliferate, going through a stage of being double-labelled as CD4+8+ cells, becomimg either CD4+ or CD8+ cells within the cortex. Cells which fail to later develop CD4 or 8 are deleted.

- 'Positive selection' for cells which can recognize MHC molecules presented on thymic epithelial cells occurs. Reacting cells survive, the rest undergo apoptosis.

- 'Negative selection' against cells which bind self MHC molecules takes place in the medulla - the antigen is carried to the thymic medulla by bone marrow-derived dendritic cells. Those cells which bind are self reactive and are deleted.

- Non-autoreactive cells which can interact with antigen displayed on an appropriate MHC molecule move to the medulla and are secreted into the blood.

Figure 6.16 Mechanisms of acquiring tolerance. These mechanisms may break down because of cross-reaction with molecules on microbes or drugs (molecular mimicry), exposure to previously sequestered antigen (for instance lens protein or spermatozoa) and 'switching on' of previously anergic cells

blood circulation. The anti-sperm antibodies, which may develop as a result, can cause infertility. Similarly, mumps may inflame the islets of Langerhans in the pancreas and has been implicated in the causation of type I diabetes mellitus.

Occasionally there is cross-reaction between a microbial antigen and normal body cells, due to a similarity in shape or structure between the self and microbial antigens; unthinkingly, the body develops an antibody or cell-mediated reaction against itself as it expunges the microbe. A person at risk of such a complication would be our 10-year-old patient, who presented at the start of this chapter with a sore throat due to a Lancefield group A streptococcal infection. This bacterium is notorious for carrying antigenic determinants which mimic the endocardium of the heart so closely that the patient develops inflammatory foci in the wall of the heart. This life-threatening condition,

which can lead to long-term cardiac damage, is known as rheumatic fever. The incidence of rheumatic fever has plummeted in recent years, possibly due to early eradication of the infection by prompt antibiotic therapy.

Following on from this point it is obvious that defects in any of the immune system's regulatory molecules may lead to aberrations in tolerance. It is thought that much of the peripheral tolerance mechanism relies on anergy on the part of self-reacting immune cells, easily lost if the system controls are tampered with.

Lastly, even anergic T or B cells may be induced to behave against their will by outside forces. An example of this is infection by Epstein–Barr virus (EBV), which can infect B cells directly, entering via their complement receptors. The presence of EBV can stimulate an infected B cell to produce antibodies. If an anergic self-reacting B cell happens to become infected, it will be switched on despite its best intentions.

The autoimmune diseases include many clinically important and potentially life-threatening conditions. They are generally divided up into those diseases which affect a single organ (organ-specific) and those which affect several organs or tissues (non-organ-specific) (Table 6.3).

You will come across some of these diseases elsewhere; for instance, the antibodies in Graves' disease stimulate the thyroid stimulating hormone receptor to secrete thyroxine and thus cause thyrotoxicosis, an example of a type II hypersensitivity reaction (page 46).

We will briefly describe systemic lupus erythematosis (SLE) to illustrate the wide-ranging effects of a non-organ-specific autoimmune disease.

Systemic lupus erythematosus is a systemic disorder in which there is chronic, relapsing and remitting damage to the skin, joints, kidneys and almost any organ. Like most immune disorders, it has a higher incidence in women. In America, it is also more common in blacks and it tends to occur in the second and third decades.

Table 6.3 Autoimmune diseases and autoantigens

Disease	Antigen(s)
Organ-specific diseases	
Hashimoto thyroiditis	Thyroid peroxidase, thyroglobulin/T4
Pernicious anaemia	Intrinsic factor
Insulin-dependent diabetes mellitus (IDDM)	Beta cells in the pancreas (tyrosine phosphatase)
Addison's disease	Adrenal cortical cells (ACTH receptor and microsomes)
Autoimmune haemolytic anaemia	RBC membrane antigens
Graves' disease	TSH receptor on thyroid cells
Pemphigus	Epidermal keratinocytes
Bullous pemphigoid	Basal keratinocytes
Guillain–Barré syndrome	Peripheral nerves (gangliosides)
Polymyositis	Muscle (histidine tRNA synthetase)
Non-organ-specific diseases	
Systemic lupus erythematosus	Double-stranded DNA, nuclear antigens
Chronic active hepatitis	Nuclei, DNA
Scleroderma	Nuclei, elastin, nucleoli, centromeres, topoisomerase 1
Primary biliary cirrhosis	Mitochondria (pyruvate dehydrogenase complex E2)
Rheumatoid arthritis	IgG (rheumatoid factor, connective tissues, collagen)
Multiple sclerosis	Brain/myelin basic protein
Sjögren syndrome	Exocrine glands, kidney, liver, thyroid
Several organs affected	
Goodpasture syndrome	Basement membrane of kidney and lung (type IV collagen)
Polyendocrine	Multiple endocrine organs (hepatic – cytochrome p450; intestinal – tryptophan hydroxylase)

From Lydyard et al., 2000: *Pathology Integrated: An A–Z of Disease and its Pathogenesis*. London: Arnold.

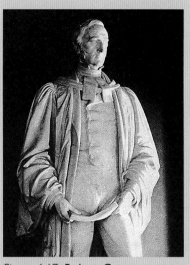
Patients may present with a characteristic 'butterfly' rash on the face, or with more subtle symptoms. Many present after their kidneys have been damaged beyond repair, in chronic renal failure.

The fundamental feature of the disease is inflammation of the small arterioles and arteries, i.e. a vasculitis, often related to the deposition of antigen–antibody complexes in the vessel walls. Involvement of the glomerular capillaries in the kidney produces a variety of types of glomerulonephritis. The other sites of involvement are joints (synovitis), heart (non-infectious endocarditis – named after Libman Sacks – and pericarditis), lungs (pleuritis and effusions) and CNS (focal neurological symptoms due to vasculitis).

The course of the illness is extremely variable and unpredictable and may range from mild skin involvement to severe renal disease leading to death.

In the auto-immune disorders, the immune response is well controlled but the initiating event of antigen recognition is wrong. There is another group of disorders in which antigen recognition proceeds normally but the body's response is exaggerated. These are called hypersensitivity reactions (page 44).

TRANSPLANTATION

We have already mentioned the role played by the MHC types I and II antigens, displayed on cell membranes, in governing the body's response to transplanted tissue or cells.

Host rejection of a tissue or organ graft may occur at various stages.

- Hyperacute rejection is mediated by pre-existing antibody or by complement. Complement damage can be a particular problem in xenografts (grafts between species). For reasons that are unclear, some organs need far more precise tissue matching than others. The most stringent requirements are for kidney and bone marrow grafts. Surprisingly, the heart and liver require little more than ABO compatibility (i.e. matching blood types).

- Acute rejection is usually mediated by antibodies. The host may already carry antibodies against the tissue transplanted into him, hence the requirement for cross-matching red blood cells and checking that the host's serum does not carry antibodies which can react with the donor's T lymphocytes. Thus, type II hypersensitivity reactions are also important in tissue transplantation.

- Chronic rejection, where T cells identify as foreign the endothelial cells of the blood vessels in the donor organ. By damaging the blood supply they cause gradually more severe ischaemic damage to the transplanted organ.

You will realize from reading the hypersensitivity sections that the body may generate either a type IV cell-mediated response, or a type II antibody response, against any tissue which fails to give the right MHC signals to the T cells.

GRAFT-VERSUS-HOST DISEASE

It is obvious but worth mentioning that, for patients who require a bone marrow transplant, it is the donor cells which react against the host, sparking off graft-versus-host disease if there is a mismatch.

IMMUNIZATION

The immune system is a natural defence mechanism but it can also be manipulated so that it will respond more quickly to a new antigen and, so hopefully, reduce the impact of the infection. This is called immunization.

Immunization may be active or passive. Active immunity involves using inactivated or attenuated live organisms or their products and the effect is reasonably long-lasting and calls up an adaptive immune response. Passive immunity results from injecting human immunoglobulin and the effect is immediate but only lasts one to two weeks.

Dictionary

Antibody is the same as immunoglobulin and makes up most of the gamma globulin fraction of the plasma proteins

Vaccination and **immunization** are the same thing. It all began with inoculation of vaccinia virus (coxpox to protect against smallpox). Vaccination generates immunity against particular antigens. Immunization may generate either humoral or cellular immunity, often both.

History   Edward Jenner (1749–1823)

It would be a crime to consider immunization without pausing for a moment to think about its history and the man responsible for developing its use. The man is Edward Jenner, a pupil of John Hunter. Jenner lived with Hunter for the first two years after coming to London and the friendship they developed continued after Jenner left London to start general practice in Berkeley, Gloucestershire. Jenner was profoundly influenced by Hunter's interest in natural history and in his methods of scientific investigation. To one of Jenner's questions, Hunter is said to have replied, '… I think your solution is just; but why think? why not try the experiment?…'

Even before Jenner, it had been noticed that an attack of smallpox protected against further disease. It was known that the epidemics varied in severity and that it was best to contract a mild form of smallpox as this resulted in life-long protection. This knowledge was widespread; in India, children were wrapped in clothing from

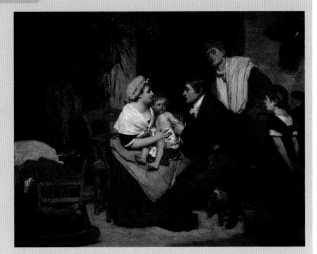

Figure 6.18 Edward Jenner (Reproduced with permission from Wellcome Library, London)

patients with smallpox; in China, scabs from smallpox patients were ground and the powder was blown into the nostrils; in Turkey, female slaves were injected under the skin with dried preparations of pus from smallpox patients. Inoculated slaves fetched a high price while pock-marked slaves were worth nothing! Lady Mary Wortley

Montagu, the wife of the British Ambassador in Constantinople, was aware of these techniques and she took the risk of having her own children inoculated. When she returned to England in 1718, she tried to convince her friend, the Prince of Wales, that he should do the same. He was worried about experimenting on the royal children but, when six orphan children were successfully immunized against smallpox, he consented and the royal children were inoculated. Medical ethics have made some advances since those days!

Jenner and others had noticed that cows suffered from a pustular disease resembling smallpox called 'variolae vaccinae' – cowpox. It was known that it could be transmitted to humans and that, apart from local symptoms, there were no ill effects. There was a widespread belief that those who had suffered from cowpox became immune to smallpox and a farmer in Dorset, Trevor Jesty, tried it out on his own children. The idea of using the cowpox virus to induce immunity to smallpox thrilled Jenner but, rather than jumping to conclusions, he followed Hunter's example and experimented. On 14 May 1796, Jenner inoculated a boy of 8 years named James Phipps with cowpox. The boy's illness took a predictable course and he recovered. On 1 July, he inoculated the boy with smallpox and no

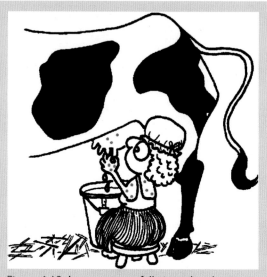

Figure 6.19 Jenner successfully inoculated against smallpox with cowpox (From Lakhani S (1992) Early clinical pathologists: Edward Jenner. *J Clin Pathol* 45. Reproduced with permission from the BMJ Publishing Group)

reaction occurred, either on this occasion or on a subsequent occasion a few months later. Jenner described this experiment to the Royal Society but it was rejected. He continued to make his observations and, in 1798, published his work entitled *An Inquiry into the Causes and Effects of the Variolae Vaccinae*. Hence, inoculation with smallpox was replaced by inoculation with cowpox. The word **'vaccination'** came into use and smallpox cases dropped in the UK as a series of laws (Vaccination Acts of 1840, 1841, 1853, 1861, 1867 and 1871) made vaccination free and compulsory, with parents liable to repeated fines until their children were vaccinated. Compulsion was withdrawn in 1948 and smallpox was eradicated globally by 1980 with the last naturally occurring case being in Somalia in October 1977.

ACTIVE IMMUNIZATION

First exposure to an antigen provokes a primary response where IgM is the major antibody. Further exposure to the antigen produces a secondary response which occurs faster, produces higher levels of antibody and the class is predominantly IgG. This is because memory B cells circulate after the first exposure and it takes far less cross-linkage of antigen to stimulate their release and extensive B cell proliferation and plasma cell formation than it did the first time that antigen was encountered.

In addition to humoral (B-cell-mediated) immunity, cell-mediated (T-cell) immunity is also induced.

The aim of *active* immunization is to give sufficient doses of antigen to ensure that, after completing the course of immunization, the person can mount a rapid effective response if exposed to the disease. The number

of doses, time intervals and need for booster doses varies with the vaccine, the natural history of the disease and the likelihood of encountering the infection.

In the United Kingdom, the present immunization schedule for children is shown in Table 6.4 and the recommendation for adults who are unimmunized or in a high-risk group is shown in Table 6.5.

Live attenuated viral vaccines, such as polio, measles, mumps and rubella, generally produce the most long-lasting immune responses and oral polio vaccine has the advantage of having maximal effect on local gut immunity, the natural portal of entry for wild polio. Non-live vaccines may be more effective when combined with adjuvants to enhance the immune response. For example, aluminium phosphate and aluminium hydroxide are used in DTP vaccine.

Table 6.4 United Kingdom immunization schedule for children (see Fig. 6.20)

Routine childhood immunization programme
Each vaccination is given as a single injection into the muscle of the thigh or upper arm

When to immunize	Diseases protected against	Vaccine given
2 months old	Diphtheria, tetanus, pertussis (whooping cough), polio and *Haemophilus influenzae* type b (Hib)	DTaP/IPV/Hib
	Pneumococcal infection	+Pneumococcal conjugate vaccine (PVC)
3 months old	Diphtheria, tetanus, pertussis, polio and *Haemophilus influenzae* type b (Hib)	DTaP/IPV/Hib
	Meningitis C	+MenC
4 months old	Diphtheria, tetanus, pertussis, polio and *Haemophilus influenzae* type b (Hib)	DTaP/IPV/Hib
	Meningitis C	+MenC
	Pneumococcal infection	+PCV
Around 12 months old	*Haemophilus influenza* type b (Hib) and meningitis C	Hib/MenC
Around 13 months old	Measles, mumps and rubella	MMR
	Pneumococcal infection	+PCV
3 years and 4 months to 5 years old	Diphtheria, tetanus, pertussis and polio Measles, mumps and rubella	DTaP/IPV or dTaP/IPV +MMR
Girls aged 12 to 13 years	Cerical cancer caused by human popillomavirus types 16 and 18	HPV
13 to 18 years old	Tetanus, diphtheria and polio	Td/IPV

Non-routine immunizations

When to immunize	Diseases protected against	Vaccine given
At birth (to babies who are more likely to come into contact with TB than the general population)	Tuberculosis	BCG
At birth (to babies whose mothers are hepatitis B positive)	Hepatitis B	Hep B

Table reproduced from www.immunisation.nhs.uk, under the terms of the Click-Use Licence.

New vaccines are being developed all the time and create interesting decisions about the best use of health funding. Recently, it has become possible to immunize against papilloma viruses that cause cervical cancer and genital warts. Clearly, prevention should be better than cure. The cervical cancer screening programmes have been so effective in reducing morbidity and mortality that, in countries where global screening systems are established, it can be difficult to justify vaccination since this will only protect those receiving the vaccine before they are infected and it will still be necessary to keep screening the majority of people who are past that age.

PASSIVE IMMUNIZATION

Passive immunity relies on using either pooled plasma containing a variety of immunoglobulins to local infectious agents or specific immunoglulin obtained from

Table 6.5 Types of vaccination appropriate to adults	
Vaccine	**Examples of relevant groups**
Rubella	Sero-negative women
D/T and polio	Previously unimmunized individuals
Hepatitis B	Healthcare workers, haemophiliacs, intravenous drug users, prison inmates
Hepatitis A	Travellers, haemophiliacs, liver disease patients, some health workers
Influenza	Elderly patients at risk of pneumonia
Pneumococcus	Splenectomized patients
Anthrax	Occupational workers, e.g. abattoir
Tick-borne encephalitis	Travellers to forests of central and eastern Europe and Scandinavia
Typhoid	
Yellow fever	Travellers to high-risk areas
Japanese encephalitis	
Cholera	No longer a requirement anywhere in the world

convalescent patients or recently immunized donors. Specific immunoglobulins are available for tetanus, hepatitis B, rabies and varicella zoster. They are most commonly used for post-exposure prophylaxis.

Key facts

The common types of vaccine

Live attenuated organisms
  Polio (oral: Sabin)
  Measles
  Mumps
  Rubella
  Tuberculosis (BCG)
Inactivated organisms
  Polio (subcutaneous: Salk)
  Pertussis
  Typhoid
  Hepatitis A
  Influenza (variable sub-type depending on prevailing strain)
Toxoid (toxin inactivated by formaldehyde)
  Tetanus
  Diphtheria
Components of the organism
  Haemophilus influenza type B (HiB) (capsular polysaccharide)
  Hepatitis B (surface protein (recombinant))
  Pneumococcus (capsular polysaccharide)

Key facts

Important pathogens for which there are no vaccines

- Rhinoviruses (colds)
- HIV/AIDS*
- Cytomegalovirus (CMV)
- Epstein–Barr virus (EBV)
- Hepatitis C virus
- Gonorrhoea
- Syphilis
- Leprosy
- Trachoma
- Malaria*
- All parasitic and protozoal infections

*Trials of possible vaccines are in progress

Figure 6.20 The effect of immunization against Hib has been dramatic: *Haemophilus influenzae* type b disease in England and Wales by age group (1990–2001) (PHLS and CDSC data). (From Public Health Laboratory Service (2002) Continuing surveillance of invasive *Haemophilus influenzae* disease. CDR weekly 12(26))

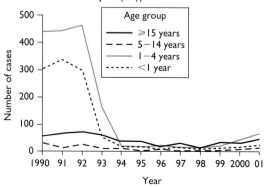

PART 3

CIRCULATORY DISORDERS

Introduction: Features of circulatory
disorders   165

Chapter 7: Vascular occlusion and
thrombosis   169
        Vascular occlusion   169
        Thrombosis   169
        Embolism   180
        Disseminated intravascular
        coagulation   186

Chapter 8: Atherosclerosis and
hypertension   189
        Clinical case: atherosclerosis   189
        Hypertension   203
        Aneurysms   207

Chapter 9: Circulatory failure   211
        Shock   211
        Clinical case: myocardial
        infarction   211
        Anaemia   220
        Organ damage due to poor
        perfusion   227
        Strokes   229
        Clinicopathological case study:
        circulatory failure   236

When I first applied my mind to observation from the many dissections of Living Creatures as they came to hand, that by that means I might find out the use of the motion of the Heart and things conducible in Creatures; I straightways found it a thing hard to be attained, and full of difficulty, so with Fracastorius I did almost believe, that the motion of the heart was known to God alone.

William Harvey (1578–1657)

It is extraordinary to think that diseases whose effects are as diverse as those of gangrene, strokes, heart attacks and divers' 'bends' are all disorders of the circulatory system. The general features of circulatory disorders are almost the opposite of the cardinal features of inflammation, which are covered in part 1: for 'calor (heat), rubor (redness), tumor (swelling) and dolor (pain)' read 'coldness, pallor/cyanosis, pain and loss of sensation'.

Why is this? The drop in temperature and change in colour are easily understood, since blood carries body heat from the core and dissipates it in the extremities and it is the red colour of the oxygenated haemoglobin pigment in the red blood cells which makes pale-skinned persons look pink. Anything decreasing blood flow to a finger or toe will decrease the tissue perfusion by warm blood, making it cold and pale, and any delay in delivery of red blood cells to the affected digit will mean that more of the haemoglobin will have given up its oxygen load, leaving blue-coloured deoxyhaemoglobin (cyanosis). Pain is a variable phenomenon, depending on the tissue affected and the type of injury. For example, a 'heart attack', or myocardial infarction, caused by sudden blockage of a coronary artery is usually associated with intense central chest pain, often radiating down the left arm, whilst a gradual 'furring up' of the arteries supplying the legs causes severe pain on walking, which disappears when the demand for oxygen by the leg muscles is removed by rest (intermittent claudication). By comparison, a 'stroke', in which the blood supply to part of the brain is suddenly interrupted, will generally cause weakness or paralysis, but no pain. Loss of sensation also varies according to the type of vascular disease and the tissue or organ affected; a stroke may destroy a sensory pathway to the brain, leading to a large area of numbness which may involve half the body, whilst blockage of the blood flow to a toe would cause numbness in just the area supplied by the vessel because of ischaemic damage to the local sensory nerves.

You will have gathered from the preceding discussion that the term 'circulatory disorders' encompasses a spectrum of symptoms and signs related to an abnormality in the blood supply. Circulatory disorders may be 'local' or 'systemic' and may gradually develop over months or years or strike suddenly and catastrophically. They may be due to a problem in the vessels, in the blood or in the heart. Perhaps the easiest way to look at these diseases is to relate them to a domestic plumbing system, the main components of which are the pipes and the pump (Fig. 1). Pipes may gradually 'fur up' (atherosclerosis), or become blocked (vascular occlusion). In plumbing, the blockage may be water freezing in the winter while our cardiovascular equivalent is thrombosis. Sometimes small fragments of thrombus may break off and be carried around the system until they lodge in a pipe with a diameter too small to let them through (embolism). Burst pipes (haemorrhage), are a nuisance and can be extremely damaging. Sometimes one can spot the area at risk, because the pipe may bulge alarmingly before it bursts (aneurysm). Pump failure for whatever reason is fairly disastrous, and in the heart this may be due to valve disease, myocardial infarction, infection, congenital abnormality, etc.

Some solutions to these problems have been found; thus affected segments of piping can be replaced (arterial bypass grafts), pumps can be tinkered with (valve grafts) or replaced (heart transplants), high pressure causing strain on the system can be relieved (antihypertensive drugs) and sometimes it is possible to remove some of the 'scale' which furs up the pipes (reaming out of arteries using balloon catheters). Of course these are usually only partial solutions and there is no doubt that prevention is the best medicine.

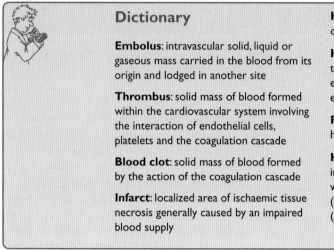

Dictionary

Embolus: intravascular solid, liquid or gaseous mass carried in the blood from its origin and lodged in another site

Thrombus: solid mass of blood formed within the cardiovascular system involving the interaction of endothelial cells, platelets and the coagulation cascade

Blood clot: solid mass of blood formed by the action of the coagulation cascade

Infarct: localized area of ischaemic tissue necrosis generally caused by an impaired blood supply

Haematoma: extravascular accumulation of clotted blood

Haemorrhage: discharge of blood from the vascular compartment into the extravascular body spaces or to the exterior

Petechiae, purpura, ecchymoses: small haemorrhages

Hyperaemia: an increased volume of intra-vascular blood in an affected tissue which may result from increased flow (active hyperaemia) or reduced drainage (passive hyperaemia = congestion)

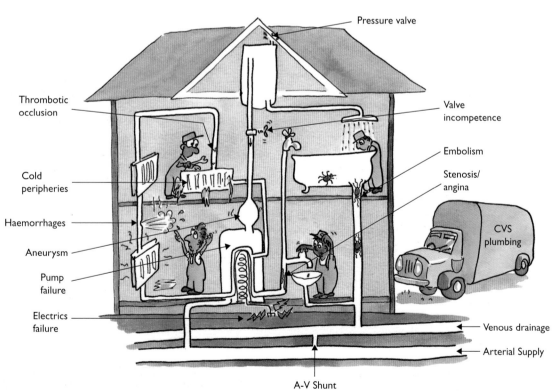

Figure 1 The cardiovascular system can be likened to a domestic plumbing system

It would be unjust to discuss circulatory disorders without a brief mention of the historical figures involved. If you had been alive in the sixteenth century, you would have been taught that blood was produced by the liver and then carried in the veins to the organs where it was consumed; this was Galen's theory of the regeneration of the blood. The portion of blood from the liver which entered the right side of the heart divided into two streams. One route was through the pulmonary artery to bathe the lungs and the other route was across the heart through 'inter-septal pores'. The left ventricle received this blood, which mixed with the 'pneuma' (air) coming to the heart through the pulmonary veins. The blood, fortified by the 'pneuma', was then ejected via the aorta towards the peripheral organs.

In 1628, this theory was challenged when Dr William Harvey published his famous work, *De Motu Cordis*, describing the dual circulation of the blood; but even in the sixteenth century people were starting to doubt Galen's theory. There were several problems with the theory. First, nobody had managed to identify 'inter-septal' pores, so Michael Servetius, the Spanish theologian and physician, suggested that blood travelled from the right to the left ventricle by circulating through the lungs; an idea for which he died a martyr's death after being denounced by John Calvin for holding heretical opinions! Second, Galen's theory proposed a mixture of air and blood in the left side of the heart, which was a difficult concept to accept once the structure of the heart valves was established. Leonardo da Vinci had drawn these accurately but it was Andrea Caselapino who described the valves' actions correctly, in 1571, and went on to use the term 'circulatio'. Thus Harvey, who studied in Padua from 1600 to 1602, would have been familiar with the Italians' ideas and was able to reach his own conclusions by 'standing on the shoulders of these giants'. Even Harvey was left with a problem: he could not demonstrate the connections between the arterial and venous sides of the circulation. The discovery of the capillaries had to wait for Marcello Malpighi's microscopical analysis of frog lung in 1661.

History — William Harvey (1578–1657)

William Harvey was born in Folkestone on 1 April 1578. It may have been April Fools day, but this man provided medicine with the boost it needed to get it out of stagnation. The value of his work is put into perspective when you realise that to be honoured as a Harveian Orator by the Royal College of Physicians is the greatest distinction that one can aspire to.

Harvey did his medical training at Caius College, Cambridge, and later at Padua, Italy. In Padua, Harvey studied with Fabricius who had succeeded Fallopio (of Fallopian tube fame). Galileo was the Professor of Mathematics at Padua at the time but does not appear to have been influential in Harvey's development.

Harvey was elected a full fellow of the College of Physicians in 1607 and soon afterwards became Assistant Physician to St. Bartholomew's Hospital. This helped to establish his private practice and, interestingly, his famous patients included King James I, King Charles I and the Lord Chancellor, Sir Francis Bacon! Although Bacon is given the credit for

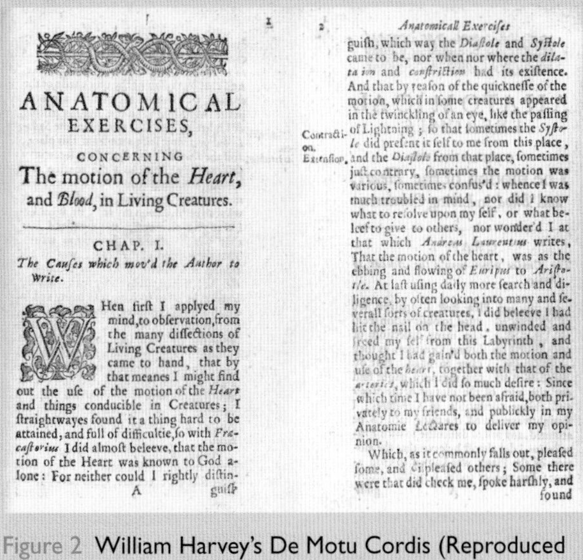

ANATOMICAL
EXERCISES,
CONCERNING
The motion of the *Heart*,
and *Blood*, in Living Creatures.

CHAP. I.

The Causes which mov'd the Author to Write.

When first I applyed my mind, to observation, from the many dissections of Living Creatures as they came to hand, that by that meanes I might find out the use of the motion of the *Heart* and things conducible in Creatures; I straightwayes found it a thing hard to be attained, and full of difficultie, so with *Fracastorius* I did almost beleeve, that the motion of the Heart was known to God alone: For neither could I rightly distin-

A guish

2 *Anatomicall Exercises*

guish, which way the *Diastole* and *Systole* came to be, nor when nor where the *dilatation* and *constriction* had its existence. And that by reason of the quicknesse of the motion, which in some creatures appeared in the twinckling of an eye, like the passing of Lightning; so that sometimes the *Systole* did present it self to me from this place, and the *Diastole* from that place, sometimes just contrary, sometimes the motion was various, sometimes confus'd: whence I was much troubled in mind, nor did I know what to resolve upon my self, or what beleef to give to others, nor wonder'd I at that which *Andreas Laurentius* writes, That the motion of the heart, was as the ebbing and flowing of *Euripus* to *Aristotle*. At last using daily more search and diligence, by often looking into many and severall sorts of creatures, I did beleeve I had hit the nail on the head, unwinded and freed my self from this Labyrinth, and thought I had gain'd both the motion and use of the *heart*, together with that of the *arteries*, which I did so much desire: Since which time I have not been afraid, both privately to my friends, and publickly in my Anatomie Lectures to deliver my opinion.

Contraction. Extension.

Which, as it commonly falls out, pleased some, and displeased others; Some there were that did check me, spoke harshly, and found

Figure 2 William Harvey's De Motu Cordis (Reproduced with permission from Wellcome Library, London)

inductive thinking, it was Harvey who applied it to his investigations of the heart. Harvey, in fact, had very little respect for Bacon and had stated that Bacon 'writes philosophy (science) like a Lord Chancellor; I have cured him of it'.

The quote at the beginning is the first paragraph of chapter 1 in his famous book *De Motu Cordis*. The movements of the heart were so fast and complicated that he often despaired at ever being able to work out the sequence of each of the movements. *De Motu Cordis* evolved in two stages; initially it was an investigation into the heart beat and the arterial pulse and only later did he include the investigation of the circulation. Together, it forms one of the most important pieces of scientific work. The book is quite small, 72 pages, and would probably fit into a white coat pocket, but the few remaining copies of the original 1628 edition would set you back a cool £200 000! That is assuming anybody is willing to sell it.

William Harvey died of a stroke on 30 June 1657.

CHAPTER 7

VASCULAR OCCLUSION AND THROMBOSIS

VASCULAR OCCLUSION

To return to the present day, we shall first consider the problems of vascular occlusion.

Vascular occlusion may be arterial or venous and the effect of any occlusion will depend on:

- the type of tissue involved
- how quickly the occlusion develops
- availability of collateral circulation.

Collateral vessels provide an alternative route for the blood and they are sometimes able to compensate completely, especially if the occlusion develops slowly. The venous system has more collaterals than the arterial system. For example, there are anastomoses between the portal and systemic veins, around the lower end of the oesophagus and also linking veins between the deep and superficial venous plexuses in the leg. This means that occlusion of a deep vein in the calf does not produce haemorrhagic infarction of the foot but only a mild oedema of the tissues and congestion of the superficial veins because of their increased flow. Unfortunately, not all veins have a collateral system. If the central vein of the retina is occluded, as may happen in thrombosis of the cavernous sinus due to local infection, the tissue of the orbit becomes oedematous and congested so that the eye is pushed forward (proptosis) and there may be local haemorrhage as the small vessels rupture because of the increased pressure. In the worst cases the venous pressure rises until it exceeds the arterial pressure and prevents arterial flow. This produces infarction, i.e. death of the tissue, and the infarcted tissue is red or purple and swollen because of the haemorrhagic oedema. The word 'infarction' actually comes from the Latin 'farcire' meaning to stuff and it is thought to have originally been used for the appearance of venous infarcts stuffed with blood.

Arterial collaterals exist in various areas such as the gut, circle of Willis and, to some extent, in the heart (see Fig. 7.10). Arterial occlusion without the benefit of collaterals will produce ischaemic infarction where the tissue is pale without any swelling. Occasionally, arterial infarcts are haemorrhagic because there is reperfusion or some limited arterial flow leading to leakage of blood from necrotic small vessels. In incomplete arterial occlusion, the effects depend on the tissue's demand for metabolites. Brain and heart tissue are highly susceptible to ischaemic injury while bone and skeletal muscle are quite resistant. It is possible to reduce a tissue's demand by cooling the tissue as is done in some types of surgery.

Vascular occlusion can be due to:

- thrombosis
- embolism
- atherosclerosis
- external compression
- spasm.

We shall discuss the first three of these causes in some depth in this chapter, starting with thrombosis.

THROMBOSIS

Patients presenting with an arterial thrombus are generally middle-aged or elderly and may have circulatory problems due to atherosclerosis. Many will be smokers and some may suffer from diabetes. Their symptoms and signs will depend entirely on which vessel is affected. In contrast, a patient with venous thrombosis may be any age but generally will be rather immobile or forced to be immobile, such as after an operation. Such patients frequently complain of pain in a calf muscle and often swelling of the foot and ankle. But why should such people suddenly develop a thrombus? Much is known now about normal haemostatic mechanisms but the most important factors influencing thrombus formation were described more than a century ago by Rudolf Ludwig Karl Virchow (Fig. 7.1).

Virchow was born on 13 October 1821. As a child he excelled at school and his examination reports were

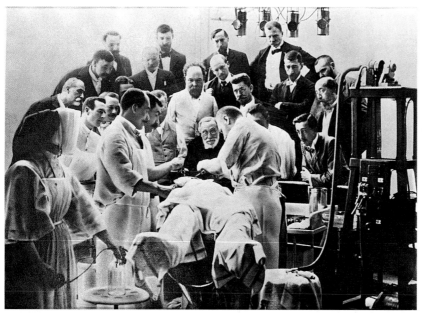

Figure 7.1 Rudolf Virchow (1821–1902) observing an operation in Berlin: he is in the dark suit at the head of the table (Reproduced with permission from Wellcome Library, London)

rather monotonous as they contained only three terms: 'excellent', 'very good' and 'most satisfactory'! Virchow attended medical school in Berlin in 1839 and, even before the existence of platelets and clotting factors was known, had suggested that the development of a thrombus depended on:

- alteration to the constituents of the blood
- damage to the endothelial layer of the blood vessel
- changes in the normal flow of blood.

These three factors are known as Virchow's triad and they are the clues which allow us to understand what has happened to our patients with venous and arterial thrombosis. But first we must revise the body's normal haemostatic mechanisms.

NORMAL HAEMOSTATIC MECHANISMS

Blood and the blood vessels perform an incredibly complex set of tasks. The blood vessels provide a conduit and the blood transports nutrients, waste products and components to defend against infection. However, the vessels are not simple tubes because it is crucial that substances can diffuse between the blood in the vessel and the surrounding tissues. This means that the small vessels (capillaries) must be permeable, ie they are designed to leak. The trick is to ensure that the leakage is under control. For larger vessels that do not need to be permeable, the potential problem occurs because

the vascular system is a closed, pressurized system and so at risk of rupture. Thirdly, we must remember that the network of blood vessels is vast and many are superficial and so susceptible to traumatic damage.

All of this means that the normal haemostatic mechanisms are crucial for stopping blood from leaking but they must also be finely controlled so that thrombus does not form under normal circumstances. There are three main components:

- platelets
- vessel wall endothelium
- soluble blood proteins involved in haemostasis.

The haemostatic blood proteins comprise:

- coagulation factors
- coagulation inhibitors
- fibrinolytic components.

Briefly, the sequence of events is as follows. Injury to the vessels causes an initial *vasoconstriction* which helps to slow the blood flow. The damaged endothelium of the vessel exposes the subendothelial connective tissue which attracts platelets and causes them to adhere to the damaged area. The activation of the platelets causes them to release soluble factors resulting in platelet aggregation called the primary haemostatic plug. Tissue factor and platelet phospholipid causes the formation of fibrin via the coagulation pathway. The fibrin acts to stabilize the platelet plug and the process is termed secondary haemostasis.

If this was all that was involved in maintaining haemostasis, could we really survive the assault on our circulation? Of course not! If the above system was set in motion with nothing to check its progress, soon the whole circulation would come to a standstill and become one big mass of thrombus. This is avoided by clearance, inhibition and inactivation of the coagulation factors as well as by digestion of fibrin.

Now if we return to Virchow's triad, we can consider both the normal physiology and pathology of each component in more detail.

Blood constituents in normal haemostasis

The most important blood constituents involved in normal haemostasis and thrombosis are platelets and the numerous components of the coagulation pathway.

Platelets

Platelets are small (3 μm) cytoplasmic fragments produced by megakaryocytes in the bone marrow under the regulation of thrombopoietin produced in the liver and kidneys. They survive for 7–10 days in the peripheral circulation and contain a variety of granules (see below).

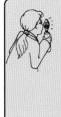

Small print

Platelets

Some diseases caused by platelet abnormalities

- von Willebrand's disease   lack of vWF
- Bernard–Soulier syndrome   lack of gpIb receptor
- 'Grey platelet' syndrome   lack of alpha granules
- Wiskott–Aldrich syndrome   lack of dense granules

All these conditions are rare but they illustrate the consequences of platelet granule abnormalities.

Platelet plasma membrane receptors

GpIb complex: binds vWF and thrombin; initiates aggregation and activation

GPIa-IIa (integrin collagen receptor $\alpha_2\beta_1$): binds type I, II, IV and IV collagen

GpIIb-IIIa (platelet integrin $\alpha_{IIb}\beta_3$): binds fibrinogen

Platelet granule contents

- *Alpha granules*
  - Platelet factor 4 (an anti-heparin)
  - Beta-thromboglobulin
  - Platelet-derived growth factor (PDGF)
  - Von Willebrand factor (vWF)
  - P-selectin
  - Thrombospondin
  - Vascular endothelial growth factor (VEGF)
  - Fibroblast growth factor (FGF)
  - Insulin-like growth factor (IGF)
  - Transforming growth factor α (TNFα)
  - Factor V and XIII
  - Fibrinogen
  - Fibronectin
  - Albumin
  - Proteoglycans
- *Dense granules*
  - CD63
  - ADP/ATP
  - Calcium
  - Magnesium
  - Histamine
  - Adrenaline
  - Serotonin
- *Lysosomes*
  - Lysosomal membrane proteins (LAMPs)
  - Acid hydrolases

Figure 7.2 Platelet adhesion, activation and aggregation. Platelet aggregates ('primary platelet plugs') can plug small breaches in the endothelium, but serious tears require the addition of a fibrin mesh (generated by the coagulation cascade) to stabilize the platelets and form thrombus while healing takes place

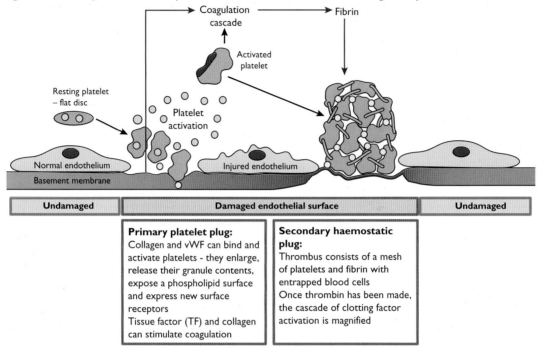

Primary platelet plug:	**Secondary haemostatic plug:**
Collagen and vWF can bind and activate platelets - they enlarge, release their granule contents, expose a phospholipid surface and express new surface receptors Tissue factor (TF) and collagen can stimulate coagulation	Thrombus consists of a mesh of platelets and fibrin with entrapped blood cells Once thrombin has been made, the cascade of clotting factor activation is magnified

Their role in thrombosis can be divided into three phases (Fig. 7.2):

- adhesion of platelets to vessel wall
- secretion of granules
- aggregation of platelets with platelets.

When the endothelium is damaged and collagen is exposed, the first event is adhesion of platelets. This is achieved via platelet surface membrane receptors:

- gp Ia, which binds to collagen
- gp Ib, which binds to von Willebrand's factor (vWF)
- gp IIb/IIIa, which binds to fibrinogen and vWF.

Following adhesion, the platelets release the contents of their granules. There are three main types of granules, the alpha granules, dense granules and lysosomes. The most important secretory products are calcium, which is needed for the coagulation pathway, and adenosine diphosphate (ADP) and thromboxane (TxA$_2$) which induce platelet aggregation. Platelet aggregation involves the gpIIb/IIIa receptor complex mentioned above. This is expressed after activation and is most important in binding fibrinogen which acts as a bridge to the adjacent platelet (Fig. 7.3). Not surprisingly,

there are 'loops' in this process to amplify the reaction. Most importantly, activated platelets express membrane phospholipid (formerly known as platelet factor 3), which stimulates the intrinsic pathway of the coagulation cascade (see below) resulting in the production of thrombin. Thrombin acts to stimulate platelets and so enhances the reaction.

The platelet has another important facet to its character; it has mechanical properties. An unstimulated platelet has a disc shape maintained by microtubules and actin and myosin filaments at the periphery. On activation, the platelet is transformed into a sphere with long pseudopods which spread over the damaged surface and then, after aggregation, the internal filaments slide so that the platelet plug contracts to stabilize and anchor it.

The most common cause of defective platelet function is aspirin therapy due to inhibition of cyclooxygenase resulting in impaired thromboxane A2 synthesis. After a single dose of aspirin, the defect lasts 7–10 days, ie. the life of the platelet.

Coagulation components

The components and pathway involved in coagulation are shown in Fig. 7.3.

Figure 7.3 Coagulation is an energy-dependent process, usually initiated by the activation of factor VII by contact with tissue factor (TF) (intrinsic pathway). Platelet phosopholipid membrane binds clotting factors so that a cascade of sequential activation can occur. Thrombin is crucial to coagulation: it catalyses the formation of fibrin from fibrinogen, exerts positive feedback on earlier stages of coagulation and initiates fibrinolytic mechanisms. The extrinsic pathway initiated by factor XII activation (Hageman factor) is closely inter-related

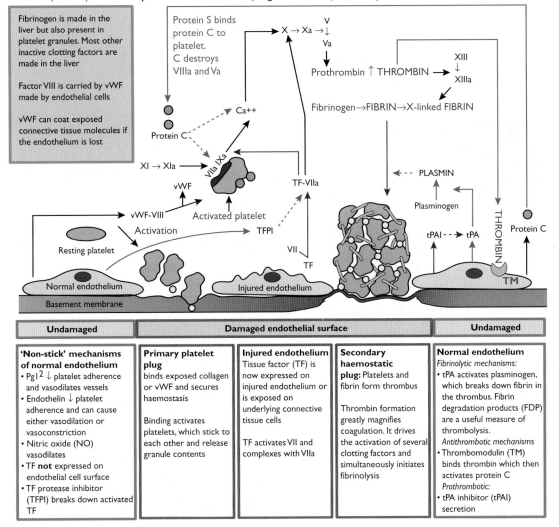

'Non-stick' mechanisms of normal endothelium	Primary platelet plug	Injured endothelium	Secondary haemostatic	Normal endothelium
• PgI^2 ↓ platelet adherence and vasodilates vessels	binds exposed collagen or vWF and secures haemostasis	Tissue factor (TF) is now expressed on injured endothelium or is exposed on underlying connective tissue cells	**plug:** Platelets and fibrin form thrombus	*Fibrinolytic mechanisms:* • tPA activates plasminogen, which breaks down fibrin in the thrombus. Fibrin degradation products (FDP) are a useful measure of thrombolysis.
• Endothelin ↓ platelet adherence and can cause either vasodilation or vasoconstriction	Binding activates platelets, which stick to each other and release granule contents	TF activates VII and complexes with VIIa	Thrombin formation greatly magnifies coagulation. It drives the activation of several clotting factors and simultaneously initiates fibrinolysis	*Antithrombotic mechanisms* • Thrombomodulin (TM) binds thrombin which then activates protein C
• Nitric oxide (NO) vasodilates				*Prothrombotic:* • tPA inhibitor (tPAI) secretion
• TF **not** expressed on endothelial cell surface				
• TF protease inhibitor (TFPI) breaks down activated TF				

This is the same system as the one we mentioned in chapter 4 when discussing inflammatory mediators. Then we were particularly interested in fibrin degradation products, now our interest focuses on fibrin, which is the final product of the pathway and acts to stabilize the plug of aggregated platelets.

The process achieves a massive amplification effect such that 1 mol of activated factor XI creates up to 2×10^8 mol of fibrin. The common pathway begins at factor X, which acts on prothrombin to produce thrombin, which itself has a variety of actions but most importantly

converts fibrinogen to fibrin. Generally, each step in this cascade involves:

- activated enzyme
- substrate for a coagulation factor
- co-factor
- calcium ions
- phospholipid surface.

Some feedback loops are included in the figure but, for simplicity, the control mechanisms which inhibit or inactivate reactions have been omitted. These mechanisms include:

- depletion of local clotting factors
- clearance of activated clotting factors by the liver and mononuclear phagocyte system
- neutralization of activated coagulation factors by forming a complex, e.g. anti-thrombin, α2 macroglobulin
- proteolytic degradation of active coagulation factors, e.g. protein C
- fibrinolysis; this is of major importance.

The most important enzyme capable of digesting fibrin is plasmin. This is produced from plasminogen either by a factor XII-dependent pathway, by therapeutic agents such as streptokinase, or by tissue-derived plasminogen activators. Plasminogen activators (PAs) fall into two classes:

- urokinase-like PA (uPA)
- tissue-type PA (tPA).

They differ in that uPA activates plasminogen in the fluid phase whereas tPA (principally produced by endothelial cells) is active only when attached to fibrin. Conveniently, some plasminogen is bound to fibrin as a thrombus is formed and so is perfectly situated for conversion by the tPA to plasmin, which can then digest the thrombus. Compounds capable of breaking down thrombi have enormous therapeutic potential for restoring blood flow before significant myocardial or cerebral infarction has occurred.

VIRCHOW POINT 1: ALTERATION IN THE CONSTITUENTS OF THE BLOOD

Blood that clots more readily than usual is termed hypercoagulable. This may be caused by a variety of different mechanisms including:

- an increase in blood cells (polycythaemia)
- loss of the plasma fraction of the blood (severe burns)
- increased numbers of platelets (thrombocythaemia)
- increased amount or aggregation of plasma proteins (myeloma, cryoglobulinaemia)
- severe trauma
- disseminated cancer
- late pregnancy
- thrombophilia.

Hypercoagulability can result from an increase in activated coagulation proteins, an increased risk of platelet aggregation or a decrease in anti-thrombotic proteins; however, the sequence of events leading to this state is complex and varied. Some mechanisms have been elucidated such as deficiencies of protein C or protein S, hereditary lack of anti-thrombin III and factor V Leiden abnormality.

> ## Dictionary
>
> **Polycythaemia:** an increase in red cells which occurs as a normal compensatory mechanism if the person has chronic hypoxaemia because of chronic cardiorespiratory problems or because they live at high altitude. It can also occur because of uncontrolled erythropoietin production by various tumours (e.g. renal cell carcinoma) or uncontrolled proliferation of the haemopoietic cells. This neoplastic proliferation is called polycythaemia rubra vera and patients often present with thrombosis.
>
> **Thrombophilia:** an inherited or acquired disorder of the haemostatic mechanisms that predispose to thrombus formation.

VIRCHOW POINT 2: CHANGES IN THE ENDOTHELIUM

Normal endothelium

The fact that the vascular tree is lined by endothelium means that the endothelial surface must be resistant to thrombus formation. The endothelium is quite remarkable, for it is capable of initiating both thrombogenic and antithrombogenic stimuli. Normally, these two groups of actions are finely balanced in favour of preventing thrombus formation. Damage to the endothelium, however, will tip the balance towards thrombosis. The endothelium also has another very important role which is to prevent the elements of blood from coming into contact with the subendothelial connective tissue, which is highly thrombogenic. This tissue normally comprises collagen, elastin, fibronectin and glycosaminoglycans. Collagen is by far the most important of these constituents and it activates the coagulation pathway as well as being a strong stimulator of platelet aggregation. In vessels affected by atheroma, not only is the endothelium more readily damaged but the subendothelial tissue consists of the components of atheroma which are extremely thrombogenic.

Damage to the endothelium

Endothelial damage is of most significance in arterial thrombosis. There may be obvious loss of endothelial cells or more subtle metabolic damage to the cells. Endothelial cells may be lost where an atheromatous plaque has ulcerated or when vessels are damaged by surgery, infection, immune-mediated damage (arteritis), indwelling vascular catheters or infusion of sclerosing chemicals in the treatment of varicose veins and haemorrhoids. Haemodynamic stress is believed to be important in producing metabolic damage to arterial endothelial cells in areas where there is turbulent flow or in patients with prolonged high blood pressure. Other potentially damaging agents include derivatives of cigarette smoke, bacterial toxins, immune complex deposition, transplant rejection and radiation.

In the heart, the endocardial surface is covered by endothelium which can be damaged in a myocardial infarction. Also, the valve surface endothelium may be damaged by inflammatory endocarditis which promotes thrombus formation on valve leaflets resulting in altered function, a variety of heart murmurs and the danger of throwing emboli into the systemic circulation (Fig. 7.4).

Clinically, the most important change is the endothelial damage related to atherosclerosis, which is discussed in the next chapter.

VIRCHOW POINT 3: CHANGES IN THE NORMAL FLOW OF BLOOD

There are two principal ways in which the normal flow can be disturbed: the normal lamellar flow pattern can be altered (turbulence) or the speed may be reduced (stasis) but both lead to similar changes.

During normal flow, red and white blood cells concentrate in the central, fast-moving stream while platelets flow nearer to the periphery and the layer closest to the endothelium is usually devoid of cells and platelets. If the blood flow slows down or turbulence produces local counter-currents, several factors increase the likelihood of thrombus formation:

- platelets come into contact with the endothelium
- turbulence may damage endothelial cells
- there is no inflow of fresh blood containing clotting factor inhibitors
- there is no clearance of blood containing activated coagulation factors.

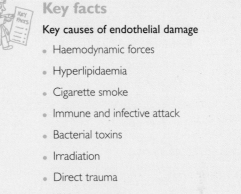

Key facts

Key causes of endothelial damage

- Haemodynamic forces
- Hyperlipidaemia
- Cigarette smoke
- Immune and infective attack
- Bacterial toxins
- Irradiation
- Direct trauma
- Various mutagens

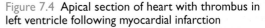

Figure 7.4 Apical section of heart with thrombus in left ventricle following myocardial infarction

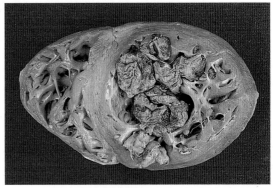

As you see, both turbulence and stasis operate in thrombosis but turbulence is most important in arteries whereas stasis is more important in veins.

Arterial thrombosis

Turbulence tends to occur where arteries branch and over the irregular surface of an atheromatous plaque. It also occurs when cardiac valves have been damaged by inflammation, as may occur with rheumatic fever and infective endocarditis, or have been replaced by artificial valves.

Stasis is generally only important in arterial thrombosis if the heart or arteries have been damaged. Abnormal dilatations of large vessels (aneurysms) will produce pockets of stagnant blood which will thrombose, and myocardial infarction may result in a localized area of damaged heart muscle, which does not move, or in an arrhythmia which will affect the contraction of a whole chamber.

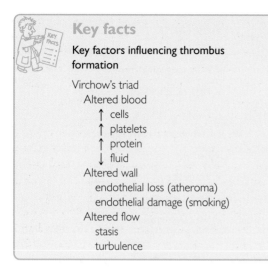

Key facts

Key factors influencing thrombus formation

Virchow's triad
  Altered blood
    ↑ cells
    ↑ platelets
    ↑ protein
    ↓ fluid
  Altered wall
    endothelial loss (atheroma)
    endothelial damage (smoking)
  Altered flow
    stasis
    turbulence

Venous thrombosis

Thrombus formation, related to stasis of blood, is more common in the venous circulation and particularly occurs in the legs or pelvic veins of immobile individuals (Fig. 7.5). Why is stasis common in the leg vessels when the patient is immobilized? If you remember the physiology of venous return from the legs, you will recall that it is contraction of skeletal muscles which pushes blood along the veins and it is the presence of valves which ensures the direction of flow. Understanding this has influenced patient management. Patients are encouraged to move their legs regularly when confined to bed, leg muscles are stimulated to contract during long operations and it is no longer common to have patients bed-bound for weeks.

Figure 7.5 Sites and clinical setting of venous thrombosis

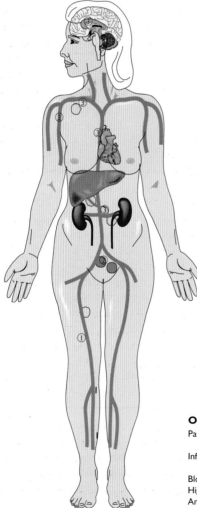

In order of frequency:	Clinical setting
① Leg veins	Immobility, post-surgery and hyper-coagulability states
② Pelvic veins	Post-childbirth, puerperal sepsis, pelvic surgery and tumours
③ **Others:**	
Inferior vena cava	Extrinsic compression by tumour, extension from leg or iliac veins
Renal vein	Tumour extension from kidney
Portal/hepatic veins	Local sepsis, tumour compression
Cavernous sinus	Facial sepsis
Superior vena cava	Extrinsic compression by mediastinal tumour
Axillary vein	Trauma from rucksack, local surgery

Other clinical settings which can predispose to thrombosis:
Patients with malignant tumours, especially carcinoma of ovary, brain and pancreas
Inflammatory disorders due to down-regulation of protein C, e.g. inflammatory bowel disease, TB, SLE
Blood disorders, e.g. polycythaemia, sickle cell, PNH
High-dose oestrogen therapy in contraceptive pills and HRT
Anti-phospholipid syndrome

Thrombus formation often begins within the venous valve pockets (Fig. 7.6). The initial cluster of platelets activates the clotting cascade to produce a small thrombus. A second phase of platelet aggregation then occurs to cover the original thrombus and promote a further wave of coagulation. This process is repeated again and again to extend the thrombus, so-called propagation. The resultant thrombus has alternate layers of platelets and a red cell–white cell–fibrin mixture which produces a rippled effect, termed 'lines of Zahn' (Fig. 7.7). The direction of the lines relates to the pattern of blood flow in the vessel. These platelet layers anchor the thrombus to the adjacent endothelium helping to stabilize it.

Once a vessel is completely occluded by thrombus, blood flow ceases and the stagnant column of blood clots without the production of any 'lines of Zahn'. This is called 'consecutive' clot and it is particularly dangerous because it is only adherent to the vessel wall through its attachment to the original focus of thrombus. This makes it especially likely to break off and embolize to another area (see later).

If the blood flow is slowed in the entire limb, then a very large consecutive clot is formed along the length of the limb's venous system (Fig. 7.8). Alternatively, the consecutive clot only extends to the point where the next venous tributary enters the main vessel. Here the blood may be flowing at a reasonable speed, but the presence of activated clotting factors will promote the adherence of a layer of platelets which may result in a fresh wave of thrombosis from this point. The involvement of platelets, however, does mean that the clot will be anchored at the points where the tributaries enter and be slightly less likely to embolize. Lines of Zahn can also be seen in arterial thrombus. These processes are illustrated in Fig. 7.6.

It is also worth emphasizing at this point that, like most phenomena in the body, the three major factors of Virchow's triad rarely work in isolation. In myocardial infarction, ischaemia damages the endocardium but the affected myocardium also fails to move normally, hence causing local stasis of blood, which is also important in formation of the thrombus within the ventricle. So, while it is imperative that one knows the basis for Virchow's triad, it is also important to remember that many factors interact to produce the final picture in any one patient.

NATURAL HISTORY AND COMPLICATIONS OF THROMBOSIS

Once a thrombus has formed, what are the possible outcomes? As you know, the body possesses many effective systems for regulating thrombus formation during normal haemostasis. The ideal solution is that these systems halt the thrombotic process and remove the debris to leave a normal blood vessel. This process is termed resolution. If the thrombus cannot be removed, it may be organized or recanalized. Alternatively, it may be cast off into the circulation, i.e. it may embolize.

Resolution is thought to occur commonly in the small veins of the lower limb. Interestingly, venous intima contains more plasminogen activator than arterial intima, which may be the reason. Drugs with a thrombolytic action, such as streptokinase, can be given to patients early after thrombosis to promote dissolution of the clot and, hence, resolution. It is important that this drug is given within hours because the drug has much less effect on polymerized fibrin, which predominates later.

Organization of a thrombus involves similar processes to the organization of inflammation described in chapter 4. When the thrombus has formed, polymorphs and macrophages begin to degrade and digest the fibrin and cell debris. Later, granulation tissue grows into the base of the thrombus so that the thrombus is converted into a mass of small vessels separated by connective tissue. These vessels originate from the vasa vasorum of the adventitia of the blood vessel and it is unlikely that the blood flowing through these is of much clinical importance (but see below for collateral circulation).

Alternatively the thrombus may occlude only part of the vessel, so that on cross-section it is attached to one side of the lumen. Organization of this mural thrombus also involves digestion by inflammatory cells, but differs in that small vessels grow in from the luminal surface rather than from the outer layers. Ultimately, the thrombus shrinks and is covered by endothelial or smooth muscle cells which produce platelet-derived growth factor (PDGF). As we shall see, this is of interest because of its potential role in the formation of atheromatous plaques (page 196).

Recanalization is a term used by clinicians to indicate that there is useful flow through a previously occluded vessel. Obviously, if streptokinase treatment has been successful, the thrombus will be dissolved, the original intimal lining will still exist and the clinician will see flow on the arteriogram; he will call this recanalization but we will not! A similar situation occurs if the clot retracts so that it is obstructing only part of the flow (Fig. 7.9). The blood flow is, at least partially, restored but through the original lumen and not through new channels.

Figure 7.6 Venous thrombosis: development, propagation and embolization

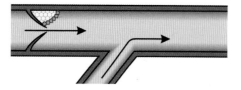

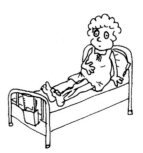

Decreased blood flow or increased coagulability
Thrombus forms in valve pocket. Platelets adhere to surface of thrombus

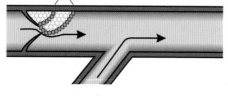

Lines of Zahn

Platelet layer propagates further thrombus formation
'Lines of Zahn' formed by alternating red and white cell and platelet deposits, orientated along blood flow.
Fibrin contracts

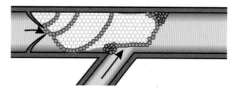

Consecutive clot

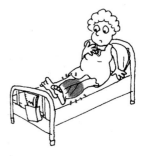

Once lumen occluded, 'consecutive' unstable, clot forms
No lines of Zahn, slow flow and no new platelets. Weakly attached to wall and easily dislodged

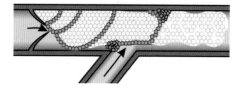

Entry of tributary
i.   may stabilize thrombus by re-attaching to wall

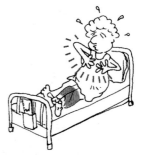

ii. permits further propagation

iii. may carry fragments of thrombus into general circulation: embolization

Figure 7.7 Splenic artery aneurysm containing thrombus showing lines of Zahn. Photomicrograph shows alternating layers of platelets (P) and blood cells (BC) trapped in a fibrin mesh

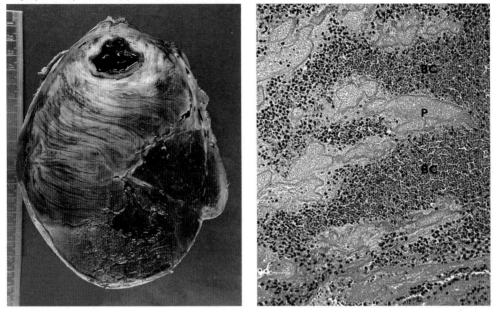

Figure 7.8 (a) Venous duplex ultrasound of the common femoral vein showing a normal right common femoral vein which compresses with probe pressure (red arrow) and demonstrates colour flow filling the entire vessel (yellow arrow). (b) Venous duplex ultrasound is the investigation of choice for the detection of deep or superficial venous thrombosis. The characteristics of an acute deep vein thrombosis are failure of the vein to completely compress on probe pressure (yellow arrow), echogenic material filling in the lumen of the vein (red arrow) and absence of colour flow in the vein (green arrow)

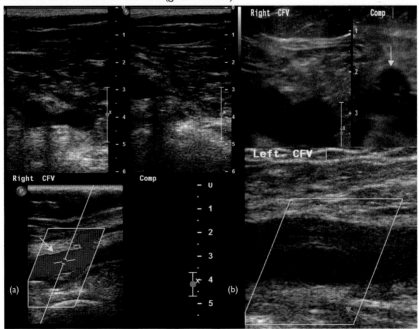

To a pathologist, recanalization involves the production of *new* endothelial-lined channels which convey blood through the occlusive thrombus. This is thought to occur by the production of clefts within the thrombus, resulting from a combination of local digestion and shrinkage. The clefts extend through the clot and become lined by endothelial cells derived from the adjacent intima. This can produce several channels separated by loose connective tissue. The amount of flow through such a segment will depend on the number and size of the conduits but the vessel will not be 'as good as new'.

This is a convenient moment to digress and discuss the way in which the cardiovascular system tries to compensate for a reduced flow through a vessel. Just as you might try to avoid a traffic jam by driving through the back roads, so the blood will search for alternative routes. The availability of such routes depends on the local anatomy. In the venous circulation, there are specific anastomoses between the systemic and portal systems around the rectum, oesophagus and umbilicus, but the penetrating veins linking the deep and superficial lower limb venous plexuses are of more relevance to our patient with a deep vein thrombosis. Thus, if a segment of the deep veins is occluded, the blood will bypass it by moving into the superficial plexus.

The arterial system has some well-characterized alternative routes like the arterial roundabout of the circle of Willis and the dual arterial supply of the lung. However, most organs do not have a dual supply and must rely on collateral vessels opening up if the main supplying vessel is occluded. If we take the heart and coronary arteries as an example, then we can often see a collateral arterial circulation in a patient who has suffered a coronary artery thrombosis (Fig. 7.10). The apparently new network of small vessels has always existed but little blood would flow through these channels because it was easier to flow down the larger artery. Once thrombosis occurs the resistance to flow increases in the main vessel, making the small channel route attractive and, hence, visible on arteriograms.

Where are these vessels? This is an area of great interest because, theoretically, any patient with a large network of connecting vessels would have some protection from suffering a large myocardial infarction. There are three main possibilities which, in probable order of clinical importance, are:

- small arterioles within the myocardium
- side branches from the large coronary arteries
- vasa vasorum.

John Hunter carried out an elegant experiment to demonstrate collateral circulation. He tied one of the carotid arteries in a stag from Richmond Park and observed the effect on the corresponding antler. The carotid pulse on that side disappeared and the antler went cold and stopped growing. Within a few weeks, however, the warmth returned and the antler started to grow again. Hunter demonstrated the collateral circulation by sacrificing the stag and injecting the carotid artery. Elegant as it was, such an experiment would not go down a bundle nowadays!

EMBOLISM

One of the complications of thrombosis is embolism and we will now go on to consider the different types of emboli and their complications.

Figure 7.9 Thrombotic obstruction of an artery or vein may be overcome by a variety of mechanisms. In some instances the vessel remains obliterated and new channels must be found for flow, or the affected tissue will die. Alternatively, thrombus may break off and embolize to distant sites. An arterial thrombus will impact in small arterioles or capillary beds and usually causes tissue infarction; a venous embolus will generally lodge within the pulmonary vasculature and may cause shock

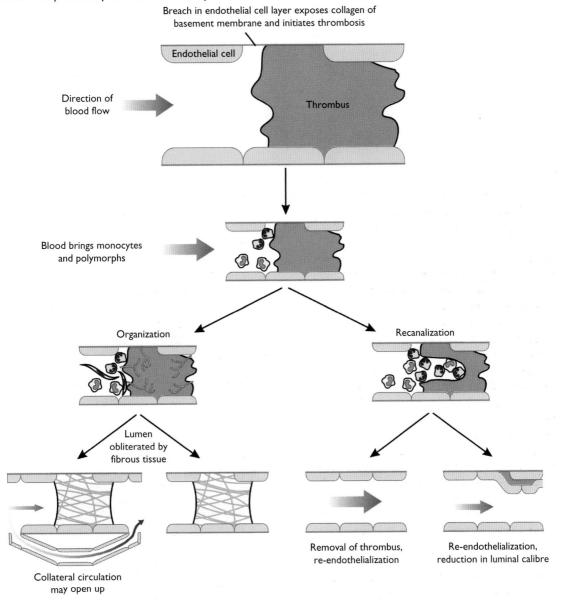

An embolus is solid, liquid or gaseous material, which is carried in the blood from one area of the circulatory system to another area.

Almost all (about 99 per cent) of emboli arise from thrombi and, thus, there is a tendency to use the term thromboembolism as synonymous with embolism. This is not strictly true as there are many other, though admittedly rarer, causes of emboli. These include:

- fragments of atheromatous plaques
- bone marrow
- fat

Figure 7.10 The development of a collateral circulation in the heart. In many patients with coronary artery atherosclerosis, luminal narrowing occurs gradually enough for the heart to adapt, by opening alternative circulatory paths. This leads to less than the expected amount of damage should a by-passed segment of coronary artery undergo sudden complete obstruction by thrombosis

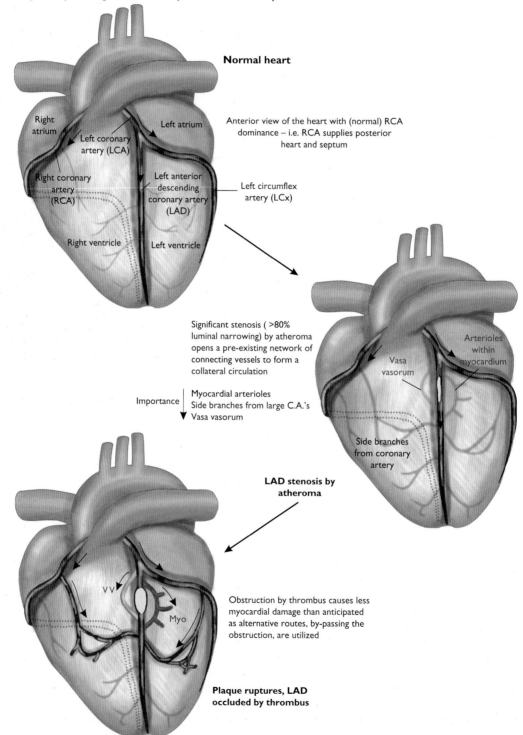

Normal heart

Right atrium

Left coronary artery (LCA)

Left atrium

Right coronary artery (RCA)

Left anterior descending coronary artery (LAD)

Left circumflex artery (LCx)

Right ventricle

Left ventricle

Anterior view of the heart with (normal) RCA dominance – i.e. RCA supplies posterior heart and septum

Significant stenosis (>80% luminal narrowing) by atheroma opens a pre-existing network of connecting vessels to form a collateral circulation

Importance

Myocardial arterioles
Side branches from large C.A.'s
Vasa vasorum

Vasa vasorum

Arterioles within myocardium

Side branches from coronary artery

LAD stenosis by atheroma

Obstruction by thrombus causes less myocardial damage than anticipated as alternative routes, by-passing the obstruction, are utilized

vv

Myo

Plaque ruptures, LAD occluded by thrombus

- air or nitrogen
- amniotic fluid
- tumour
- foreign material, e.g. intravenous catheter.

Since the majority of the emboli come from thrombi, we shall start our discussion with this particular type.

Where emboli lodge depends on their size, origin and the relevant cardiovascular anatomy. Those that arise in the venous system can travel through the right side of the heart to end up in the pulmonary circulation. Those that arise in the left side of the circulation will block systemic arteries and the clinical effect will depend on the organ involved, be it brain, kidneys, spleen or the periphery of limbs.

Emboli to the lungs from venous thrombosis represents an important preventable cause of morbidity in hospitalized patients and we shall consider this first.

PULMONARY EMBOLISM

The lungs are very interesting organs because they have a dual blood supply. Not only does the lung receive deoxygenated blood via the pulmonary arteries but also oxygenated blood from bronchial arteries feeding directly from the aorta. Hence, the lungs have an established collateral arterial circulation. This means that occlusion of a branch of the pulmonary artery rarely causes infarction of the lung parenchyma and because the alveolar walls are intact, resolution is possible. The effects of a pulmonary embolus will depend on three factors:

- the size of the occluded vessel
- the number of emboli
- the adequacy of the bronchial blood supply.

The size of the occluded vessel (Figs 7.11 and 7.12)

If a large embolus occludes a main pulmonary artery or even sits astride the bifurcation of the pulmonary trunk, a so-called saddle embolus, the patient's blood pressure will suddenly drop and there may even be instant death. If the patient survives and reaches the hospital, it may be possible to lyse the embolus using medical therapy or remove it surgically (embolectomy). It is tempting to postulate that the circulatory collapse is due to acute strain put on the right heart by sudden obstruction to the outflow tract. However, this cannot be the whole story because patients tolerate ligation of the pulmonary artery during removal of a lung

Figure 7.11 | CT pulmonary angiography has become the investigation of choice for detecting pulmonary embolism. The technique relies on a bolus of intravenous iodinated contrast given through a large cannula in a proximal arm vein with the scan being timed to start during maximal opacification of the pulmonary arterial tree. CT pulmonary angiography became possible because of the advent of the helical or spiral CT scanners which appeared in the 1990s and which are capable of acquiring very thin slices very quickly, allowing an image to be produced in any anatomical plane. The CTPA shows a saddle embolus (red arrow) from a deep vein thrombosis of the leg lying across the bifurcation of the pulmonary outflow tract.

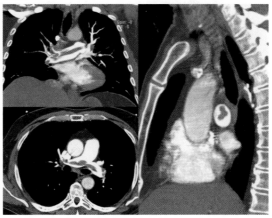

at surgery. Possibly the left ventricular outflow drops because the left atrial filling has been reduced or perhaps there is a reflex vasoconstriction of the entire pulmonary vasculature.

Around 95 per cent of emboli originate in the ileofemoral venous system with a small number coming from the pelvic veins, calf muscle veins and superficial veins of the legs. Obviously, the diameter of these emboli will correspond with the diameter of the vessel of origin, which is less than the size of the major pulmonary arteries. So how does an embolus block a vessel larger than itself? It becomes coiled, as illustrated in Fig. 7.12.

Not infrequently, a long single embolus may fragment in the circulation to produce numerous small emboli. These may reach the small pulmonary arteries as a 'shower' to occlude several vessels at the same time, producing similar sudden, severe clinical effects to a single large embolus.

If a medium-sized pulmonary artery becomes blocked, this may produce no clinical effect because the bronchial circulation is able to supply the lung parenchyma.

Figure 7.12 The effects of pulmonary embolism range from catastrophic shock with circulatory collapse, through moderate or mild respiratory impairment with pleuritic chest pain, to virtually no symptoms at all. The size, number and timing of the emboli and the quality of the bronchial artery circulation all influence the outcome. If small embolic events are sufficiently separated by time, thrombolytic mechanisms may clear them and restore normal circulation. The type of embolus also influences the sites affected and the clinical outcome. Here we illustrate three patterns of pulmonary thromboembolism

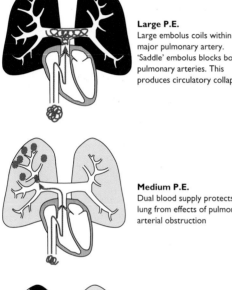

Large P.E.
Large embolus coils within major pulmonary artery. 'Saddle' embolus blocks both pulmonary arteries. This produces circulatory collapse

Medium P.E.
Dual blood supply protects lung from effects of pulmonary arterial obstruction

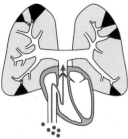

Multiple emboli combined with poor bronchial blood supply
Leads to pulmonary infarction
Bronchial artery not shown

Generally, there will be local haemorrhage but no damage to the framework of the lung and so complete resolution can occur. If the haemorrhage is small, the patient may be asymptomatic but, if large, the patient may have some shortness of breath or haemoptysis.

If the small peripheral pulmonary arteries are involved, there may be infarction because the area is beyond the territory of the bronchial collateral supply so the pulmonary arteries are, in effect, end arteries. Generally the area

affected will be quite small but may produce symptoms, especially if there are multiple emboli.

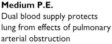

> ### Dictionary
>
> **Dyspnoea**: sensation of shortness of breath. When associated with cardiac failure, it may be due to pulmonary oedema interfering with gaseous exchange and lung stretch reflexes. If worse on lying flat, it is called orthopnoea.
>
> **Haemoptysis**: coughing up blood from the respiratory tract.

The number of emboli

Multiple emboli may be thrown into the lungs as a single event or there may be successive embolic episodes. The first situation occurs when a single large embolus fragments into smaller emboli before reaching the lungs. The second scenario happens when initially only part of the thrombus breaks off but, hours or days later, a second piece follows. If a patient survives the initial pulmonary embolus, there is a 30 per cent risk of suffering from a further embolus. This makes it extremely important that the patient receives prompt and effective anticoagulant therapy to reduce the risk. However, the anticoagulant therapy will not remove the existing embolus; that requires fibrinolytic treatment as described earlier. Sometimes a patient will remain in 'shock' despite complete lysis of the embolus and this is possibly due to intense vasoconstriction of the peripheral pulmonary vessels.

The adequacy of the bronchial blood supply

If a patient suffers from heart failure or has pre-existing pulmonary disease, the bronchial blood supply will be impaired and emboli lodging in medium-sized pulmonary arteries will result in infarction. Since the blockage is relatively proximal, the infarct will be large, extending as a cone with the apex at the blocked vessel and the base on the pleura (Fig. 7.12). Initially, the area will be firm and purple because of the haemorrhage and congestion but later it will be replaced by pale fibrous tissue and the area will shrink. Infarcts are most common in the lower lobes of the lungs and are multiple in 50 per cent of cases.

These patients tend to get chest pain related to inflammation of adjacent pleura and shortness of breath due both to a reduction in lung volume and humoral and neural factors leading to vasoconstriction and bronchoconstriction.

A typical clinical scenario is that of an elderly patient in hospital who has cardiac failure and a fractured neck of femur following a fall. The combination of recumbency, cardiac failure and postoperative dehydration combine to create an ideal situation for the formation of a deep vein thrombosis in the leg veins. A moderate sized embolus, over a background of an inadequate collateral supply due to cardiac failure, results in significant ischaemia of the lung parenchyma and infarction.

THE FATE OF THE EMBOLUS

In some ways this is similar to that of a thrombus. Ideally, it will be lysed by the fibrinolytic system to restore patency of the vessel. If not, organization takes place and the mass will be incorporated into the wall with possible recanalization of the vessel. Spontaneous lysis is often very good so it is important to support the patient to allow 'nature' to do the healing.

If there are multiple emboli or repeated episodes of embolization and organization, the pulmonary vessel wall will thicken, resulting in a rise in pulmonary arterial pressure (pulmonary hypertension). This in turn means an increased work load for the right ventricle, which tries to compensate by becoming thicker (hypertrophy). Eventually, the right ventricle may not be able to compensate and cardiac failure will ensue. Right ventricular enlargement due to pulmonary disease is called cor pulmonale.

SYSTEMIC EMBOLISM

Systemic emboli travel in the internal circulation and commonly originate in the left side of the heart from thrombi forming on areas of myocardial infarction or thrombus forming on atheromatous plaques in the aorta or carotid arteries. Other causes include fragments of atheromatous plaques that result from fissuring or ulceration of a plaque and release lipid and cholesterol mixture into the circulation.

Arterial emboli, unless very small, nearly always cause infarction. Emboli to the lower limbs may produce gangrene of a few toes or of the entire limb. Cerebral emboli cause death or infarction unless the embolus lodges in an area which receives adequate collateral supply through the circle of Willis. Alternative sites are the upper limb and the vessels supplying the gut, kidney and spleen. A special type of systemic embolus is the infected material from vegetations on the heart valves in infective endocarditis. These produce septic infarcts and large abscesses in the affected tissues.

OTHER TYPES OF EMBOLI

The other types of emboli generally enter veins rather than arteries because veins have thinner walls and a lower pressure. Therefore, most are venous emboli which lodge in the lungs.

> **Key facts**
>
> **Key sources of thromboemboli**
>
> *Heart*
> - Left ventricle secondary to myocardial infarction
> - Left atria secondary to fibrillation
> - Rheumatic heart disease
> - Cardiomyopathy
> - Infective endocarditis
> - Valve prosthesis
>
> *Vessels*
> - Ulcerated arteriosclerotic plaques
> - Aortic aneurysm
> - Arterial prosthesis

Bone marrow emboli

Bone marrow emboli are occasionally seen in histological sections of lungs at autopsy. This is especially likely if the patient has suffered major trauma, such as a road traffic accident, but can even occur with the 'trauma' of attempted cardiac resuscitation, particularly in elderly people whose costal cartilages have ossified. Anything which fractures bone can release bone and bone marrow into the venous circulation with resultant pulmonary emboli but the clinical significance of this type of embolization is unclear.

Fat emboli

Fat from the marrow cavities of long bones or from soft tissue also can enter the circulation as a result of severe trauma. However, they even form without any trauma (as listed below) and so alternative mechanisms must operate. Fortunately, although fat globules are found in the lungs of most victims of severe trauma, less than

5 per cent will suffer from the 'fat embolism syndrome', which is characterized by respiratory problems, a haemorrhagic skin rash and mental deterioration 24–72 hours after the injury. The syndrome is unlikely to result merely from mechanical blockage of vessels but probably involves chemical injury to the small vessels of the lungs, producing pulmonary oedema and activation of the coagulation pathway to cause disseminated intravascular coagulation (DIC). However, the exact mediators have not been identified. The origin of the fat in the non-trauma cases may be chylomicrons and fatty acids in the circulation coalescing to form droplets: the emulsion instability theory.

Air and nitrogen emboli

Large quantities of air within the circulation can act as emboli by forming a frothy mass which can block vessels or become trapped in the right heart chambers to

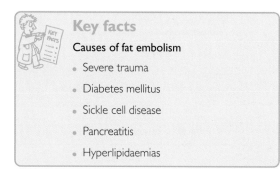

Key facts

Causes of fat embolism

- Severe trauma
- Diabetes mellitus
- Sickle cell disease
- Pancreatitis
- Hyperlipidaemias

impede its pumping. Air can either enter the circulation from the atmosphere or it can be produced within the circulation by alteration of pressure.

Severe trauma to the thorax may open large vessels (e.g. internal jugular veins) allowing air to be sucked in during inspiration, or air may be forced into the uterine vessels during badly performed abortions or deliveries. Fortunately, small quantities of air, as may be introduced during venesection, dissolve in the plasma and it probably takes about 100 mL to produce problems.

A special type of air embolism occurs in deep sea divers. Normally insoluble gases, such as nitrogen or helium in the diver's breathing mixture, will dissolve in the blood and tissues at the high pressures which occur deep beneath the sea surface. As the diver surfaces, the pressure is reduced and the gas begins to come out of solution as minute bubbles. If the reduction of pressure is rapid then these bubbles form emboli which are

particularly likely to lodge in the skeletal and cerebral circulation. The situation is slightly more complicated because platelets adhere to the nitrogen bubbles, activate the coagulation system and produce disseminated intravascular coagulation (see below). The acute form of decompression sickness or 'bends' involves pain around joints and in skeletal muscle, respiratory distress and, sometimes, coma and death. In the early stages, it can be treated by putting the victim in a 'decompression' chamber where the high pressure will redissolve the bubbles and allow a slow, controlled decompression. The chronic form or Caisson disease produces multiple areas of ischaemic necrosis in the long bones. (Caissons are high-pressure underwater chambers.)

Amniotic fluid emboli

This is an uncommon, but life-threatening form of embolization. Basically, amniotic fluid is forced into the circulation due to tearing of the placental membranes and rupture of the uterine or cervical veins. These emboli are a mixture of fat, hair, mucus, meconium and squamous cells from the fetus and they most commonly lodge in the mother's alveolar capillaries. Clinically, there is sudden onset of respiratory failure often followed by cerebral convulsions and coma. There is also excessive bleeding as a result of disseminated intravascular coagulation (DIC) and the consumption of clotting factors (Fig. 7.13). Over 80 per cent of the patients who develop amniotic fluid emboli will die. The exact mechanism is still unclear but it is not due simply to blockage of the pulmonary vasculature; it is postulated that some factor, such as prostaglandin $F_{2\alpha}$, in the amniotic fluid may be involved.

Tumour emboli

Embolization of tumour is an important mechanism of tumour spread but it is unlikely to have any immediate cardiovascular effects. The mechanisms involved in this process will be discussed in chapter 14.

DISSEMINATED INTRAVASCULAR COAGULATION

This is a convenient moment to discuss DIC. We have just mentioned amniotic fluid embolism and we are about to move on to 'shock'; both conditions which can produce DIC. Furthermore, DIC results from a loss of

Figure 7.13 Disseminated intravascular coagulation: clinical settings and effects

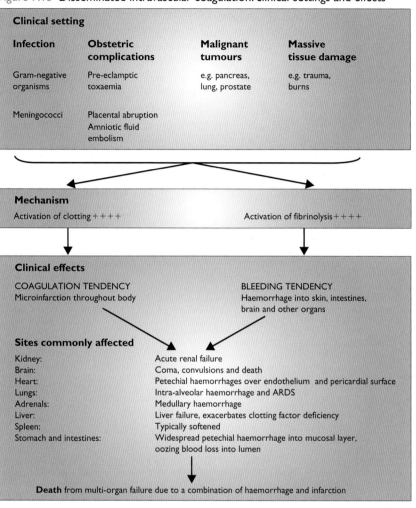

control in the clotting and fibrinolytic systems, which should still be fresh in your memory!

There is no typical clinical presentation because any organ may be affected and the major problem may be excessive clotting, which blocks numerous vessels, or inadequate clotting resulting in haemorrhage. As a general rule, sudden-onset DIC presents with bleeding problems, is particularly associated with obstetrical complications and may resolve once the obstetric situation improves. In contrast, chronic DIC is commoner in patients with carcinomatosis and the thrombotic manifestations dominate.

Small thrombi form anywhere in the circulation and produce microinfarcts. In the brain this may result in convulsions and coma, lung damage produces dyspnoea and cyanosis and renal changes cause oliguria and acute renal failure. Fibrin deposition not only produces thrombi but also results in a haemolytic anaemia as the red cells fragment whilst squeezing through the narrowed vasculature (microangiopathic haemolytic anaemia).

The fundamental problem is that there is excessive activation of coagulation, which ultimately is complicated by consumption of the coagulation factors and overactivity of the fibrinolytic system. Clotting activation occurs through increased activity of tissue factor, either released from damaged tissues or upregulated on circulating monocytes or endothelial cells in response to pro-inflammatory cytokines. It also occurs in widespread endothelial damage (e.g. by endotoxaemia), which exposes underlying collagen. Ultimately, intense fibrinolysis results in excess fibrin-degradation products that inhibit fibrin production. These latter mechanisms will predominate in haemorrhagic DIC.

Not surprisingly, the prognosis is very variable and the management extremely difficult because you are trying to balance a see-saw which is out of control. If you inhibit the clotting system too much, the patient will bleed, but any bleeding tendency may require fresh frozen plasma, which may contribute to microthrombus formation.

So far we have concentrated on thrombosis, embolism and shock, all conditions which may suddenly affect healthy people of any age. Now we will move on to the major cardiovascular problems of later life, namely hypertension, myocardial infarction and strokes (Fig. 8.1). These are overwhelming causes of morbidity and mortality in developed countries and all are associated with atherosclerosis of arteries, so it is of great importance to try to identify the causes and mechanisms of atherosclerosis.

CLINICAL CASE: ATHEROSCLEROSIS

Let us briefly consider a possible clinical picture in a patient debilitated by vascular problems.

A 48-year-old man complains of blurring of his vision. He is known to suffer from diabetes which is a complex metabolic disorder characterized by hyperglycaemia (raised blood glucose). At the age of 14 years, he presented with the typical diabetic symptoms of tiredness, weight loss, polyuria (increased urine production) and polydypsia (increased thirst). His blood glucose was raised, glucose was found in his urine and he has been on insulin therapy since that time.

His present complaint of blurred vision started 3 months ago. On questioning, he also complained of shortness of breath, especially on exertion, and cramps in his calf muscles on exercise. On examination, he was found to have a raised blood pressure, a mild degree of cardiac failure with pulmonary oedema, small haemorrhages and small blood vessel proliferation in his retina

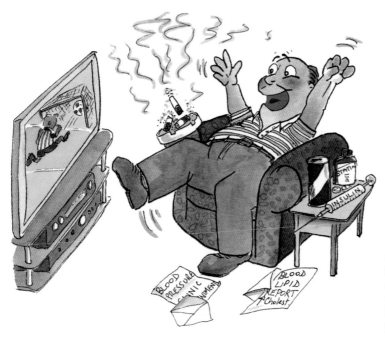

Figure 8.1 **The arteriopath.** Risk factors include: age, gender (male), obesity, smoking, diabetes, lack of exercise, hypertension, hyperlipidaemia and type 'A' personality (impatient, workaholic)

and systolic bruits in his neck (abnormal sounds, heard through the stethoscope, caused by turbulent blood flow). His blood tests showed a small rise in urea and creatinine indicating a degree of renal impairment.

This unfortunate man has widespread disease related to arterial pathology. The arterial pathology comes under the general heading of arteriosclerosis, commonly referred to as 'hardening of the arteries', although this does not relate to a specific pathologically recognized entity. His large and medium-sized arteries are likely to be narrowed by fibro-lipid atherosclerotic lesions (see next section) and his small arteries and arterioles will show the proliferative or hyaline changes of arteriolosclerosis. Atherosclerosis is principally a disease of the intima and may result in narrowing of the vessel, obstruction or thrombosis. Arteriosclerosis, on the other hand, affects the media with a resultant increase in wall thickness and decreased elasticity which may lead to hypertension (see Fig. 8.14).

Let's look at his symptoms to see if we can suggest a cause for each problem.

- His long-standing diabetes makes him much more likely to develop atherosclerosis than non-diabetic people of the same age.
- Fibro-lipid atheromatous plaques in his coronary arteries will reduce the perfusion of the cardiac muscle resulting in chronic ischaemia which damages the heart muscle so that it pumps less efficiently. Because the left side of the heart generally fails first this will result in pulmonary oedema.
- Atheroma in the carotid arteries produces the bruit heard on auscultation and may lead to cerebral infarction.
- The combination of poor cardiac function and atheromatous plaques in the abdominal aorta and femoral vessels will explain the pain and cramp in his calf muscle, which is secondary to poor perfusion.
- Hyaline arteriolosclerosis will affect small renal vessels leading to glomerular damage which will induce hypertension through a complicated mechanism involving the hormones renin and angiotensin. This exacerbates the atheroma and worsens the cardiac failure.
- The cause of his blurred vision may be of vascular origin as the retina is frequently damaged by small haemorrhages, microaneurysms and new vessel formation, although diabetes can also produce a host of other ocular changes.

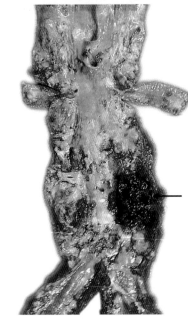

Figure 8.2 **Descending aorta with atheroma and thrombus in an aneurysm (arrow)**

The next stage in understanding this man's disease is to consider the actual appearance of his vessels (Figs 8.2 and 8.3).

WHAT DOES THE VESSEL LOOK LIKE?

The lesion of atherosclerosis is not one specific entity but a spectrum of arterial changes that have been classified by the American Heart Association into six types. The most important ones are those that can cause symptoms and these are:

- atheromatous lesions
- fibro-fatty lesions
- complicated lesions.

The earlier asymptomatic lesions include fatty streaks, which occur as early as the first decade and are seen in all parts of the world but are uncommon in older people.

Atheromatous and fibro-fatty lesion

This is raised above the surrounding intima and protrudes into the lumen. It is whitish-yellow in colour and varies in size from 0.5 to 1.5 cm and may even become bigger if adjacent plaques coalesce. On slicing, the plaque is composed of a fibrous cap covering a soft yellow lipid centre, which reminded the early pathologists of porridge or gruel and so was termed atheroma.

Figure 8.3 The arteries most commonly affected by atheroma

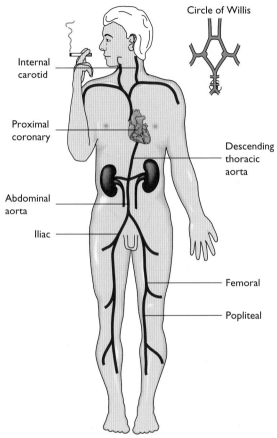

Circle of Willis

Internal carotid

Proximal coronary

Descending thoracic aorta

Abdominal aorta

Iliac

Femoral

Popliteal

The intima is greatly thickened by the fibro-fatty deposition and the media may be thinned due to a loss of smooth muscle cells resulting in both a loss of elasticity and a weakening of the wall. The adventitia may show new vessels budding off the vasa vasorum and providing the potential for a collateral circulation if obstruction occurs (Fig. 8.4).

Generally, the fibrous cap is composed of smooth muscle cells, collagen, elastin and proteoglycans. Beneath this there is a more cellular region of macrophages, T lymphocytes and smooth muscle cells covering the soft gruel-like mass of lipid, cellular debris, cholesterol clefts, plasma proteins and lipid-laden cells (foam cells) derived from macrophages and smooth muscle cells. At the edges of the lesion, there may be new vessel formation.

These plaques are commoner in the aorta, femoral, carotid and coronary arteries where they may produce clinical problems by causing partial or complete occlusion, thrombosis, embolism or aneurysm formation (see later). Areas of turbulent flow are worst affected so that lesions often occur around the ostia of vessels. However, the abdominal aorta is more liable to atheroma than the thoracic aorta but the explanation for this is unknown.

From the clinical standpoint, it would be nice to know which lesions are fairly stable and which are liable to cause problems. This led to classifying plaques as lipid- or fibrous-rich depending on the predominant

Figure 8.4 The key components of the atheromatous plaque

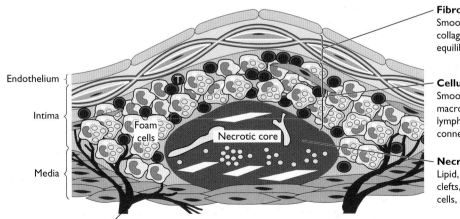

Fibrous cap
Smooth muscle and collagen in dynamic equilibrium

Cellular layer
Smooth muscle, macrophages, lymphocytes, less connective tissue

Necrotic core
Lipid, cholesterol clefts, fibrin, foam cells, cell debris

Endothelium

Intima

Media

Foam cells

Necrotic core

Neovascularization at base of plaque

feature, and, in the American Heart Association classification, are 'type IV atheromatous lesions' and 'type V fibro-fatty lesions' Also the plaque can be concentric or eccentric, with the eccentric plaque retaining some active media capable of responding to vasomotor signals. About 12 per cent of atherosclerotic plaques in coronary arteries are both eccentric and lipid-rich and it is these that are most likely to undergo acute thrombosis because of plaque injury. In around 25 per cent of cases of plaque injury, the damage is superficial involving only surface endothelium and superficial collagen. Some believe that these result from vasospasm and are more common in cigarette smokers. In the remainder, there is deep plaque fissure leading down to the lipid pool which is a powerful stimulant for platelets and the clotting cascade.

There is much interest in the 'unstable' plaques and whether it is possible to make them more stable. Unstable plaques are known to have fewer smooth muscle cells, less extracellular matrix, more extracellular lipid and many lipid-filled macrophages. Plaque stability is seen as a balance between damage and repair in the intima (Fig. 8.5). The damage is due to inflammation mediated by macrophages and T cells, and the repair involves smooth muscle cells producing matrix and fibres. It is hoped that influencing the macrophage activity might reduce the incidence of acute coronary events. A number of proteases have been implicated in thinning of the fibrous cap, in particular the matrix metalloproteinase (MMP), stromelysin 3. Other important factors may be interferon-γ through its action inhibiting collagen synthesis, and increased macrophage apoptosis. As well as improving the stability of the plaques, reducing thrombus formation is likely to be important and so stopping smoking or taking low-dose aspirin is beneficial. To summarize, plaques are not static lesions but can change in a gradual or abrupt way and also be influenced by changes in other layers of the vessel wall. In the coronary arteries, if there is a slow increase in plaque volume it is likely to lead to stable angina. Deep

Figure 8.5 **The dynamics of plaque stability**

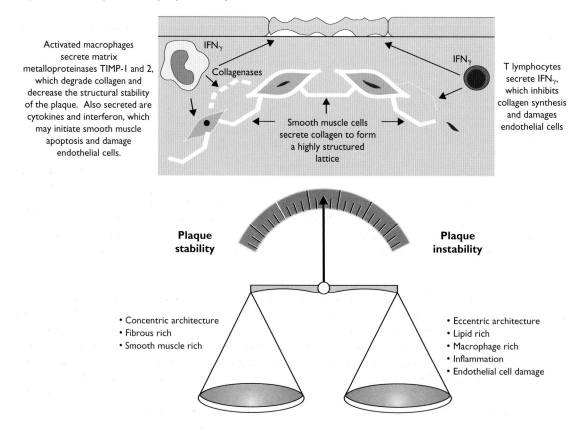

Figure 8.6 (a) Atheromatous plaque with fissuring (F) and thrombus (T) formation. (b) Angiogram showing narrowing (arrow) of the coronary artery corresponding to (a)

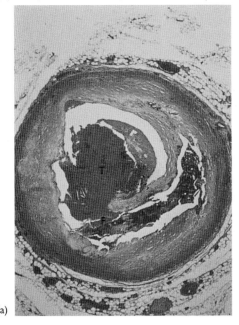

(a)

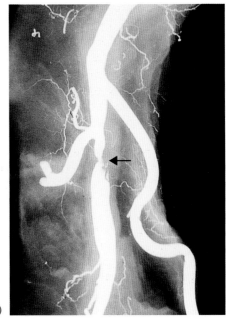

(b)

plaque fissuring will produce acute thrombosis and episodes of unstable angina, myocardial infarction or sudden death (Fig. 8.6). Endothelial dysfunction or superficial plaque injury may lead to inappropriate vasoconstriction. Atrophy of the media can result in aneurysm formation, and vessel proliferation in the adventitia can provide a network of collateral vessels. Ruptured plaques can heal and plaques, in general, may remodel or calcify.

Fatty streaks

Fatty streaks, like atheromatous plaques, occur in large muscular and elastic arteries but differ in that they are commonest in the region of the aortic ring and the thoracic aorta. They do not affect blood flow but could represent a precursor lesion for atheromatous plaques. They first appear as tiny, round or oval flat yellow dots, which become arranged in rows and finally coalesce to form a streak. The aortic surface area covered by streaks increases up to the third decade but then declines as atheromatous plaques occupy the intima. Interestingly, they occur proximal to branch points and ostia in areas of low haemodynamic stress and so are not correctly sited to be forerunners of fibrolipid plaques. The population distribution is also very different with fibrolipid plaques commoner in males in developed countries

whereas fatty streaks are found from a very early age and are independent of sex, race or geography.

RISK FACTORS FOR ATHEROSCLEROSIS

Now that we have a mental image of the appearance and distribution of atherosclerosis, we shall consider the risk factors which are believed to be important.

Age

Deaths from ischaemic heart disease increase with advancing age. Interestingly, initial involvement by atheroma affects different vessels at different ages. Thus, small aortic lesions appear in the first decade, coronary artery lesions in the second decade and cerebral arterial lesions in the third decade.

Gender

The death rate from ischaemic heart disease is higher in men than in women up to the age of 75 years, after which the incidence is similar. Myocardial infarction is extremely rare in premenopausal women suggesting that endocrine differences may be important and that the effect of oestrogens on lipid metabolism is a possible mechanism. However, initial evidence suggesting that hormone replacement therapy protects against cardiovascular disease has not been confirmed and the lifetime burden for cardiovascular disease is greater in women because they live longer and have an increased risk of stroke over the age of 75 years.

Genes

As our knowledge of the genome increases, we find more associations with particular diseases and can try to unravel the likely mechanism in order to consider possible interventions. Genetic influences on cardiovascular disease include:

- genes affecting cholesterol levels through changes to LDL receptor, apolipoprotein B and apolipoprotein C
- variants in angiotensinogen associated with hypertension
- predisposition to type 2 diabetes
- altered inactivation of nicotine which decreases the likelihood of smoking
- altered ion channel proteins influencing rare causes of arrhythmias.

Racial differences exist with blacks and South-East Asians having a higher risk than whites.

Smoking

Smoking one packet of cigarettes a day increases the likelihood of having a myocardial infarction by 300 per cent. Traditionally, more men than women have smoked but, as women have taken up the habit, their risk has risen. Fortunately, giving up smoking reduces the risk which means it is likely that smoking does not only promote atheroma but may also cause occlusion of vessels. This could be due to an increased local clotting tendency because of altered platelet function. Stopping smoking for 1–2 years reduces the risk of myocardial infarction to 'only' twice that of non-smokers. So-called 'safer' cigarettes, which have a lower tar and nicotine content, reduce the risk of bronchial carcinoma but do not appear to reduce the risk of coronary heart disease. How smoking damages vessels is not known but suggestions include increased free-radical activity, raised carbon monoxide levels or a direct effect of nicotine.

Hypertension

Hypertension significantly increases the risk of ischaemic heart disease and 'strokes'. The diastolic blood pressure level is considered more important than the systolic level and a diastolic pressure consistently greater than 95 mmHg is deemed harmful. Drug treatment to reduce the blood pressure decreases the risk in patients with moderate to severe hypertension but it is unclear whether it benefits patients with mild hypertension. Most of the evidence suggesting the role of hypertension as a risk factor involves complex multifactorial analysis of large studies which, although the proper method for assessing the evidence, is not as easy to grasp as some simpler observations. Evidence of the direct role of hypertension in producing atheroma comes from two examples of congenital abnormalities of the cardiovascular system. Patients with congenital narrowing of part of the aorta (coarctation) develop atheroma in the proximal hypertensive segment but not in the distal region, where the pressure is lower. The other example is the rare abnormality of having one coronary artery originating from the low-pressure pulmonary artery. The coronary artery linked to the aorta develops atheromatous changes with age but the artery linked to the pulmonary supply remains atheroma free.

Hyperlipidaemia

Evidence for the role of fats in atheroma comes from a variety of sources and the literature on the role of lipids in atherosclerosis would fill a library so we shall just highlight some of the more important points.

- Atheromatous lesions contain far more lipid than the adjacent intima.
- Atheromatous plaques are rich in cholesterol and cholesterol esters (65–80 per cent), derived from blood lipoproteins.
- Intimal lesions can be produced in some animals by increasing the plasma concentration of certain lipids through drug or diet manipulation.
- Macrophages accumulate cholesterol (LDL) and this is increased if there is endothelial damage.
- In populations with a high incidence of atherosclerosis, there are high plasma concentrations of certain lipids (low density lipoproteins (LDL) rich in cholesterol appear most harmful, very low density lipoproteins (VLDL) do some harm but high density lipoproteins (HDL) appear cardioprotective).
- In families with genetic disorders causing hypercholesterolaemia or in groups with acquired hypercholesterolaemia (e.g. hypothyroidism and nephrotic syndrome), atherosclerosis is increased.
- Cardiovascular mortality can be reduced by lowering the plasma cholesterol with diet or drugs (e.g. statins).

Diabetes

The risk of a myocardial infarction in a diabetic patient is twice that of a non-diabetic patient and, as our clinical scenario illustrated, their arterial disease is widespread. Arterial disease accounts for around 70 per cent of the deaths of diabetics in Western countries. A possible mechanism is change in lipids so that HDL may be decreased and LDL increased because receptor-mediated catabolism is reduced.

Other possible risk factors

- lack of regular exercise
- obesity
- low weight at 1 year of age
- 'type A' personality/stress
- low socio-economic group
- *C. pneumoniae* infection.

It has been suggested that infection, especially with *Chlamydia pneumoniae* or cytomegalovirus, might increase the risk of atheroma. The potential mechanisms could include altering the response of the vascular wall cells to injury and promoting chronic inflammation within the wall. Although seroepidemiological studies and direct detection of bacterial components in atherosclerotic lesions provides some evidence, the hypothesis is far from accepted. Fetal origin of adult disease is more widely accepted, especially the association between low birth weight or low infant weight and

Key facts

Risk factors for atherosclerosis

Unmodifiable	age, gender, personality
Modifiable	diabetes, hyperlipidaemia
Preventable	smoking, obesity

subsequent development of hypertension and cardiovascular disease.

Metabolic syndrome

With the increasing availability and effectiveness of interventions, it is crucially important to identify those at increased risk of cardiovascular disease so that they can be appropriately treated and their risk reduced (Fig. 8.7). The conventional risk factors (see above) have been used to construct models used in clinical practice and many of these are derived from Framingham data. There has been interest in recent years as to whether the 'metabolic syndrome' is an independent risk factor. Definitions of the metabolic syndrome vary but are based on the combination of impaired glucose metabolism, hypertension, dyslipidaemia and central obesity. Studies conflict on its clinical usefulness with a recent large community-based study in middle-aged men demonstrating a 1.4 increased risk for total mortality and 1.6 increased risk for cardiovascular mortality after accounting for conventional risk factors.

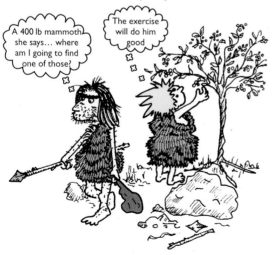

Figure 8.7 Lifestyle changes: a lot could be said to recommend a return to the low-fat, fibre-rich dietary habits of our forbears, with plenty of exercise

Key facts

Metabolic syndrome

Definition	Indicative measurement
Impaired glucose tolerance	Fasting glucose >6.1 mmol/L
Hypertension	BP $> 130/85$
Dyslipidaemia	Triglycerides >1.7 mmol/L HDL cholesterol <1.04 mmol/L
Central obesity	BMI > 29.4 kg/m²
	Waist circumference >102 cm

Figure 8.8 The development of the atheromatous plaque. Endothelial cells may be damaged by cigarette smoke, flow disturbances and hyperlipidaemia. This increases their permeability to low-density lipoproteins, which enter the arterial intima by insudation. See Fig. 8.4 for the structure of the established plaque

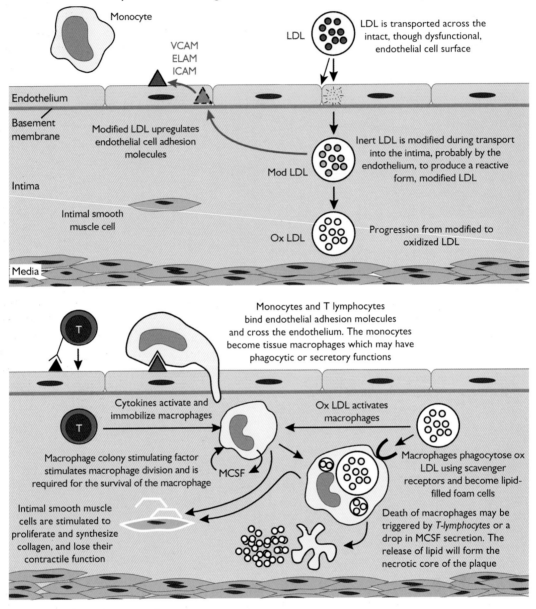

HOW IS THE ATHEROMATOUS PLAQUE PRODUCED?

Now that we know who is most likely to suffer from atherosclerosis, we need to look at the theory of how atheroma is produced. The 'reaction to injury' theory has its origin deep within the history books as it incorporates the ideas of Virchow, Duguid and Rokitansky.

Reaction to injury theory (Fig. 8.8)

Virchow believed that leakage of plasma proteins and lipid from the blood to the subendothelial tissue stimulated intimal cell proliferation. He regarded the cell proliferation as a form of low-grade inflammation and termed it the 'imbibition hypothesis'; later often called the 'insudation' or 'infiltration' hypothesis. Rokitansky is credited with the 'encrustation' theory, which suggested that thrombi forming on damaged endothelium could become organized to form a plaque. The modern 'reaction to injury' theory was proposed by Ross and Glomset in 1976 and modified in 1993. Essentially, they suggest that some change or damage to the vascular endothelium causes increased permeability to proteins and lipid and also leads to the aggregation of platelets and monocytes. These leucocytes release various enzymes and growth factors which promote smooth muscle cell proliferation Monocytes migrate from the blood into the sub-endothelial layers, where they become macrophages and ingest the lipid. A short, sharp injury can be completely repaired but chronic repeated injury leads to the formation of an atheromatous plaque.

Stable atheromatous plaques may not produce any clinical effect but problems occur if a lipid lesion covered by a thin fibrous capsule is disrupted releasing material that promotes local thrombosis. The thrombosis may cause an acute occlusion of the vessel with potentially devastating effects or only cause a partial occlusion. Partially occlusive thrombus undergoes organization and becomes incorporated into the plaque to increase its size. The factors involved can be thought of as atherogenic factors important in producing the early plaque and thrombotic factors important in its progression.

Endothelial cell damage is known to be produced by a variety of factors such as haemodynamic forces, hyperlipidaemia, cigarette smoke, immune mechanisms, certain viral antigens, irradiation and various mutagens. This damage plays an atherogenic and thrombogenic role. The next stage required in the reaction to injury theory is that the aggregated platelets and monocytes release substances to promote smooth muscle proliferation and the influx of more leucocytes.

Platelet-derived growth factor (PDGF) is believed to be important because smooth muscle proliferation is observed *in vivo* in zones where platelets adhere to damaged endothelium and *in vitro* PDGF can promote both proliferation and migration of smooth muscle cells. Interestingly, there are two animal models which provide supporting evidence. In one, the platelets lack the granules that contain PDGF and the animals do not develop atheroma. In the other, pigs lacking von Willebrand factor, which is necessary for platelet adherence and aggregation, are resistant both to thrombosis and spontaneous atherosclerosis. Other growth factors, such as fibroblast growth factor and endothelial cell growth factor are probably involved as well as a reduction in the growth inhibitors (TGF-β and endothelial-derived relaxing factor (EDRF)) produced by macrophages and endothelial cells. The end result is that smooth muscle cells migrate from the media to the intima, they proliferate, they accumulate cholesterol and cholesterol esters to become one of the types of foam cells (the other is macrophage derived) and they also manufacture extracellular matrix.

The influx of leucocytes is apparent from simple observation, i.e. by counting the number of macrophages and lymphocytes in the atheromatous lesions and comparing this with the very small number present in non-atheromatous intima. Once lymphocytes and macrophages are involved, the whole complex army of cytokines can be called into action to promote chemotaxis, cell proliferation, altered permeability etc.

Oxidized lipoproteins (OLPs) deserve a mention because of the clear association between LDL blood levels and coronary artery disease. It appears that OLPs may be produced by reactive oxygen species altering the lipoprotein present in plaques. The altered LDL is then recognized by the 'scavenger' receptor on macrophages and phagocytosed so that the macrophage becomes a foam cell. The OLPs may ultimately contribute to the death of the macrophage.

OLPs are thought to be able to cause:

- endothelial cell damage
- smooth muscle cell injury leading to central necrosis of the plaque
- foam cell formation, as the OLP are taken up by the receptor for modified LDL
- recruitment and retention of macrophages.

Can 'lifestyle' changes prevent cardiovascular disease?

This is what your patients really want to know! Should they be losing weight, taking regular exercise, stopping drinking, stopping smoking and altering their diet? The epidemiological studies suggest that these are risk factors but does intervention make a difference and who should do it?

First, what is the ideal diet? You should be a reasonable weight because in patients who are very overweight, weight reduction of about 10 kg reduces low density lipoprotein (LDL) cholesterol by 7 per cent and raises high density lipoprotein (HDL) cholesterol by 13 per cent. Regular exercise appears to enhance this effect. The standard teaching is that diets should restrict total fat intake to less than 30 per cent of all calories with no more than 10 per cent of this fat being from saturated fat, cholesterol intake should be limited to less than 300 mg/day and fibre intake should be increased. Unfortunately, this only produces a drop in total cholesterol of about 2 per cent and, although greater reduction can be achieved with more stringent diets, they are generally too unpalatable. Eating two portions of oily fish per week appears to reduce mortality but adding β-carotene, vitamin C or E supplements (i.e. similar to a high fruit and vegetable diet) has not been demonstrated to have an effect. Moderate alcohol consumption may actually help reduce strokes but heavy drinking increases the risk by raising blood pressure. Exercise appears to have a good impact in both primary and secondary prevention but 30 minutes per day for at least 5 days per week is probably required.

The alternative is to use drugs such as statins which inhibit the enzyme HMG CoA reductase and so reduce endogenous production of cholesterol. The statins also produce some lowering of triglyceride (TG) and a rise in HDL levels. The current recommendation in the UK for the use of statins depends on whether it is primary or secondary prevention (i.e. patients with or without clinically overt atherosclerotic disease). For patients with overt atherosclerotic disease, both lifestyle changes and statin therapy are recommended. For primary prevention, the current approach is to use statins if the 10-year CHD risk is greater than 20 per cent (approx equivalent to a CV risk of 40 per cent). Lifestyle changes are recommended even if the risk is less than 20 per cent and may eliminate the need for statins. There are various tables and software for calculating the 10-year risk of coronary heart disease (CHD = fatal or non-fatal myocardial infarction and angina) or cardiovascular disease (CV = CHD plus stroke, heart failure and peripheral vascular disease).

It is important to remember that you are trying to influence two different pathological mechanisms: the production of an atheromatous lesion and the occlusive event, such as thrombosis or vasoconstriction, therefore there may be different dietary factors affecting the processes, i.e. 'atherogenic' and 'thrombogenic' dietary factors. Obviously, it is likely that any atherogenic factors operate over decades and starting on a low-fat diet as you retire will cause little change to your plaques.

However, the likelihood of thrombosis could be affected by an alteration of diet in later life.

LIPIDS AND CORONARY HEART DISEASE

The first stage in our discussion needs to establish which dietary-derived blood levels correlate with coronary heart disease (CHD). Then we need to review the biochemical pathways involved so that we can try to understand the complex interplay between dietary intake of a substance and the blood levels. Finally, we can consider the observed effects of altering diets.

Risk of coronary heart disease increases with:

- raised serum total cholesterol concentration
- raised LDL cholesterol concentration
- reduced HDL cholesterol concentration.

Lipid metabolism

There are two important pathways for lipid metabolism: the exogenous and the endogenous (see Figs 8.9 and 8.10). Exogenous (i.e. dietary) lipids are digested to release triglycerides (TGs) and cholesterol esters. These combine with phospholipids and specific apoproteins to make them water soluble and are called chylomicrons. The TG component of the chylomicron can move from the circulation into cells by lipoprotein lipase activity on the endothelial surface of cells. Once inside the cell, it may be converted to glycerol and non-esterified fatty acids which are a major energy source.

Once the chylomicron has lost TG, it is called a chylomicron remnant particle (CMR) and it is rich in cholesterol. This particle attaches to liver receptors via apo-B48 and apo-E and enters the hepatocyte.

Endogenous lipid refers to the various lipids produced by the liver. The building blocks are glycerol and fatty acids reaching the liver from fat stores or synthesized from glucose, and cholesterol derived from lipoproteins (such as the CMR) or synthesized locally from acetate and mevalonic acid using the enzyme hydroxy methyl glutaryl coenzyme A (HMG Co A). Glycerol and fatty acids combine to produce TG. The liver releases VLDL, rich in TGs and with about 25 per cent cholesterol. Loss of some TGs produces IDL, and further loss of TG results in cholesterol-rich LDL. This LDL is removed from the circulation by attachment to high-affinity LDL receptors via apoprotein B100 on the liver and peripheral cells, and the LDL is broken down to amino acids and cholesterol. The alternative route is through low-affinity LDL receptors and it is these

Figure 8.9 Exogenous lipid pathway (see also Table 8.1)

- Pancreatic lipases break down dietary fat into fatty acids (FA) and cholesterol. Bile salts render them hydrophilic and they are absorbed in the duodenum and jejunum, where FAs are re-esterified into triglycerides (TGs). ACAT, an enzyme in the wall, maximizes cholesterol uptake and esterification.
- Chylomicrons form, containing TG and cholesterol inside a hydrophilic phospholipid (PL) shell. They enter lacteals, which are lymphatics, which finally reach the blood via the thoracic duct; thus they do not enter the portal venous drainage.
- In the blood HDL donate apoproteins E and C2 to the chylomicron. Chylomicrons release their triglyceride into the tissues when C2 activates lipoprotein lipase (LL) on capillary endothelial cells.
- The chylomicron remnant binds to a liver receptor for ApoE/B48 and is taken up, broken down and its components recycled.

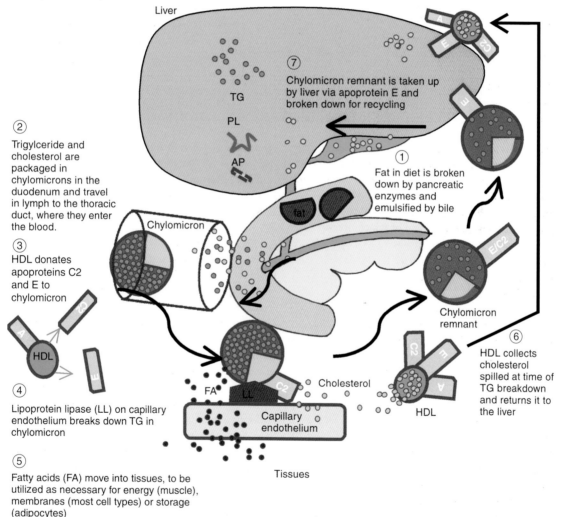

receptors that are thought to be important in atherosclerosis. If there are high levels of LDL, the liver and peripheral cells accumulate some intracellular cholesterol that inhibits endogenous synthesis of cholesterol and suppresses the production of their LDL receptors so reducing LDL uptake from the blood and probably diverting more LDL to cells with low-affinity receptors.

A really encouraging feature has been the recognition of a reverse cholesterol transport mechanism that may remove cholesterol from the plaques into the

cation of lipoproteins

	ite of production	Major lipid	Major apoprotein	Role/fate
	ntestinal mucosal cell	TG	B48	Transport of dietary TG
	Removal of TG from chylomicron	Cholesterol	B48	Transport dietary cholesterol to liver
VLDL	Liver	TG	B100, C11, E	Transport endogenous TG
IDL	Partial removal of TG from VLDL	TG and cholesterol	B100, E	Taken up by liver or converted to LDL
LDL	Further removal of TG from IDL	Cholesterol	B100	Transport endogenous cholesterol to liver and tissues
HDL	Liver and intestinal mucosal cell	Phospholipid	A, D	Complex

CMR, chylomicron remnant particle; IDL, intermediate density lipoprotein; LDL, low density lipoprotein; TG, triglyceride; VLDL, very low density lipoprotein.

serum. This involves HDL secreted by the liver and is initiated by the ATP binding cassette transporter A1 (ABC A1) and then esterified by lecithin–cholesterol acyltransferase (LCAT).

There are a variety of conditions that produce secondary hyperlipidaemia, several of which overlap with the risk factors for atherosclerosis.

Key facts

Causes of secondary hyperlipidaemia

Nutritional	obesity
	alcohol abuse
Hormonal	diabetes
	hypothyroidism
Drugs	beta blockers
	high-dose steroids
Miscellaneous	stress
	bile duct obstruction and primary biliary cirrhosis
	nephrotic syndrome and chronic renal failure

HOW DO WE REDUCE THE POPULATION'S RISK OF CORONARY ARTERY DISEASE?

Of course, it is good to observe the factors that increase the risk but it is even more important to discover whether manipulating the factor can reduce the risk. We now know that in people with no other specific risk factors (primary prevention studies), the risk of CHD reduces by 10 per cent and the risk of non-fatal myocardial infarction reduces by about 20 per cent if a 10 per cent fall in serum total cholesterol is achieved. Similar figures are available for secondary prevention studies (i.e. patients who already have CHD) to support altering the levels of LDL and HDL cholesterol. Medical science has come a long way in the last 20 years and now has more knowledge and better drugs for combating heart disease, but which interventions are most effective for improving a nation's health? A key decision is whether to aim at the whole population, identify and target only high-risk people or concentrate only on those with a specified single risk, such as raised cholesterol level. History suggests that 20 years ago, the population strategy was the best and, in the United States between 1976–80 and 1988–94, blood cholesterol levels fell by about 5 per cent; predominantly related to replacing saturated with unsaturated fats in processed food. Since then there has been little decrease in the US population's cholesterol level and patient-based strategies are more effective now it is recognized that about 35 per cent of predicted cardiovascular deaths occur in 4 per cent of the population. The advent of effective lipid-lowering medication and ideas on dietary supplements have also been factors.

The literature on diets is complex and often contradictory but it is worth discussing the role of trans fatty acids, omega 3 fatty acids and some factors influencing HDL levels because they are topics of popular debate.

Trans fatty acids are present in margarine and manufactured foods, which use vegetable oil that has been

Figure 8.10 Endogenous lipid pathway (see also Table 8.1)

- VLDL transport endogenously generated fatty acids (FAs) in triglyceride (TG) to the tissues.
- As lipoprotein lipase (LL) on capillaries liberates fatty acids from triglyceride, the protein concentration in the particle increases and the remnant becomes IDL then LDL.
- Both IDL and LDL can be taken up and endocytosed by the B100 receptor on the liver, then broken down.
- LDL is rich in cholesterol and passively crosses the endothelium, which may oxidize it en route (important in atherogenesis). Tissues which require cholesterol synthesize LDL receptors and take it up. There is often a surplus. LDL levels can be reduced by the use of statins.
- HDL has two main roles: first, it donates and receives apoprotein C2 and E to the other lipoproteins; and second, it removes excess cholesterol from the blood and tissues, taking it to the liver for excretion via bile. HDL levels increase with exercise.

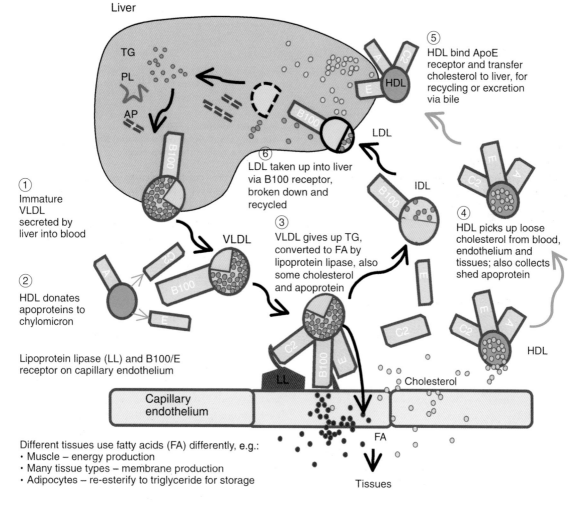

partially hydrogenated to make it semi-solid. They have no known nutritional value and, in 2004, Denmark virtually eliminated them from Danish diets by making it illegal for oils and fats to contain more than 2 per cent industrially produced trans fatty acids. A trans fatty acid is an unsaturated fatty acid with at least one double bond in the trans molecular configuration.

Polyunsaturated fats lower LDL concentration, mono-unsaturated fats have no effect on LDL and removing trans fatty acids reduces total cholesterol. Dietary trans fatty acids increase LDL cholesterol and reduce HDL cholesterol and have a more adverse effect than saturated fats on the ratio of total cholesterol to HDL cholesterol. A 2 per cent increase in trans fatty

Figure 8.11 Endothelial cell function in health and disease

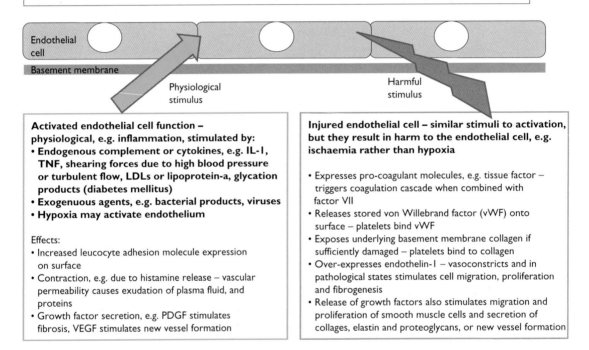

Normal endothelial cell function is as follows:
- Barrier, contains blood
- Anti-thrombotic activity due to prostacyclin (pg12), heparin-like molecules, plasminogen activator, thrombomodulin (binds thrombin, activates protein C)
- Maintains vascular tone: balance between nitric oxide and prostacyclin (Pg12) which vasodilate and endothelin and ACE which vascoconstrict
- Metabolizes hormones and lipoproteins
- Diffusion of oxygen, carbon dioxide
- Active or passive roles in delivery of nutrients, e.g. glucose, or hormones to tissues and removal of waste/unwanted substances from the tissues

Endothelial cell

Basement membrane

Physiological stimulus

Harmful stimulus

Activated endothelial cell function – physiological, e.g. inflammation, stimulated by:
- **Endogenous complement or cytokines, e.g. IL-1, TNF, shearing forces due to high blood pressure or turbulent flow, LDLs or lipoprotein-a, glycation products (diabetes mellitus)**
- **Exogenuous agents, e.g. bacterial products, viruses**
- **Hypoxia may activate endothelium**

Effects:
- Increased leucocyte adhesion molecule expression on surface
- Contraction, e.g. due to histamine release – vascular permeability causes exudation of plasma fluid, and proteins
- Growth factor secretion, e.g. PDGF stimulates fibrosis, VEGF stimulates new vessel formation

Injured endothelial cell – similar stimuli to activation, but they result in harm to the endothelial cell, e.g. ischaemia rather than hypoxia

- Expresses pro-coagulant molecules, e.g. tissue factor – triggers coagulation cascade when combined with factor VII
- Releases stored von Willebrand factor (vWF) onto surface – platelets bind vWF
- Exposes underlying basement membrane collagen if sufficiently damaged – platelets bind to collagen
- Over-expresses endothelin-1 – vasoconstricts and in pathological states stimulates cell migration, proliferation and fibrogenesis
- Release of growth factors also stimulates migration and proliferation of smooth muscle cells and secretion of collages, elastin and proteoglycans, or new vessel formation

acids has been associated with a 23 per cent increase in the incidence of coronary artery disease and occurred when the intake was very low (2–7 g/day, i.e. 3 per cent of total energy intake).

Essential polyunsaturated fatty acids include omega 3 and omega 6 fatty acids. Omega 6 fatty acids are plentiful in Western diets because they are found in many vegetable oils but they cannot be converted, by humans, into omega 3 fatty acids, most of which are obtained from fish oils. Some of the possible actions of omega 3 fatty acids are speculative but it is now recommended that dietary changes to increase omega 3 fatty acid intake should be used in secondary prevention after myocardial infarction.

They have an anti-arrhythmic action in animal models and cultured cardiac myocytes, appear to have an anti-thrombotic effect, and may influence the atherosclerotic

process. When patients awaiting carotid endarterectomy were fed fish oils, the atherosclerotic plaques contained more omega 3 fatty acids, had thicker fibrous caps and less inflammation than those from patients not receiving fish oil. They also may have a direct effect on endothelial cell function to improve dilatation and a modest reduction in blood pressure (Figs 8.11 and 8.12).

What influences your HDL level? Genes, environment and lifestyle all play a part, but almost 40 per cent of the variation in HDL cholesterol levels may be genetic, with polymorphisms of the cholesterol ester transfer protein (CETP) gene being most important, and roughly half of the environmental variation in men is attributed to increased alcohol consumption, which decreases CETP activity. Hormone replacement therapy raises HDL but is not cardioprotective, whereas exercise and stopping smoking raise HDL and are

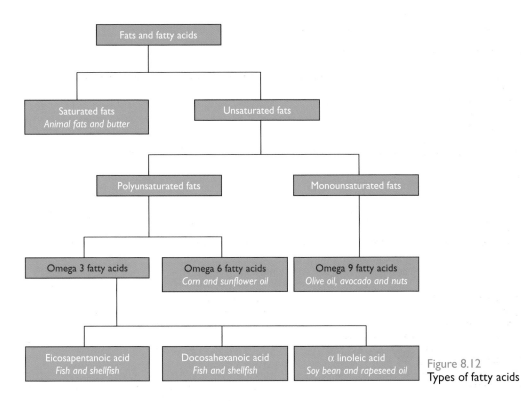

Figure 8.12
Types of fatty acids

beneficial, so simply achieving a higher HDL level is not a guarantee of better cardiac outcomes. A low CETP increases the concentration of HDL; thus, there is much interest in modifying CETP activity. However, early results with CETP inhibitors have been disappointing and this probably makes it best to regard HDL as an important molecule in some beneficial cholesterol pathways but not to see raising HDL levels as an end in itself. It is possible that blocking a key enzyme in the reverse cholesterol transport mechanism could actually be harmful.

The polypill contains aspirin, a statin and an ACE inhibitor; thus, it should reduce platelet stickiness, LDL and blood pressure and so some people believe it should be widely available as a preventative measure but the research is incomplete.

HYPERTENSION

Many of the circulatory diseases we have discussed are related to hypertension (Fig. 8.13). Atheroma, arteri-olosclerosis, myocardial infarction, left ventricular hypertrophy and aneurysms are linked by their association with hypertension, so we should discuss some of

what is known about the aetiology and pathogenesis of hypertension.

Hypertension is extremely common, affecting around 25 per cent of adults if a blood pressure of greater than 140/90 mmHg is regarded as abnormal. Unfortunately, organ damage may be irreversible by the time a patient presents with symptoms so it is important to screen the people who are most susceptible. So you will need to know about the factors influencing blood pressure. Hypertension is predominantly a condition of

Key facts

Factors that may raise blood pressure

- High salt intake
- High alcohol intake
- Coffee
- Smoking
- Stress
- Cold environment

Figure 8.13 **Complications of hypertension**

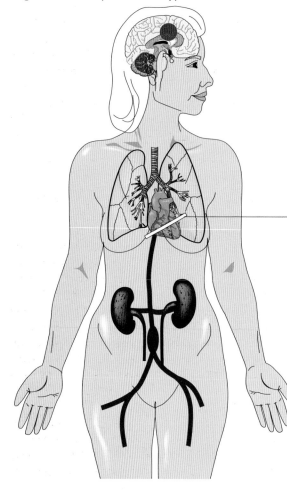

Brain
Microaneurysms and intracerebral haemorrhage

Lungs
Pulmonary oedema due to left ventricular failure

Heart
Left ventricular hypertrophy and failure; myocardial infarction

Kidneys
Ischaemic cortical damage

Blood vessels
Atherosclerosis and aneurysm formation

middle and later life and is classified as 'benign' or 'malignant'. Fortunately, 'benign' hypertension is much commoner, is relatively stable and is treatable with long-term anti-hypertensive drugs. 'Malignant' hypertension only affects 5 per cent of hypertensive patients but it is more severe and is liable to affect men under 50 years of age. It is defined as a diastolic pressure of more than 120 mmHg. The major dangers of hypertension are coronary heart disease, cerebrovascular accidents, congestive heart failure and chronic renal failure.

In 95 per cent of cases, there is no obvious cause and this is termed primary, essential or idiopathic hypertension. Most of the remainder are due to renal disease, with a small number due to endocrine abnormalities (secondary hypertension: see box).

WHAT MECHANISMS MAY OPERATE IN HYPERTENSION?

We will have to be content with describing some of the theories concerning hypertension, as nobody knows the answers. First, it is useful to review the factors influencing the control of blood pressure. In simple terms, the arterial pressure will depend on the cardiac output and the total peripheral resistance. The cardiac output depends on the heart rate, its contractility and the blood volume. It may increase in the early stages of hypertension but is more usually normal. Thus chronic hypertension appears to be due to increased tone in small arteries and arterioles. The resistance is determined by the arteriolar lumen, which may expand or contract depending on the state of the smooth muscle cells in the vessel wall. This is called local vascular tone and is influenced by a

> **Key facts**
>
> **Mediators that influence vascular tone**
>
> | Constrictors | Angiotensin I |
> |---|---|
> | | Endothelin I |
> | | Catecholamines |
> | | Thromboxane |
> | | Leukotrienes |
> | Dilators | Prostaglandins |
> | | Kinins |
> | | PAF |
> | | Endothelium-derived |
> | | relaxing factor |
> | | (nitrous oxide) |

variety of mediators (see box), which may act throughout the body or be produced and have their action locally, i.e. autoregulation.

It is suggested that essential hypertension could result from a primary defect in renal sodium excretion, possibly combined with abnormalities in sodium or calcium transport in other cells. Patients can be divided into those with high renin (20 per cent), low renin (30 per cent) and those with intermediate renin levels (50 per cent). The 'high-renin, salt-resistant, dry' ones are thought to have some well-perfused nephrons and some poorly perfused. The under-perfused nephrons secrete renin and retain sodium while the well-perfused ones respond by increasing salt excretion. The high renin causes angiotensin II production resulting in vasoconstriction and vascular smooth muscle hypertrophy and hyperplasia. This type of hypertension responds best to inhibitors of the renin–angiotensin II system (e.g. ACE inhibitors and angiotensin II antagonists).

'Low-renin, salt-sensitive, wet' cases have renal sodium and water retention of unknown origin but made worse by high salt intake. The retention suppresses renin secretion, and excess sodium probably causes vasoconstriction in smooth muscle by altering calcium transport. This hypertension is responsive to sodium restriction, diuretics and calcium channel blockers. The patients with intermediate renin levels probably have a mixture of both types of mechanism operating. The high-renin patients are the most likely to suffer tissue and organ ischaemia.

Most now accept that the salt intake in Western countries contributes to hypertension and salt intake should be reduced from a daily average of 9 g to 5 g or less. The evidence for this comes from randomized controlled trials of reducing salt intake, which showed a dose-dependent cause–effect relationship and no threshold effect. Even more important has been the confirmation that reducing dietary salt intake lowers cardiovascular events by around 30 per cent over the next 10–15 years. This was irrespective of sex, ethnicity, age, body mass and blood pressure. Unfortunately, only the minority (up to 20 per cent) of intake is under our control because most is in manufactured products, such as bread and processed food.

Secondary hypertension is most often related to renal disease and results from abnormalities in the renin–angiotensin system, abnormal salt and water balance and renal vasodepressor substances. Angiotensin II is increased in response to raised renin levels and will increase vascular resistance, by causing vascular smooth muscle contraction, and increase blood volume through aldosterone, which promotes distal tubular reabsorption of sodium. Negative feedback is provided through a lowering of renin levels secondary to the increase in angiotensin II, the raised pressure in the glomerular afferent arteriole and decreased proximal tubule sodium reabsorption which influences the macula densa. Increased renin secretion occurs in all of the renal causes of hypertension listed in the box on page 206, except for many cases of chronic renal failure. In chronic renal failure, there is sodium and water retention which is probably related to a reduced glomerular filtration rate influencing tubular sodium handling. Theoretically, renal disease might produce hypertension through a reduction in its secretion of vasodepressor substances such as prostaglandins or platelet activating factor. A group of powerful vasoconstricters are the endothelins. Endothelin I is the most potent vasoconstrictor yet discovered. Its plasma level is not raised in hypertensive individuals but it is produced by endothelium and primarily acts locally on vascular smooth muscle. Production is increased by changes in sheer stress, hypoxia and inflammatory mediators. It may have an important role in maintaining the blood pressure following a myocardial infarction and in endotoxic shock but may be detrimental by producing local ischaemia in heart muscle or in Raynaud's disease. Already antagonists are being tried in clinical trials. It is also mitogenic for smooth muscle cells and so may have a role in the formation of atheroma. It is interesting to note the overlap between substances that vasoconstrict and substances that promote growth. Vasoconstrictors, such

Key facts

Causes of secondary hypertension

Renal disease
    Acute or chronic glomerulonephritis
    Vasculitis, e.g. systemic lupus
      erythematosus
    Renal artery stenosis
    Chronic pyelonephritis
    Diabetic nephropathy
Cardiovascular disease
    Coarctation of aorta (hypertension in
      upper half of body)
    High cardiac output states
Hormonal
    Phaeochromocytoma: excess
      catecholamines from tumour
    Cushing's syndrome: excess
      corticosteroids
    Primary
      Adrenal cortical
        adenoma/hyperplasia
    Secondary
      Pituitary basophil adenoma
      Corticosteroid therapy
      Paraneoplastic, e.g. oat cell tumour
    Conn's syndrome: excess aldosterone
    Adrenal cortical adenoma/hyperplasia
    Adrenogenital syndrome
    Acromegaly: excess growth hormone
    Pituitary acidophil adenoma
Neurological
    Raised intracranial pressure
    Haemorrhage
    Tumour
    Abscess
    Hypothalamic or brainstem lesion
Pre-eclampsia in pregnancy

as noradrenaline and angiotensin II, promote smooth muscle growth while growth factors, such as platelet-derived growth factor and epidermal growth factor, can cause vasoconstriction.

WHAT DO THE VESSELS LOOK LIKE?

Hyaline and hyperplastic arteriolosclerotic changes are very different to atheromatous damage. They only affect small vessels, do not have any increase in lipid and primarily affect the media, whereas atheroma is initially an

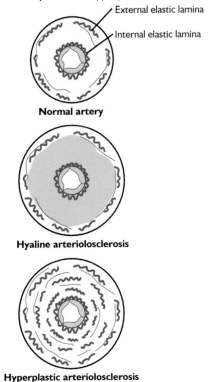

Figure 8.14 Hyaline and hyperplastic arteriolosclerosis

External elastic lamina
Internal elastic lamina

Normal artery

Hyaline arteriolosclerosis

Hyperplastic arteriolosclerosis

intimal problem. Both are very important because of their strong association with hypertension (Fig. 8.14).

Hyaline arteriolosclerosis generally occurs in elderly or diabetic patients and involves the deposition of homogenous, pink material which thickens the media, resulting in a narrowed vessel. This material is probably a combination of increased extracellular matrix, produced by smooth muscle cells, and plasma components which have leaked through a damaged endothelium.

Hyperplastic arteriolosclerosis is found in patients who have a rather sudden or severe prolonged increase in blood pressure. The media of the vessel wall is thickened by a concentric proliferation of smooth muscle cells and an increase in basement membrane material. In the worst cases (malignant hypertension), there may be fibrinoid necrosis of the vessel walls.

Does wall thickness return to normal if blood pressure is lowered? This is an important question because if vascular resistance was the result of morphological change, then reversal of these changes might produce a normotensive patient who did not require continuous antihypertensive therapy. At present, it is not possible to give a complete answer but, in humans, some

Figure 8.15 Types of aneurysm and their complications

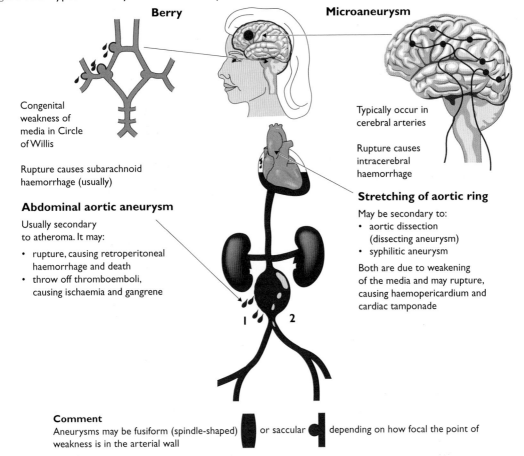

Berry

Congenital weakness of media in Circle of Willis

Rupture causes subarachnoid haemorrhage (usually)

Microaneurysm

Typically occur in cerebral arteries

Rupture causes intracerebral haemorrhage

Abdominal aortic aneurysm

Usually secondary to atheroma. It may:

- rupture, causing retroperitoneal haemorrhage and death
- throw off thromboemboli, causing ischaemia and gangrene

Stretching of aortic ring

May be secondary to:
- aortic dissection (dissecting aneurysm)
- syphilitic aneurysm

Both are due to weakening of the media and may rupture, causing haemopericardium and cardiac tamponade

Comment
Aneurysms may be fusiform (spindle-shaped) or saccular depending on how focal the point of weakness is in the arterial wall

antihypertensive drugs do produce some reduction in wall thickness and, in animals, the angiotensin converting enzyme (ACE) inhibitors are clearly effective while thiazide and hydralazine-like vasodilators have only a minor effect. Thus, simply lowering the blood pressure is not enough and, maybe, some antihypertensives are achieving the morphological changes through other actions on smooth muscle cells.

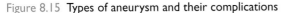

ANEURYSMS

An aneurysm is a localized dilatation in a blood vessel which may produce no symptoms, may cause problems through pressing on adjacent structures, can become occluded by thrombus or may rupture with potentially devastating effects.

Let us start with berry aneurysms. As the name suggests, these are more than just a dilatation and appear like a cherry stuck on the side of a vessel. Berry aneurysms are usually small, less than 1.5 centimetres in diameter and are globular in shape. Although referred to as congenital, they are not present at birth but develop because there is a defect in the media of the blood vessels at sites of bifurcation. These occur most commonly around the circle of Willis. Patients with berry aneurysms generally present with a sudden severe headache and some lose consciousness because the aneurysm has leaked. Occasionally, a patient will have ocular problems or facial pain because of pressure on the cranial nerves by an unruptured aneurysm. Frequently, these patients are young or middle-aged and are not normally hypertensive but are assumed to have raised their blood pressure by acute exertion.

History Thomas Willis (1621–1675)

Thomas Willis was the son of a Wiltshire farmer who fought with Charles I's army until it was defeated. He then went into medical practice in Oxford where, with others, he formed the Royal Society. Both an anatomist and a clinician, he wrote descriptions of the nervous system that were illustrated by Christopher Wren and made many original observations; but he was not the first to recognize or describe the circle of Willis. Key achievements were his first description of the 11th cranial nerve, recognizing the sweetness of urine in diabetes mellitus but not in diabetes insipidus, and appreciating that hysteria was not a disease of the uterus but a disease of the brain!

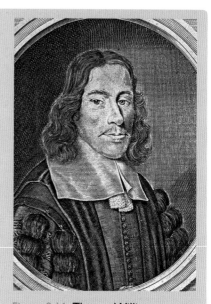

Figure 8.16 Thomas Willis (Reproduced with permission from Wellcome Library, London)

The other important type of aneurysm affecting cerebral vessels is the microaneurysm or Charcot–Bouchard aneurysm (Fig. 8.17). These are generally multiple small aneurysms only a few millimetres in diameter present on small arteries within the cerebral hemispheres. They occur in older, hypertensive individuals and are a common cause of intracerebral haemorrhage, a form of 'stroke'.

Atherosclerotic aneurysms are commonest in the abdominal portion of the aorta and they may present with massive haemorrhage or as a pulsatile mass in the abdomen, which may compress structures such as the ureters. Often they become complicated by thrombosis with the risk of shedding emboli into lower limb vessels. These aneurysms occur in individuals with risk factors for atheroma and they develop due to thinning of the media exacerbated by hypertension. It is not known how atheroma, an intimal disease, produces medial damage. The aneurysms are generally fusiform in shape and often extend for several centimetres along the aorta. Aneurysms greater than 6 centimetres in diameter are likely to rupture so it is recommended that these are replaced by prosthetic grafts as replacement after rupture carries a high mortality.

Cystic medial necrosis is a descriptive term for necrosis of the media associated with the formation of mucoid cystic lakes. The cause of cystic medial necrosis is unknown but it is associated with hypertension and may involve production of abnormal collagen, elastin and proteoglycans in the media, as occurs in Marfan's syndrome. It is important as a possible aetiological factor in aortic dissection, in which blood tracks down through the media. Unfortunately, aortic dissection is often referred to as an aortic dissecting aneurysm despite the vessel not being dilated.

Figure 8.17 Photomicrograph showing microaneurysm with a thrombus (Courtesy of Dr S. Edwards, SGHMS)

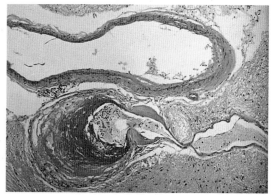

Antoine Marfan was a French paediatrician whose major contribution is not the syndrome named after him but his studies on pulmonary tuberculosis which recognized the immunity conferred by healed local lesions; this became known as Marfan's Law and inspired Calmette to develop the BCG vaccination. He was the pioneer of clinical paediatrics in France, specializing in infections and nutrition.

'In medicine it is always necessary to start with the observation of the sick and to always return to this as this is the paramount means of verification. Observe methodically and vigorously without neglecting any exploratory procedure using all that can be provided by physical examination, chemical studies, bacteriological findings and experiment, one must compare the facts observed during life and the lesions revealed by autopsy.'

Aortic dissection usually occurs in the 40–60-year-old group and affects men more commonly than women, although it does occur in pregnant women, possibly because of generalized hormonal actions, which soften connective tissue. Patients complain of sudden severe pain in the centre of the chest, similar to that felt in myocardial infarction but this often radiates to the back and moves as the dissection progresses. The first event in aortic dissection is a tear in the intima so that blood enters the media and tracks down between the middle and outer thirds of the media (Figs 8.18 and 8.19). The tear often occurs in the ascending aorta and is thought to be due to shearing forces on the intima because of turbulent blood flow. Any hypertension will exacerbate both the turbulence and the forces splitting the media. Once the blood begins to track along the media, it can travel in either direction and it can rupture back into the aorta or it can rupture out into the peritoneal cavity, pericardial sac or pleural cavity. Rupture outwards is catastrophic and common. Rupture into the aorta is rare but has a good prognosis and will produce a double-barrelled aorta. Extension of the dissection will occlude the mouths of any tributaries which become involved and this commonly affects the coronary, renal, mesenteric, iliac or cerebral vessels. More recently, dissection of the vertebro-basilar vessels has been described.

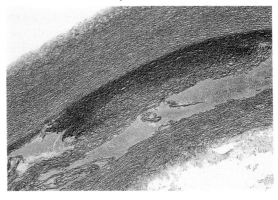

Figure 8.18 Elastin stain of aorta showing dissection of the wall by blood (stained yellow) (Courtesy of Dr S. Edwards, SGHMS)

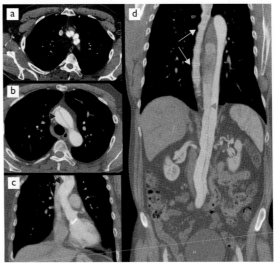

Figure 8.19 (a–d) Computed tomography (CT) scan image series in a 34-year-old man with Marfan syndrome which illustrates a life-threatening complication of the disease: aortic dissection. The dissection raises an intimal flap which can be identified on cross-sectional imaging as a low-density line running through the origin of the brachiocephalic, carotid and subclavian arteries (blue arrow), the aortic arch (red arrow) and the descending thoracic and abdominal aorta (green arrow). Note the aortic valve replacement (blue arrow) a consequence of aortic regurgitation and the scoliosis of the thoracic spine (yellow arrow), all features of Marfan syndrome.

Aneurysms secondary to inflammation will include those due to syphilis, arteritis and infection. Syphilitic aneurysms tend to occur in the ascending and arch of the aorta where they are ideally situated to cause mischief. Those that arise close to the aortic valve ring lead to dilatation of the ring and hence to aortic incompetence, the result of which is overload of the left ventricle and cardiac failure.

Aneurysms may rupture into the trachea or oesophagus to produce haemoptysis (coughing up blood), haematemesis (vomiting blood) or death. Any cause of aortic expansion within the chest can produce difficulty in breathing or swallowing due to compression, persistent cough due to irritation of the recurrent laryngeal nerves, or problems of bone erosion. Fortunately, untreated syphilis is now less common in the Western world and these complications are rare.

Aneurysms secondary to vasculitis, such as polyarteritis nodosa, tend to occur in the renal and mesenteric vessels where they lead to local ischaemia. Patients, therefore, may present with renal failure or with intestinal infarction and peritonitis, all of which have a significant mortality. Aneurysms secondary to infection are called mycotic aneurysms. Such aneurysms tend to be 'saccular', i.e. the wall is weakened in a particular focus that 'blows out' to form a sac. Most of the other conditions we have mentioned cause more diffuse weakening of the arterial wall, which dilates to form a 'fusiform' or spindle-shaped aneurysm.

SHOCK

Shock is a wonderful word! It means such different things to medical and lay people. How often we hear news reports that someone has suffered from shock after witnessing some tragic event. No doubt that person is surprised and possibly emotionally disturbed but they are not in a state of circulatory collapse, which is what a doctor regards as shock.

The 'shocked' patient is desperately ill and requires intensive treatment both to correct the condition that has produced the circulatory collapse and also to cope with the widespread ischaemic damage resulting from shock. By definition, the patient will have hypoperfusion of many tissues. Blood pressure may be low but need not be, as the patient may either have compensated by increasing peripheral vasoconstriction to keep the pressure normal or may have had a high blood pressure which has now dropped. There may be pallor, cold extremities, sweating and a tachycardia; the first two signs due to poor perfusion and the other two resulting from the attempt to compensate, which includes the release of adrenaline.

What has happened to precipitate this disastrous state? Well, logically, there will be a sudden generalized poor perfusion if the pump fails or if there is insufficient blood, so-called cardiogenic and hypovolaemic shock (Fig. 9.1). Abrupt heart failure may result from myocardial infarction, arrhythmias and cardiac tamponade while hypovolaemic shock follows fluid loss due to haemorrhage, severe burns, diarrhoea or vomiting. Shock following pulmonary embolism mimics cardiogenic shock but the heart is normal and the reduced output is because the left atrial filling has dropped (Fig. 9.2). A rather special but clinically very important form of shock is 'septic shock' due to overwhelming infection, especially those caused by Gram-negative bacteria which have endotoxic lipopolysaccharides (see page 33).

Key facts

Important mediators of vascular dilatation and increased permeability in septic shock

- Histamine
- Thromboxane
- Serotonin
- Prostaglandins
- Leukotrienes
- TNF-α
- IL-1α
- C3a and C5a

Here the pathogenesis is complicated because of the varied effects of the bacterial products on endothelial cells, platelets and leucocytes which leads to a veritable web of interactions resulting in disseminated intravascular coagulation (DIC) and reduced blood volume because of vasodilatation and increased vascular permeability. Similar mechanisms probably operate in anaphylactic shock and neurogenic shock.

Let us concentrate first on cardiogenic shock as this follows naturally from the previous chapter on atherosclerosis and hypertension.

CLINICAL CASE: MYOCARDIAL INFARCTION

Let us consider the clinical aspects. A typical scenario may be as follows. A 63-year-old man presented to the Accident and Emergency department complaining of chest pain. He had had central chest pain for 1–2 hours and the pain radiated down the left arm and into his

Figure 9.1 The pathogenesis and clinical effects of shock. Shock may be due to pump failure (cardiogenic shock) or loss of blood volume (hypovolaemic shock) but, if treatment is unsuccessful, the clinical outcome is much the same. ARDS, adult respiratory distress syndrome; DIC, disseminated intravascular coagulation (see pages 228–229)

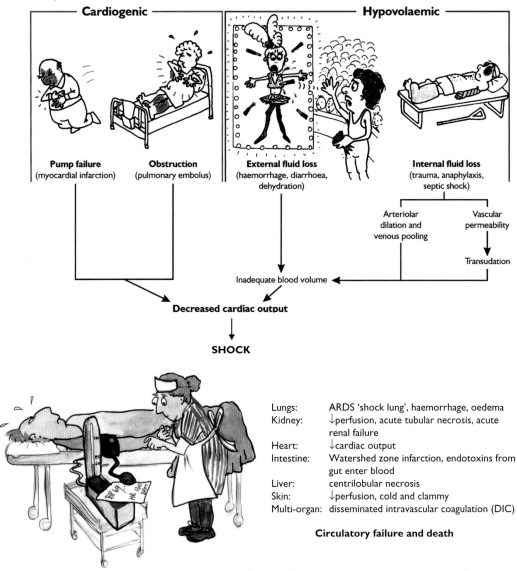

Lungs:	ARDS 'shock lung', haemorrhage, oedema
Kidney:	↓perfusion, acute tubular necrosis, acute renal failure
Heart:	↓cardiac output
Intestine:	Watershed zone infarction, endotoxins from gut enter blood
Liver:	centrilobular necrosis
Skin:	↓perfusion, cold and clammy
Multi-organ:	disseminated intravascular coagulation (DIC)

Circulatory failure and death

neck. He was feeling nauseated and also complained of shortness of breath. He had a history of hypertension for the last 5 years and had been receiving treatment. He also smoked 25 cigarettes per day and was obese. His father died at the age of 55 of a 'heart attack'.

On examination he was found to have a pulse rate of 40 beats/min, blood pressure of 110/80 and he was in cardiac failure. An electrocardiogram (ECG) suggests an inferior myocardial infarction and he was found to be in complete heart block. This man has acute coronary syndrome and, as house physicians and residents, you will encounter this sort of situation with alarming regularity. The first priority is to make the correct diagnosis, recognize the type of acute coronary syndrome

Figure 9.2 **The pathogenesis of shock in pulmonary embolism**

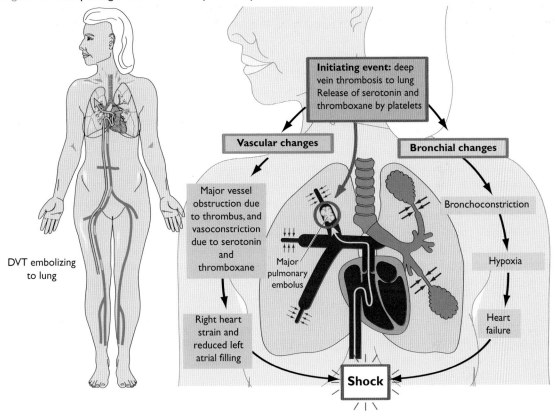

DVT embolizing to lung

Initiating event: deep vein thrombosis to lung Release of serotonin and thromboxane by platelets

Vascular changes

Bronchial changes

Major vessel obstruction due to thrombus, and vasoconstriction due to serotonin and thromboxane

Bronchoconstriction

Major pulmonary embolus

Hypoxia

Right heart strain and reduced left atrial filling

Heart failure

Shock

and instigate urgent treatment. Acute coronary syndrome takes one of three forms:

- crescendo angina
- unstable angina
- myocardial infarction.

Myocardial infaction is diagnosed when two of the following criteria are present:

- prolonged cardiac pain at rest and unresponsive to GTN
- characteristic ECG changes
- detectable T or I troponin or creatine kinase MB isoenzyme in the blood 12 hours after the onset of symptoms.

Because urgent therapy is crucial, it is not sensible to wait 12 hours for the rise in serum markers of myocyte damage and so, on admission, acute coronary syndromes are divided into those with and without ST segment

Figure 9.3 **Risk of death from admission to hospital to 6 months after discharge** (Redrawn from Fox *et al* (2006), *BMJ* 333, 1091. With permission from BMJ Publishing Ltd)

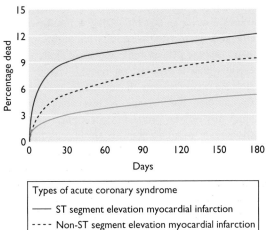

Types of acute coronary syndrome

— ST segment elevation myocardial infarction

- - - Non-ST segment elevation myocardial infarction

— Unstable angina

elevation. ST segment elevation suggests that there is transmural ischaemia and these patients require urgent reperfusion therapy (thrombolysis or PCI; see page 219). For those with non-ST segment elevation, anti-thrombotic treatment is appropriate with a combination of anti-platelet agents (aspirin and a platelet membrane ADP receptor antagonist) and anticoagulants. In high-risk patients, early coronary angiography to assess the state of the vessels and revascularization, if indicated, is used.

Figure 9.3 shows the risk of death from admission to 6 months after discharge for patients with different acute coronary syndromes. It should be remembered that approximately 20 per cent die before they reach the hospital.

In our patient, the cardiac markers were raised after 12 hours and so he is classified as having a myocardial infarction. So what is the pathological sequence of events that leads to a myocardial infarction and what are the complications that may arise as a consequence?

WHAT MECHANISMS LEAD TO MYOCARDIAL INFARCTION?

In myocardial infarction, the cardiac muscle cells die because of a lack of nutrients, most importantly oxygen. Generally, this results from poor blood flow to the myocardium because of narrowing or total occlusion of one or more coronary arteries. The extent of the infarction will depend on the amount of collateral flow, the metabolic requirements of the cells and the duration of the insult. Atheroma of the coronary vessels accounts for the majority of cases but rarer causes include vascular spasm, emboli, arteritis and anaemia.

We have stated in the previous chapter that plaques can be stable or unstable. The stable plaques narrow the coronary arteries so that blood flow is insufficient for even a moderate increase in cardiac work, such as walking upstairs, and the patient will complain of chest pain on exercise which is relieved on resting. This is called angina and occurs because the myocardial cells become ischaemic but the damage is reversible. Unstable plaques may not be producing any clinical problems until an 'acute' event occurs when the fibrous cap of the plaque splits so that blood can reach the soft necrotic centre. This can distort and enlarge the plaque but, most significantly, the plaque contents activate the thrombotic cascade. Platelets and fibrin will aggregate to block the lumen and the platelet constituents (thromboxane A2, histamine and serotonin) may worsen the situation by promoting spasm in the vessel

wall. It is not known why the plaque fissures but it may be influenced by macrophage activity in the soft atheromatous centre, by vasospasm in the wall, by bending and twisting of the vessel as the heart contracts or by altered distribution of stresses on the wall. It is often stated that coronary artery stenosis is not likely to produce clinical symptoms unless the cross-sectional area is reduced by 75 per cent. This is true for long-standing fibrosed areas of atheroma, but the majority of plaques which fissure to produce occlusion are fairly small and have an abundance of soft lipid. You will recall that soft plaques are more likely to fissure than hard, fibrous plaques.

Vasospasm is an elusive mechanism for a pathologist to identify because there will be nothing to see at autopsy. However, it may be seen on angiography in some patients with angina or infarction and principally occurs in areas damaged by atheroma. It is potentially of great therapeutic importance because it may be influenced by drugs. Nitric oxide (NO) (originally called endothelin-derived relaxing factor) may be important in vasospasm either through reduced local production, reduced responsiveness of the smooth muscle cells or early neutralization.

PATTERNS OF INFARCTION

Occlusion of a single vessel, as described above, will produce a regional infarct, occupying the segment of myocardium that is normally supplied by a particular coronary artery (Fig. 9.4). The infarct may involve a variable thickness of the myocardial wall, but when it involves the full thickness of the wall it is referred to as a transmural infarction. Ninety per cent of transmural infarctions result from thrombosis complicating atheroma. Myocardial infarction is much commoner in the left ventricle and interventricular septum but approximately 25 per cent of posterior infarctions will extend into the adjacent right ventricle or even into the atria. Occasionally, the infarcted region does not correlate with the thrombosed vessel and this is termed 'infarction at a distance'. It occurs because the patient has had previous coronary artery problems and has developed a collateral circulation so that, for example, long-standing poor flow through the left anterior descending coronary artery may make the anterior wall of the left ventricle dependent on collateral flow from the right coronary artery. Thus sudden occlusion of the right coronary artery may result in infarction of the region normally associated with the left anterior descending artery.

Figure 9.4 **Patterns of myocardial infarction.** The region of myocardium affected by coronary artery (CA) thrombosis is reasonably predictable, generally following the patterns illustrated here. The patterns may vary, however: some people are 'right CA dominant' when much of the left CA territory is supplied by the right CA. Other modifying factors include the presence of a collateral circulation (see Fig. 7.10)

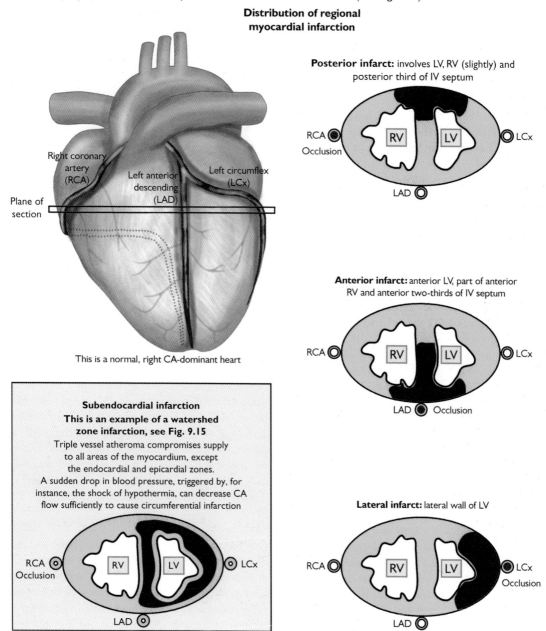

Distribution of regional myocardial infarction

This is a normal, right CA-dominant heart

Posterior infarct: involves LV, RV (slightly) and posterior third of IV septum

Anterior infarct: anterior LV, part of anterior RV and anterior two-thirds of IV septum

Lateral infarct: lateral wall of LV

Subendocardial infarction
This is an example of a watershed zone infarction, see Fig. 9.15
Triple vessel atheroma compromises supply to all areas of the myocardium, except the endocardial and epicardial zones. A sudden drop in blood pressure, triggered by, for instance, the shock of hypothermia, can decrease CA flow sufficiently to cause circumferential infarction

The other important pattern of myocardial damage is the subendocardial infarction. The pathogenesis of this type of infarction is different from the regional infarction as there is generally widespread atherosclerosis in all coronary vessels but no specific occlusion. The subendocardial region is the most vulnerable part of the myocardium for two reasons. First, any collateral supply that is developed tends to supply the subepicardial part of the myocardium; and second, the subendocardium is under the greatest tension from the compressive forces of the myocardium and, hence, most likely to be ischaemic. Normally, blood will flow into the myocardium when the aortic root pressure exceeds the left ventricular cavity pressure as occurs during diastole. Generalized reduction in myocardial perfusion results from any combination of coronary stenosis, reduction in aortic root pressure, increase in left ventricular cavity pressure, myocardial thickening and shortening of diastole.

Subendocardial infarction is much less common than transmural infarction. It is confined to the inner half of the myocardium and may be regional or circumferential. A very thin layer of subendocardial muscle remains viable because it receives nutrients and oxygen from the ventricular luminal blood. It should be noted, however, that even a transmural, regional infarct probably begins in the subendocardial region and then spreads to the rest of the wall.

WHAT ARE THE APPEARANCES OF INFARCTION?

Let us consider the clinical example described earlier in which the patient's ECG showed him to have had an inferior infarction.

If he had died within a few hours, autopsy would have revealed a thrombus within the right coronary artery. This artery supplies the posterior wall of the left ventricle and the posterior third of the interventricular septum. Ischaemia of the septum would explain his complete heart block as this would damage the conduction pathway. No macroscopical abnormality would be seen in the myocardium, as the infarction would be only 6 hours old, but the area of infarction could be highlighted using histochemical techniques. Normal heart muscle contains dehydrogenases which leak out of fibres that have been damaged by ischaemia. If a 1 cm slice of myocardium is dipped into a solution of the yellow dye nitroblue tetrazolium (NBTZ), the normal myocardium will appear blue due to the reduction of the dye by the dehydrogenase enzymes while the ischaemic myocardium will be pale and unstained. If the patient had died at 24 hours, the infarcted area would either appear pale or be red–blue due to the trapped blood. Later the dead myocardium becomes pale yellow, softened and better defined with a rim of hyperaemic tissue at the periphery.

Over the next few weeks, the necrotic muscle is replaced by fibrous scar tissue and this is usually complete by 6 weeks. The exact time course depends on the size of

Figure 9.5 Heart slice through the right and left ventricles stained with NBTZ to demonstrate infarction in the area supplied by the left anterior descending artery. The left ventricular wall has ruptured (arrow), allowing blood into the pericardial space (Slice viewed from below; right ventricle at the right of photograph)

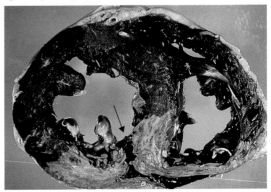

the infarct and any complications that may occur. See Fig. 9.5.

Under the light or electron microscope, the cardiac muscle will show the typical changes of reversible and irreversible ischaemic damage, which was described in chapter 1.

In clinical practice, substances that leak from the ischaemic cells can be measured in the blood and used as indicators of myocyte damage. Troponin T and I are cardiac markers that are not normally present in the blood but are released from myocardial cells when damaged. These rise 12 hours after the symptoms commence and persist for up to a fortnight. Other cardiac enzymes (creatinine phosphokinase, hydroxybutyrate dehydrogenase and aspartate and alanine transferase) are also released but are no longer commonly measured.

WHAT COMPLICATIONS MAY OCCUR?

Our 63-year-old man was in cardiac failure and complete heart block, two of the commonest complications of myocardial infarction (Fig. 9.6). First, we will consider arrhythmias. This may be a type of heart block, ventricular tachycardia or bradycardia, ventricular fibrillation or asystole. Arrhythmias are responsible for many cases of sudden death following myocardial infarction and their prompt diagnosis is of crucial importance in the management of these patients. The arrhythmias occur either because of ischaemia or death of the specialized conducting tissue of the heart, or are due to the interruption of the conduction of impulses

Figure 9.6 Patients who survive an acute myocardial infarction may develop subsequent cardiac problems. Those which tend to occur acutely are arrowed red, more chronic problems are arrowed purple. Arrhythmias may occur at any time

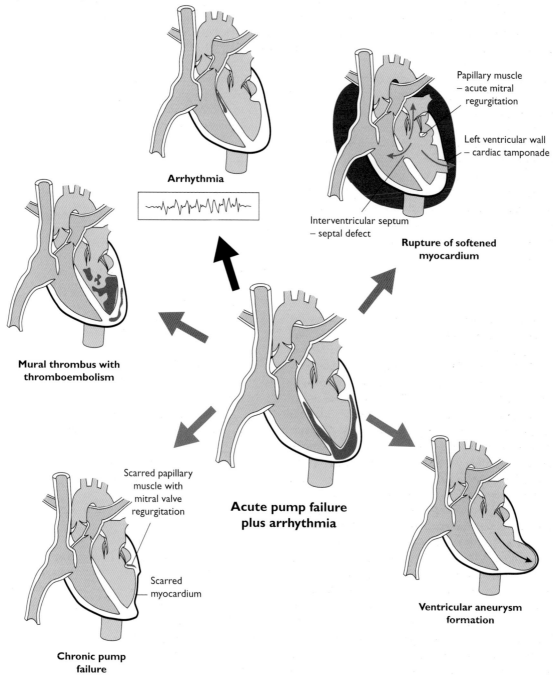

Arrhythmia

Papillary muscle
– acute mitral
regurgitation

Left ventricular wall
– cardiac tamponade

Interventricular septum
– septal defect

**Rupture of softened
myocardium**

**Mural thrombus with
thromboembolism**

**Acute pump failure
plus arrhythmia**

Scarred papillary
muscle with
mitral valve
regurgitation

Scarred
myocardium

**Ventricular aneurysm
formation**

**Chronic pump
failure**

within the damaged myocardium. A damaged atrioventricular node, for instance, may lead to complete heart block while damage to the conducting fibres within the ventricles will produce left or right bundle branch block. Damaged myocardial fibres may also be 'arrhythmogenic' and so initiate abnormal impulses which may terminate in ventricular fibrillation. It is interesting that many of the drugs used to treat arrhythmias, which act by altering the action potential, are capable also of inducing them. Potentially fatal ventricular arrhythmias without specific myocardial damage can also occur as a result of an acute thrombosis linked to plaque fissuring, and probably represents the extreme end of the spectrum of unstable angina.

The second complication mentioned was cardiac failure. His cardiac failure could be due to complete heart block, so restoring normal sinus rhythm will be important in his treatment. Cardiac failure may also occur because of extensive death of muscle cells in the left ventricular wall or because they have been 'stunned' by a short period of ischaemia and are temporarily unable to contract, but may recover over a few days. If a papillary muscle is damaged then mitral valve incompetence will produce cardiac failure. Initially, the papillary muscle is likely to be intact but incapable of contraction. After 4–5 days, the infarction has softened and the muscle may rupture, allowing the valve leaflet to prolapse, i.e. to float upwards into the left atrium. Similar softening occurs in infarcted tissue in the left ventricular wall so that it may rupture. This occurs in transmural infarction (i.e. full thickness) but not in subendocardial infarction. Within 24–48 hours of transmural infarction, the damaged ventricular muscle stretches, i.e. it becomes thinner, and is liable to aneurysm formation or rupture. This is often referred to as 'infarct expansion' but it should be appreciated that the amount of tissue damage is not increasing. It is merely a stretching of the damaged area. Rupture may take place in the interventricular septum, which creates a ventricular septal defect (VSD), or through the ventricular wall so that the blood leaks into the pericardial cavity, producing a haemopericardium which inhibits the normal action of the heart, so-called cardiac tamponade. Generally, either of these complications is fatal and is most likely to occur 5–7 days after a myocardial infarction.

The body's immune system responds to the infarction so that the pericardial surface overlying the infarcted area usually becomes inflamed (pericarditis) by the second or third day. In most cases, this is self-limiting, but the friction between the pericardial surfaces produces a pericardial rub which may be heard through a stethoscope. Similar changes occur on the endocardial surface of the infarct which, in combination with stasis, predispose it to mural thrombosis. Whenever there is thrombosis, there is a risk of embolism. In this case, these would be systemic emboli affecting organs such as the brain or kidneys.

Finally, the healed and fibrotic wall may balloon out to produce a cardiac aneurysm, which itself can be a site of thrombus because of stasis.

Dictionary

Tachycardia: increase in pulse rate

Bradycardia: abnormally slow heart rate

Arrhythmia: abnormal cardiac electrical rhythm

Asystole: absence of cardiac electrical activity

Fibrillation: uncoordinated and ineffective muscle contraction

---

Extreme circulatory failure, as in shock, is a consequence of decreased cardiac output due to pump failure or blood volume loss. Lesser degrees of poor tissue perfusion can occur through any combination of pump failure, blood abnormalities and peripheral vascular disease. We have discussed heart and vessels quite extensively and should now turn our attention to the blood.

HOW SHOULD MYOCARDIAL INFARCTION BE TREATED?

Almost a quarter of a million people in England and Wales have a myocardial infarction each year and around half will be dead within a month. Morbidity and mortality are related to the extent of the myocardial damage and clinical outlook depends on the rapidity with which normal coronary artery flow can be re-established. The blockage is usually a consequence of fissure or rupture of the fibrous cap of an atherosclerotic plaque resulting in local platelet aggregation and thrombus formation, which can rapidly narrow or block the artery. Thus, reperfusion requires removing or bypassing the obstruction and most commonly involves:

- thrombolysis to dissolve the clot
- percutaneous coronary intervention (PCI) using balloon catheterization and stenting to physically remove the obstruction and try to prevent its reformation
- bypass surgery, most commonly using the internal mammary artery, to provide an alternative route.

Research is also under way looking at whether infusing the patients' own stem cells into their coronary arteries might facilitate myocardial regeneration in the area of damage.

The key factors for success are how quickly the treatment can be started and whether it achieves normal blood flow. This is assessed angiographically (Fig. 9.7) and recorded as normal (grade 3), impaired flow (grade 2), nearly occluded (grade 1) or fully occluded (grade 0).

Thrombolysis is not suitable for patients with uncontrolled hypertension, haemostatic disorders or recent surgery, trauma or stroke, but has the advantage of being easy to administer and so capable of being started as soon as the diagnosis is made, even before the patient reaches hospital. It is generally demonstrated to be as effective as percutaneous coronary intervention if started within 3 hours but significantly less effective in the 3–12 hour period. PCI is better than conservative

Figure 9.7 **CT coronary angiography uses several post-processing computer techniques to display the coronary arteries to greater advantage, including unfolding of the arteries. Note the calcified plaque producing stenoses (red arrows). LM, left main artery; LAD, left anterior descending artery; RCA, right coronary artery; PLV, posterior left ventricular artery (posterior descending artery)**

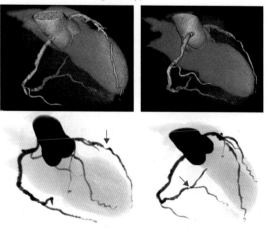

management in the 12–48 hours after symptom onset but the major benefits are when the 'door to balloon' time is less than 2 hours. In real life, there is often a delay in organizing PCI and even greater delay if considering bypass surgery. Bypass surgery is generally regarded as the treatment of choice for unstable angina and acute myocardial infarction, if the option is available.

PCI is the main treatment in the UK with 73 000 procedures in 2005 compared with 25 000 bypass operations; however, in-stent restenosis requires a further intervention in 12–20 per cent. This is a consequence of injury-induced cell proliferation and led to the development of drug-eluting stents coated with agents that inhibit smooth muscle cell proliferation. These drugs, unfortunately, also inhibit endothelial cell proliferation so that endothelial recovery can take several months with drug-eluting stents, rather than 1 month for bare stents and there is a need to treat patients with a platelet inhibitor to prevent late thrombosis. You will appreciate that knowledge of thrombosis, platelets, arterial smooth muscle cells and the endothelium helps you to understand the need for poly-pharmacy in these patients and to make sensible treatment decisions if problems arise.

Assuming that your patient has survived the initial phase, they will need further treatment (so-called 'secondary prevention') to minimize the risk of another cardiac event. You will not be surprised that this is multi-pronged to influence all the alterable harmful factors. Patients will modify their lifestyle to stop smoking, take exercise and maintain a healthy weight and diet. Drug treatment will include reducing the load

Key facts

Antiplatelet agents and anticoagulants

Three classes of antiplatelet agents are:

- aspirin
- platelet membrane ADP receptor antagonists, e.g. clopidogrel
- platelet glycoprotein 2b/3a receptor inhibitor, e.g. abciximab

Four classes of anticoagulants are:

- unfractionated heparin
- low molecular weight heparin
- pentasaccharides (inhibitors of factor X)
- direct thrombin inhibitors

on the cardiac muscle (ACE inhibitor and beta blocker), decreasing the likelihood of thrombosis (aspirin) and optimizing serum lipids (statin). Any complications, such as heart failure, must be treated and the possibility of coronary revascularization should be considered.

ANAEMIA

It is beyond the scope of this book to describe the whole of haematology but we can provide a framework for thinking about blood disorders and help you to appreciate that abnormalities in the blood can manifest as symptoms and signs in almost any organ, i.e. it is a common mechanism of disease.

The key components of blood (excluding platelets and clotting factors) are the fluid, the red cells with their haemoglobin for oxygen transport, and the white cells with their defence functions. What can go wrong with each of these? The simple answer is too much, too little or the wrong sort. Abnormalities of white cells are discussed in chapters 4 and 5 (inflammation) and chapters 11 and 12 (malignancy). Derangements of fluid balance are best looked up in a physiology or renal book. This leaves us to consider the red cells, but first a brief overview may help.

WHAT IS ANAEMIA?

> *The modern haematologist, instead of describing in English what he can see, prefers to describe in Greek what he can't.*
>
>   Richard Asher, 1959 (in the *Lancet*)

A few key words or parts of words will help us through the maze of blood disorders. Any word ending in '...aemia' relates to the blood (e.g. polycythaemia, hypoalbuminaemia) just as words ending in '...uria' relate to the urine (e.g. haematuria, blood in the urine; anuria, not passing urine). A prefix of 'hypo' indicates too little, 'micro' means too small, 'hyper' is too much and 'macro' is too big. *Leuk*aemia literally means white blood but has become synonymous with a malignancy of blood cells. *Ana*emia strictly means a lack of blood, which is not really correct because there is a reduction in red blood cells rather than an absence. The term is now used to indicate a reduction in haemoglobin concentration in the blood, so what are the possible causes?

Dictionary
Glossary of haematological terms

Anaemia: reduction in haemoglobin in blood

Pancytopenia: reduction in all blood cell types

Neutropenia: reduction in neutrophils

Thrombocytopenia: reduction in platelets

Polycythaemia: increase in red cells

Thrombocythaemia: increase in platelets

Leucocytosis: increase in white cells

Leukaemia: malignant haemopoietic cells in blood

Aplastic marrow: no haemopoiesis in marrow

Hypoplastic marrow: reduced haemopoiesis in marrow

Hyperplastic marrow: increased haemopoiesis in marrow

Leucoerythroblastic: red and white cell precursors in peripheral blood may indicate marrow replacement by fibrosis, tumour, abscesses

Red cell changes

Normocytic: normal cell size

Macrocytic: increased mean corpuscular volume (MCV)

Microcytic: decreased mean corpuscular volume (MCV)

Normochromic: normal haemoglobin (Hb) concentration

Hypochromic: Decreased mean corpuscular haemoglobin (MCH)

Poikilocytosis: variation in shape

Anisocytosis: variation in size

Howell–Jolly bodies: nuclear remnants in delayed maturation

The red blood cells contain haemoglobin, which is important in the transport of oxygen. The haemoglobin level may drop because the number of red cells is low (reduced red cell mass) or the content of haemoglobin is reduced. Red cell numbers may be reduced because of impaired production, acute or chronic blood loss through bleeding or a reduced life span for a variety of reasons.

Table 9.1 Morphological classification of anaemia

Type	MCV	MCH	Common causes
Normocytic/normochromic	Normal	Normal	Anaemia of chronic disease; chronic renal failure
Microcytic/hypochromic	↓	↓	Iron deficiency; β-thalassaemia trait; anaemia of chronic disease (severe)
Macrocytic (megaloblastic)	↑	Normal	Folic acid deficiency; vitamin B12 deficiency
Macrocytic (non-megaloblastic)	↑	Normal	Liver disease; alcohol ingestion; hypothyroidism
Leucoerythroblastic anaemia	Normal	Normal	Replacement or infiltration of marrow

Megaloblastic refers to abnormal maturation of erythroid cells detectable on examination of the marrow

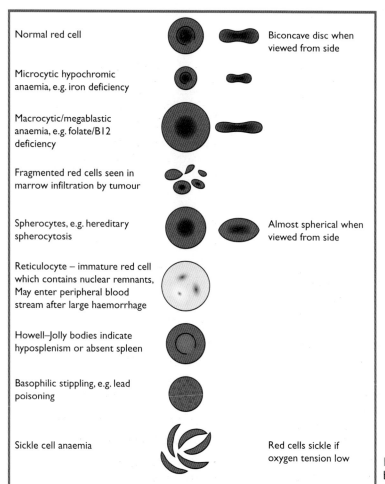

Normal red cell — Biconcave disc when viewed from side

Microcytic hypochromic anaemia, e.g. iron deficiency

Macrocytic/megablastic anaemia, e.g. folate/B12 deficiency

Fragmented red cells seen in marrow infiltration by tumour

Spherocytes, e.g. hereditary spherocytosis — Almost spherical when viewed from side

Reticulocyte – immature red cell which contains nuclear remnants, May enter peripheral blood stream after large haemorrhage

Howell–Jolly bodies indicate hyposplenism or absent spleen

Basophilic stippling, e.g. lead poisoning

Sickle cell anaemia — Red cells sickle if oxygen tension low

Figure 9.8 The morphology of red blood cells in different types of anaemia

Table 9.2 Causes of anaemia

Decreased red cell production

Defective haemoglobin production
  Iron deficiency
  Anaemia of chronic disease
  Sideroblastic anaemia
Defective DNA synthesis (megaloblastic anaemia)
  Vitamin B12 deficiency
  Folic acid deficiency
Stem cell failure, e.g. aplastic anaemia
Bone marrow replacement, e.g. infiltration by malignant
  disease
Inadequate erythropoietin stimulation, e.g. chronic renal
  failure
Other nutritional and toxic factors
  Scurvy
  Protein malnutrition
  Chronic liver disease
  Hypothyroidism

Increased red cell destruction, i.e. haemolytic anaemias

Intrinsic defect of erythrocytes
Congenital
  Haemoglobinopathies, e.g. sickle cell anaemia and
    thalassaemias
  Membrane defects, e.g. hereditary spherocytosis
  Enzyme deficiency, e.g. glucose 6-phosphate
    dehydrogenase deficiency (G6PD)
Acquired, e.g. paroxysmal nocturnal haemoglobinuria

Extrinsic cause for haemolysis
Immune-mediated
  Autoimmune haemolytic anaemia
  Haemolytic disease of the newborn
  Blood transfusion-related haemolysis
  Drug-induced immune haemolytic anaemia
Direct acting
  Infections, e.g. malaria
  Snake venom
  Physical trauma, e.g. microangiopathy
  Hypersplenism

Blood loss

Anaemia can be classified according to its cause (Tables 9.1 and 9.2) or according to the appearance of the blood (Figs 9.8 and 9.9). It is important to know both because the first investigation of a pale patient is to perform a full blood count which will detail the haemoglobin level in the blood, the number of red blood cells, the size of the red cells (mean corpuscular volume) and

Figure 9.9 (a) Microcytosis and hypochromia in a case of iron-deficiency anaemia. (b) Oval macrocytes in a case of pernicious anaemia

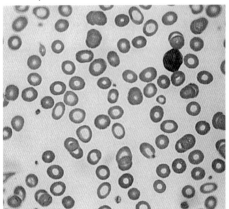

(a)

(b)

the haemoglobin in a red cell (mean corpuscular haemoglobin). If the haemoglobin level indicates that the patient is anaemic, then you can use the MCV and MCH to classify the anaemia on cell size and haemoglobin concentration and also look up the possible causes in Table 9.2. Let us try it for an imaginary patient. Remember '...cytic' refers to the cell and '...chromic' refers to the haemoglobin concentration.

A 21-year-old woman goes to see her general practitioner for a prenatal health check as she wishes to become pregnant for the first time. The doctor advises her about the risks of smoking and alcohol on the fetus and performs a physical examination and finds no abnormalities. Her blood pressure is normal and he takes a blood sample for further analysis. The blood result and normal values are shown in Table 9.3.

Table 9.3 Normal peripheral blood values and those from a patient		
	Normal	Patient
Haemoglobin (g/dL)	Male, 13.5–17.5; female, 11.5–15.5	8.2
Erythrocytes ($\times 10^{12}$/L)	Male, 4.5–6.5; female, 3.9–5.6	4.7
Haematocrit (PCV) (%)	Male, 40–52; female, 36–48	31
MCV (fL)	80–95	69
MCH (pg)	27–34	24.5
Reticulocytes ($\times 10^9$/L)	25–125	96

When the patient returns to the surgery the following week, the doctor explains that she has a minor problem because she is anaemic and probably has iron deficiency. How do you classify her anaemia?

Hopefully, you have concluded that our woman has small red cells with a reduced haemoglobin concentration, i.e. a microcytic hypochromic anaemia. To search further for a cause, you need more information. The commonest causes of anaemia can be identified through a combination of:

- reticulocyte count
- morphological appearance of the cells in the peripheral blood
- haemoglobin electrophoresis
- serum iron
- bone marrow examination
- serum ferritin (serum iron and iron binding capacity were originally used)
- serum B12 and folate levels
- Schilling test
- antibody screens (e.g. parietal cell and intrinsic factor antibodies).

Reticulocytes are newly released red cells that are slightly larger than mature red cells and have a more basophilic (blue) cytoplasm on routine Giemsa staining. Approximately 1 per cent is the normal level (giving a count of 25×10^9/L to 125×10^9/L) and an increased number indicates increased red cell turnover. Normally, the reticulocytes become mature red cells in the marrow and it is only when demand for red blood cells exceeds supply that these immature forms are released in significant numbers. Our woman has a normal reticulocyte count so the most likely diagnosis is iron-deficiency anaemia, which is a common finding in premenopausal and pregnant women and easily treated with iron tablets. The doctor is not likely to investigate any further unless the pregnant woman has other problems, but we shall digress to discuss the causes of iron deficiency and iron overload. Iron deficiency is important to understand because it is common. Iron overload is worth remembering as an example where homeostasis cannot be achieved through increased excretion. Think about it! You drink too much water and the kidney responds. Take too much salt or vitamin C and you excrete what you do not need. However, there is no controllable excretion method for iron. Is this a unique situation? No, just consider calorie intake!

IRON-DEFICIENCY ANAEMIA

Iron is an important element with well-known roles in haemoglobin, myoglobin, cytochromes and various

Key facts

Causes of iron-deficiency anaemia

Inadequate intake
Deficient diet
Malabsorption
    Generalized malabsorption, e.g. coeliac disease
    Post-gastrectomy (rapid gastrojejunal transit)

Increased iron loss
Reproductive tract
    Heavy menstruation
    Pregnancies and miscarriages
Gastrointestinal tract
    Oesophageal varices
    Peptic ulcer disease
    Chronic aspirin ingestion
    Hookworm infestation
    Haemorrhoids
    Tumours
Miscellaneous
    Epistaxis
    Haematuria
    Haemoptysis

Increased demand for iron
Early childhood
Pregnancy and lactation
Erythropoietin therapy

enzyme systems in the cells. Approximately 80 per cent of the body's iron is in one of these functional forms while the remaining 20 per cent is stored as ferritin or haemosiderin. Iron is absorbed in the upper small intestine and transported in the blood bound to the glycoprotein transferrin. There is no control over the excretion of iron and iron loss from the body is through loss in secretions, exfoliated cells and menstrual blood. There is some control over the absorption of iron with between 10 and 20 per cent of dietary iron being absorbed. This does not leave much of a safety margin so iron deficiency is the commonest cause of anaemia and occurs because of an imbalance between absorption and loss. In developed countries, an average diet contains about 15 mg of iron and the daily requirement for *absorbed* iron is 0.5–1.0 mg for men and 0.7–2.0 mg for women. This means that any reduction in dietary iron, problem with absorption or increased requirement for iron will lead to deficiency (see box on page 223). Iron balance is particularly precarious in premenopausal women because of menstrual blood loss. Fifty millilitres of whole blood contains about 25 mg of iron, which would require an extra 250 mg of iron in the diet to be back in balance.

There are no immediate problems for the person developing iron deficiency because red cell production continues but the iron stores in the marrow become depleted. Once the iron stores are inadequate, red cells are still produced but they are small (microcytic) with too little haemoglobin (hypochromic) and the patient will become tired and lethargic, breathless on exertion and appear pale. They may also have problems due to the effects of iron deficiency on epithelial cells if they do not receive treatment but remain chronically iron deficient. This complication, however, is rare in most countries. The mucous membranes of the mouth, tongue, pharynx, oesophagus and stomach become thin (atrophic) which may cause difficulty in swallowing (dysphagia) and produce mucosal webs in the upper oesophagus. Fingernails become spoon-shaped (koilonychia) and split easily and the thinned stomach wall does not produce a normal amount of acid. This combination of problems in severe iron deficiency is called the Plummer–Vinson syndrome and is cured by giving iron.

MEGALOBLASTIC ANAEMIA

The next woman in our prenatal clinic has Crohn's disease, which is an inflammatory disease that can affect any area of the gastrointestinal tract. The terminal

---

Small print

Paterson–Kelly–Plummer–Vinson syndrome

This syndrome was first described in 1909 by Donald R. Patterson (ear, nose and throat surgeon in Cardiff) and Adam B. Kelly (ENT surgeon in Glasgow). It was also described by Henry S. Plummer (physician, Mayo Clinic, USA) and Porter P. Vinson (physician in Virginia, USA). In medical textbooks, you may come across a variety of combinations of these names.

Key facts

Features specific to certain types of anaemia

Feature	Type of anaemia
Koilonychia ('spoon nails')	Iron deficiency
Jaundice	Haemolytic or megaloblastic
Leg ulcers	Sickle cell and other haemolytic anaemias
Bone deformities	Thalassaemia major and other severe congenital haemolytic anaemias
Infection and/or bruising	Bone marrow failure

---

ileum is commonly involved and this can result in anaemia due to vitamin B12 deficiency. Her blood results are shown below.

Haemoglobin (g/dL)	5.0
Erythrocytes ($\times 10^{12}$/L)	1.7
Haematocrit (PCV) (per cent)	21
MCV (fL)	128
MCH (pg)	33
Reticulocytes ($\times 10^9$/L)	40

The MCV is increased and the MCH is normal consistent with a macrocytic anaemia. We are going to concentrate on the subset of macrocytic anaemias that have abnormal erythroid maturation in the bone marrow resulting in large precursors and called 'megaloblastic'. Megaloblastic anaemia is most commonly due to

Table 9.4 Causes of megaloblastic anaemia

Vitamin B12 deficiency
Inadequate diet
   Strict vegans excluding milk, eggs and cheese
Absorption problem
   Intrinsic factor deficiency
      Pernicious anaemia
      Total and subtotal gastrectomy
   Terminal ileal disease
      Crohn's disease
      Surgical removal
Competition by microorganisms
   Bacterial overgrowth in blind loops
   Fish tapeworm infection

Folic acid deficiency
Inadequate diet
   Malnutrition
   Chronic alcoholism
Absorption problem
   Generalized malabsorption
   Tropical sprue
   Gluten-induced enteropathy (coeliac)
Increased demand
   Early childhood
   Pregnancy
   Erythroid hyperplasia in severe haemolytic
     anaemias
Use of folic acid antagonists
   Anticonvulsants, e.g. phenytoin
   Anticancer drugs, e.g. methotrexate

Defects of DNA synthesis
Congenital enzyme deficiency, e.g. orotic aciduria
Acquired enzyme deficiency
   Alcohol
   Therapy with hydroxyurea

vitamin B12 or folate deficiency (see Table 9.4). Both are co-factors for the conversion of deoxyuridine to deoxythymidine, an essential step in the synthesis of DNA.

Working down our list of investigations, we first ask for a reticulocyte count and a peripheral blood film. The laboratory tells us that there are few or no reticulocytes but the red cells contain Howell–Jolly bodies which are nuclear remnants due to delayed maturation. The red cells are large (macrocytic) and of variable shape (poikilocytosis) and the neutrophils are hypersegmented (most normal neutrophils have three or four lobes whereas hypersegmented cells have more). These are all features of megaloblastic anaemia. The next step is to measure the serum vitamin B12 level and serum and red cell folate levels. If the folate level is low, we have a diagnosis of folate deficiency whose cause should be identified by taking a good history. If the vitamin B12 is low, we can investigate further and need to understand a little more about B12 absorption. Vitamin B12 is absorbed in the terminal ileum as a complex bound to intrinsic factor. Intrinsic factor (IF) is produced by the parietal cells in the stomach. This means that you need an adequate diet and a normal stomach and terminal ileum to avoid B12 deficiency. We assume that our woman with Crohn's disease will fail to absorb the B12/intrinsic factor complex because she has a diseased terminal ileum, but how could we prove this? We could demonstrate that her bone marrow is vitamin B12 deficient by *injecting* some vitamin B12 and observing an almost immediate increase in reticulocytes. In people with a normal terminal ileum but a damaged stomach, the parietal cells are unable to produce intrinsic factor and so no absorption occurs. This can be detected by performing a Schilling test when radiolabelled vitamin B12 is given *orally* and the amount of radioactivity absorbed into the blood and excreted in the urine is measured. If lack of intrinsic factor is a problem, then absorption will be low unless intrinsic factor is also given *orally*. If absorption is low when vitamin B12 and intrinsic factor are given together, then the terminal ileum is likely to be damaged or there is something else blocking absorption of the B12/IF complex.

The commonest cause of B12 deficiency in Britain is pernicious anaemia (Fig. 9.10). This is aptly named because patients with megaloblastic anaemia can have a very severe anaemia and may even die without treatment. Pernicious anaemia or Addison's anaemia is when the vitamin B12 deficiency is due to autoimmune damage to the stomach resulting in chronic atrophic gastritis where an inflamed and thinned stomach mucosa fails to produce adequate intrinsic factor or acid. This disease occurs predominantly after the age of 50 years and is commoner in men. As well as severe anaemia, the sufferers may have neurological problems such as subacute combined degeneration of the cord and segmental demyelination of peripheral nerves. These are due to the lack of vitamin B12 and do not occur in folate deficiency. They are also at an increased risk of stomach carcinoma. *Helicobacter pylori* infection may initiate an autoimmune gastritis, which presents in younger people as iron deficiency and in the elderly as pernicious anaemia.

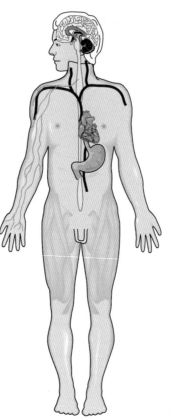

Clinical features of pernicious anaemia
Severe megaloblastic, macrocytic anaemia
Peripheral neuropathy
Subacute combined degeneration of the cord
  • demyelination of posterior and lateral columns
  • paraesthesia
  • loss of position and vibration sense
  • ataxia
  • weakness
  • spasticity
Increased risk of gastric carcinoma

Figure 9.10 Clinical features of pernicious anaemia

Key facts

Clinical features of megaloblastic anaemia

- Slow onset

- Gradually progressive

- Mild jaundice due to excess breakdown of RBC in ineffective erythropoiesis

- Glossitis

- Angular stomatitis

- Mild malabsorption due to epithelial abnormalities

- Purpura due to thrombocytopenia

- Excess apoptosis

- Sterility

- Increased melanin

What would have happened to our women if their anaemia had not been discovered at prenatal testing? Let us discuss the effects of anaemia first. The anaemic patient has too little haemoglobin and hence a potential problem with the transport of oxygen to the tissues. The demand from the tissues will depend on the person's level of activity so that an anaemic person may be asymptomatic when sitting at a desk but would have problems running a marathon; pregnancy can be regarded as a 9-month marathon (with a sprint finish!). An anaemic person can often compensate for the reduced amount of haemoglobin in the blood by pushing the blood round faster, i.e. increasing the cardiac output. The pregnant woman has the problem that in a normal pregnancy cardiac output needs to increase by around 30 per cent so compensation for anaemia may not be possible. So what will suffer? The mother will suffer with breathlessness, tiredness, weakness and possibly dizziness or fainting. The baby will suffer because nutrition through the placenta may be inadequate leading to a 'small for dates'

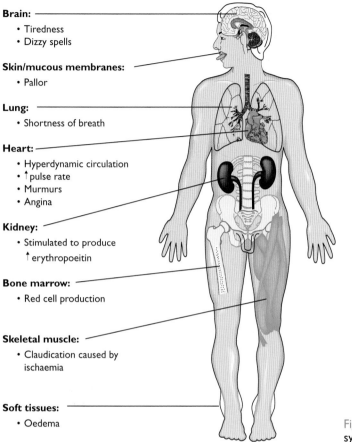

Brain:
- Tiredness
- Dizzy spells

Skin/mucous membranes:
- Pallor

Lung:
- Shortness of breath

Heart:
- Hyperdynamic circulation
- ↑pulse rate
- Murmurs
- Angina

Kidney:
- Stimulated to produce
  ↑erythropoeitin

Bone marrow:
- Red cell production

Skeletal muscle:
- Claudication caused by
  ischaemia

Soft tissues:
- Oedema

Figure 9.11 **Presenting symptoms and systemic effects of anaemia**

baby lacking the normal stores of nutrients transferred between mother and baby in the last trimester.

If we think about patients in general with anaemia, their problems will depend on how low the haemoglobin is, how quickly the anaemia has developed and how well they can compensate. Older people are usually less able to adapt and, in addition to problems of shortness of breath, weakness, lethargy, palpitations and headaches, may have symptoms of cardiac failure, angina, intermittent claudication or confusion (Fig. 9.11).

ORGAN DAMAGE DUE TO POOR PERFUSION

Whatever the cause of poor perfusion, the effect at tissue level is similar with a reduced delivery of oxygen and nutrients so that cells' normal functions are disturbed. The details of reversible and irreversible cell

Key facts

Organs damaged in a patient with shock

Organ	Damage
Kidney	Acute tubular necrosis
Lung	ARDS
Heart	Ischaemic damage
Brain	Watershed infarcts
Liver	Fatty change/necrosis
Adrenal	Focal haemorrhagic necrosis
Pancreas	Pancreatitis
Stomach	Erosive gastritis
Duodenum	Ulceration
Small and large bowel	Haemorrhagic gastroenteropathy/ infarction

injury was discussed in chapter 1, so here we will concentrate on the clinical effects. The most important organs for immediate survival are the heart and brain, so the body has mechanisms for shunting blood from other tissues to protect these two organs. Frequently the kidneys and lungs will be underperfused and sufficiently damaged to be the immediate cause of death.

ADULT RESPIRATORY DISTRESS SYNDROME

The lungs are fairly resistant to short periods of ischaemia but, if prolonged, the patient may develop 'shock lung' or 'adult respiratory distress syndrome' (ARDS) which can be life-threatening, as it is difficult to maintain adequate ventilation, even with a mechanical ventilator. For oxygen to reach the alveolar blood, air must move in and out of the lungs and be able to diffuse across the alveolar septae. In 'shock lung' there is severe oedema affecting peribronchial connective tissue and alveolar septae and spaces. This both reduces the lung compliance and impairs alveolar diffusion; that means double trouble and a mortality rate of around 50 per cent.

The probable sequence of events (Fig. 9.12) is that the 'shock' causes the release of mediators, such as activated complement (C5a), leukotriene B4 and platelet activating factor, which promote leucocyte aggregation and activation in the lung. The neutrophils produce arachidonic acid metabolites, such as thromboxane, which cause pulmonary vasoconstriction, oxygen-derived free radicals which injure the endothelial and epithelial cells, and lysosomal enzymes which digest local structural proteins.

The damaged alveolar capillary *endothelial* cells are leaky, which leads to interstitial alveolar oedema and fibrin exudation. The damaged alveolar *epithelial* cells, particularly the type I pneumocytes, desquamate to form the characteristic hyaline membranes in combination with surfactant and protein-rich oedema fluid (Fig. 9.13). These are the same as the hyaline membranes in neonatal hyaline membrane disease and in both situations indicate severe epithelial injury with lack of surfactant. The lack of surfactant leads to collapse of alveolar air spaces (atelectasis) and so further reduces compliance and gas transfer.

RENAL DAMAGE

Impaired renal blood flow results in acute tubular necrosis, a major cause of acute renal failure. This is not apparent immediately in a 'shocked' patient but will become evident once their 'shocked' state is under control and there is no circulatory reason for poor urine output. Then the patient will be noted to have oliguria (urine output of 40–400 mL/day; normal, 1500 mL/day), salt and water overload, a high plasma potassium and urea, and a metabolic acidosis. At this stage a renal biopsy would show numerous foci of tubular epithelial cell loss, affecting any area of the nephron, and epithelial 'casts', i.e. dead epithelial cells, present in the tubular lumens. The important clinical point is that the patient can make a complete recovery if appropriately managed, e.g. by dialysis, and rectifying the cause of the shock. After a few days, the tubular epithelium will regenerate and the urine volume will increase, often to above normal values because the tubules are unable to concentrate the urine, and there may be excessive loss of water, sodium and potassium; the so-called diuretic phase. Slowly the tubular epithelium returns to normal and reasonable renal function is restored.

BRAIN AND CARDIAC DAMAGE

Despite the body's best efforts to protect the heart and brain, these organs may become underperfused.

Damage to the brain may be mild or devastating. The neurons are most vulnerable to ischaemia, particularly the large Purkinje cells of the cerebellum and the pyramidal cells in the hippocampus. A short episode of hypoperfusion may not cause any irreversible neuronal damage, or the number of neurons damaged may be too few to produce any clinical effect beyond temporary confusion. However, prolonged ischaemia will result in infarction which most commonly affects the 'water-shed' areas at the junctional zones between the main

---

Key facts

Key causes of ARDS

- Sock
- Diffuse pulmonary infection, especially viral
- Oxygen toxicity
- Aspiration pneumonitis
- Cardiac surgery involving extra-corporeal pumps
- Inhalation of toxins or organic solvents
- Paraquat

Figure 9.12 Pathogenesis of adult respiratory distress syndrome (ARDS). An initiating event causes shock (see Fig. 9.1). Acute inflammatory mediators damage vascular endothelium, the alveolar walls and lining epithelium and cause pulmonary vasoconstriction, oedema, collapse and the formation of membranes over the alveolar surface

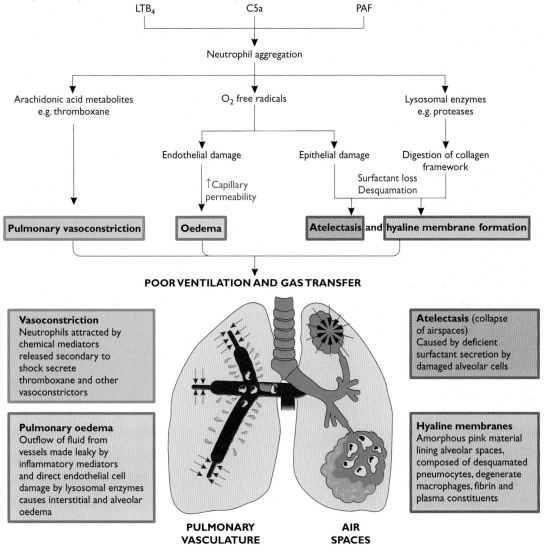

arterial territories (Fig. 9.15). This may result in severe permanent cerebral damage or coma and death. It is important to remember that the 'watershed' effect operates in many organs if there is poor perfusion. In the heart, this is the subendothelial zone because the endocardium is nourished by direct diffusion from the blood in the cardiac chambers and the outer myocardium is supplied by arterioles penetrating from the outside. In the gut, areas such as the splenic flexure of the colon are at the boundary between arterial supplies and vulnerable to poor perfusion.

STROKES

As we reach the end of the section on cardiovascular disorders, it is a good moment to discuss 'strokes'. To understand 'strokes', you need to pull together the topics we have covered in these three sections: namely, thrombosis, embolism, atherosclerosis, hypertension, aneurysms and circulatory failure. So what is the clinical picture? Very variable is the answer because different areas of the brain perform very distinct functions and

Figure 9.13 Lung photomicrograph showing adult respiratory distress syndrome. There is irregular ventilation due to the presence of hyaline membranes, exudate and cell debris within the alveolar spaces

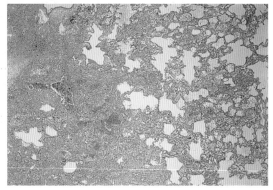

the patient's symptoms and signs will depend on the location of the damage.

First, a definition: *A stroke is a sudden loss of some cerebral function due to a vascular lesion.* It is usual to exclude haemorrhage caused by trauma (subdural and extradural haemorrhage) and to exclude global loss of function as might occur with generalized hypoxia or hypoperfusion (e.g. brain damage secondary to a cardiac arrest). If the loss of function lasts for less than 24 hours, it is called a transient ischaemic attack (TIA).

Second: *Are strokes a significant cause of death and disability?*

Approximately 10 per cent of deaths are due to stroke, which puts it in the top five causes of death. In the USA, there are approximately half a million cases of stroke each year. Roughly half will die and, of the remainder, half will have permanent significant disability. Around a third of strokes occur in people under 65 years of age. Thus, any intervention that can reduce the incidence or severity of strokes can have a major impact.

Third: *What is the commonest type of stroke?*

Strokes occur when cerebral tissue is deprived of its blood supply. This is most commonly *ischaemic* in nature (80 per cent or more) due to blockage of an artery by thrombus (50 per cent or more) or embolus (30 per cent or more). You already know about the causes of thrombosis and the importance of unstable atheromatous plaques (see page 214) and the types and sources of emboli (see page 180). Most other strokes are due to *haemorrhage*, which can be intracerebral (about 10 per cent) or subarachnoid (about 5 per cent) and are associated with aneurysms (see page 207). Around 80 per cent of intracerebral haemorrhages occur in the presence of hypertension. See Fig. 9.16.

History   Johannes Purkinje (1787–1869)

Johannes Purkinje was a Bohemian physiologist who, while still a medical student, produced classical descriptions of acute poisoning with belladonna, camphor and ipecac after experimenting on himself! He became interested in all aspects of sight and developed animated cartoons that were the forerunner of movies, described the visual hallucinations of digitalis and belladonna, recognized the value of dreams as an indicator of personality and used the swings and merry-go-rounds of Prague amusement park to investigate vertigo. Outside of work, he translated the works of Shakespeare, Tasso and Schiller into Czech.

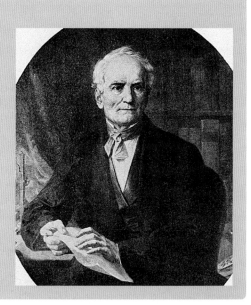

Figure 9.14 Johannes Purkinje (Reproduced with permission from Wellcome Library, London)

Figure 9.15 **Watershed zones.** The brain, heart and colon are particularly at risk of ischaemic damage as they receive oxygenated blood from the most peripheral branches of supplying arteries with no territorial overlap. This supply can be compromised by hypotension, often due to shock. The regions affected in the brain are shown here. In the heart, subendocardial infarction may occur at the boundary between the peripheral myocardial blood supply from the coronary arteries and direct diffusion from the endocardial side (see Fig. 8.4). In the colon, the splenic flexure lies at the boundary between the inferior mesenteric and superior rectal arteries

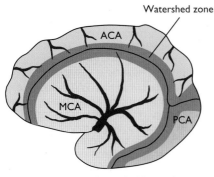

Lateral aspect of left cerebral hemisphere

Key:

MCA   Middle cerebral artery
ACA   Anterior cerebral artery
PCA   Posterior cerebral artery

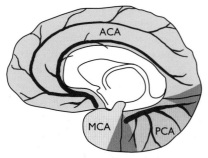

Medial aspect of right cerebral hemisphere

CEREBRAL BLOOD SUPPLY AND STROKES

The clinical effect of a disease process will depend on how well the body can respond to the insult. With vascular problems affecting the brain, this is influenced by the vascular anatomy and so it is time to revise some basic facts. You will recall that some vessels are end arteries and blockage will lead to infarction of a clearly defined tissue segment (see Fig. 1.10 for kidney and

Fig. 1.13 for heart). In the brain, the small cerebral vessels are end arteries but the others are not and, to a greater or lesser extent, may compensate for blockage through being part of a collateral circulation.

The brain receives blood through two internal carotid arteries and two vertebral arteries. The two vertebral arteries join to become the basilar artery which, with the two internal carotid arteries, feeds the Circle of Willis at the base of the brain (Fig. 9.17). If the Circle of Willis is anatomically normal and free from significant atheroma, it can be an effective collateral route, such that one internal carotid artery can be totally blocked without causing damage. Blockage of the vertebro-basilar system, however, is less easy to compensate for.

The blood supply to the brain has two other unusual features. One is the effect of brain swelling (cerebral oedema) and the other is the ability to respond to and protect the brain from the effects of high or low blood pressure (autoregulation). The brain is encased in a hard, non-elastic structure (the bony skull) which has some fibrous internal dividing walls (tentorium cerebelli and falx cerebri) and one significant opening (foramen magnum). If a part of the brain increases in size, a so-called space-occupying lesion, then it presses on adjacent structures and may interrupt the blood supply directly or by herniation. For example, tentorial herniation can stop flow in the posterior cerebral or superior cerebellar arteries. The swelling that accompanies infarction can cause this. See Fig. 9.18.

> **Dictionary**
> **Hernia:** a protrusion of part of an organ through an aperture

Autoregulation refers to changes in the resistance of cerebral arterioles in response to changes in blood pressure. This is believed to be able to compensate for systolic blood pressures as low as 50 mmHg (as in 'shock') or as high as 160 mmHg in normal individuals and is an example of effective homeostasis. However, this mechanism is disturbed after strokes, head injury or anaesthesia.

Transient ischaemic attacks have similar causes to ischaemic strokes and indicate an increased likelihood of having a stroke of anything from 10 to 50 per cent. The main mechanisms are poor perfusion due to sudden cardiac problems or thromboembolism. Their

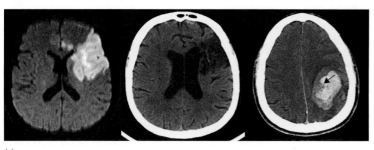

(a)

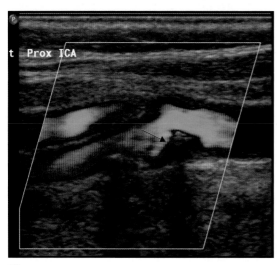

(b)

Figure 9.16 (a) Brain scans from patients with two types of stroke. Left: MRI scan showing an acute thromboembolic stroke, viewed within 2 hours of the event, which shows multifocal areas of infarction. This is diffusion weighted imaging (DWI) which looks at the mobility of water molecules in tissue. The bright areas on the image reflect areas of restricted water movement, in effect mapping areas of cytotoxic oedema. Middle: A CT scan from this patient 2 weeks later shows the area of infarction as a dark area with loss of volume in that part of the brain. Right: CT scan in a different patient with acute right hemiplegia showing a haemorrhagic infarct in the left middle cerebral artery territory. Acute haemorrhage is bright on CT (blue arrow). (b) A colour Doppler ultrasound of the left internal carotid artery (ICA) origin shows plaque at the origin of the ICA (black arrow)

recognition is particularly important now that preventative treatment is becoming more effective (see below).

WHO IS MOST LIKELY TO HAVE A STROKE AND HOW CAN THEY BE PREVENTED?

You have already worked through the risk factors and preventative measures for coronary artery disease (page 198) and you should not be surprised to learn that they are similar for cerebrovascular disease. That is the advantage of understanding the key mechanisms of disease; once the principles are appreciated they can be applied to other situations. Combining the factors for thromboembolism, hypertension and atherosclerosis will give you the main pointers for stroke. For example, there is correlation between non-haemorrhagic stroke and raised serum total cholesterol, LDL cholesterol and triglycerides and lowered HDL cholesterol, i.e. the factors important in atherosclerosis. The treatment is, predictably, a combination of lifestyle, diet, exercise,

smoking cessation, statins, anti-thrombotic agents and anti-hypertensive therapy. For the acute event, prompt revascularization is important but may be difficult to achieve.

Ischaemic strokes are predominantly a consequence of acute events in unstable atheromatous plaques, with the important factors being the same as those for acute coronary syndromes, i.e. fibrous cap stability, size of lipid core and degree of inflammation. Ruptured carotid plaques are more likely than smooth plaques to be associated with future *coronary* events, which suggests that plaque instability is a systemic phenomenon. Thus, assessment of the carotid arteries with modern imaging techniques could allow us to identify and treat those most at risk of acute vascular events in any area of the body. Possibilities include ulceration of the plaque surface on conventional arterial angiography, ultrasound to identify lipid-rich echolucent plaques, magnetic resonance imaging to assess the lipid core and

Figure 9.17 The Circle of Willis is an anastomosing complex of arteries at the base of the brain, derived from the right and left internal carotid and vertebral arteries, linked by the anterior and posterior communicating arteries. Three major branches, the anterior, posterior and middle cerebral arteries, supply each side of the brain. Despite the anastomoses proximally, the distal branches have no alternative routes for blood flow so obstruction of small vessels by thromboembolus leads to ischaemic stroke. Patients with hypertension are at risk of haemorrhagic stroke, related to intracerebral haemorrhage from a microaneurysm. Microaneurysms differ from berry aneurysms, which cause subarachnoid haemorrhage

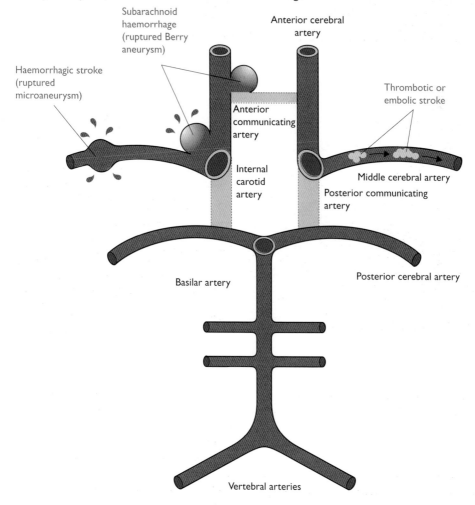

intra-plaque haemorrhage and positron emission tomography and molecular radiolabelling to quantify macrophage infiltration.

That brings us nearly to the end of this section on circulatory disorders. We started with the words of William Harvey, conveying his despair at trying to understand the physiology of the motions of the heart. Physiology and pathology are of fundamental importance in clinical medicine and the words of Sir William

Osler, perhaps the greatest physician of recent times, provide an appropriate ending:

A man cannot become a competent surgeon without the full knowledge of human anatomy and physiology, and the physician without physiology and chemistry flounders along in an aimless fashion, never able to gain any accurate conception of disease, practising a sort of popgun pharmacy, hitting now the malady and again the patient, he himself not knowing which.

Figure 9.18 **Sites of herniation in the brain**

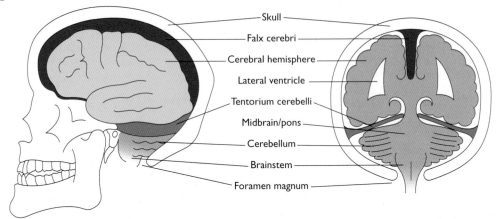

Skull
Falx cerebri
Cerebral hemisphere
Lateral ventricle
Tentorium cerebelli
Midbrain/pons
Cerebellum
Brainstem
Foramen magnum

(a) Sagittal section of a skull with a slightly shrunken brain, revealing part of the falx cerebri and tentorium cerebelli

(b) Coronal section through the skull

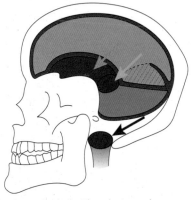

(c) Sagittal section of a skull with no brain, to show dural folds and possible sites of herniation

There are three main sites at which herniation of the brain can occur in response to a space occupying lesion in the brain

Beneath the FALX CEREBRI (pink arrow)

Through the TENTORIUM CEREBELLI (yellow arrow)

Through the FORAMEN MAGNUM (red arrow)

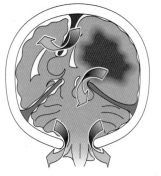

(d) Coronal section through a head containing a space occupying lesion in one cerebral hemisphere

The **falx cerebri** separates the cerebral hemispheres. Superior and inferior sagittal veins run within the fixed and free borders respectively. The corpus callosum passes beneath the falx to unite the hemispheres. The cingulate gyrus may be displaced laterally. The free edge is usually also displaced and the ventricles compressed.

The **tentorium cerebelli** separates the cerebellum from the cerebral hemispheres. The midbrain passes through the space anterior to the free border and may be displaced inferiorly.

The **forum magnum** provides the exit hole for the spinal cord, which is sheathed in tough dura mater in the spinal canal. Tonsillar herniation occurs when the cerebellar tonsils are pushed through the skull and death by 'coning' occurs when the vital centres in the brainstem are compressed.

History   William Osler (1849–1919)

Many people believe that Sir William Osler was the most loved and the greatest physician of recent times. This was not for his scientific contribution but for his ability to fascinate the young students and for completely transforming medical education and clinical medical training.

Osler was born at Bond Head, Ontario, Canada. His parents were English missionaries who had migrated to Canada. He was the youngest of nine children. His initial intention was to follow his father into the church and he started his studies at Trinity College, Toronto. He changed his mind, however, and enrolled at the Toronto Medical School in 1868. He finished his medical education at McGill University. Having qualified, he spent the next 2 years travelling around Europe, the longest period being spent with Sir John Burdon-Sanderson at University College, London.

He returned to Canada with the intention of entering general practice but within a few months was appointed lecturer in medicine at McGill. He taught physiology and pathology to the medical students. The following year he was appointed professor. After a decade in Montreal, he went as Professor of Medicine to Pennsylvania and in 1888, he accepted a post at the new John Hopkins Hospital in Baltimore. He was the second of the famous 'Hopkins four', the others being William Welch, chief of pathology, Howard Kelley, chief of obstetrics and gynaecology and William Halstead, chief of surgery. It was with these three colleagues that Osler revolutionized the medical curriculum.

Figure 9.19 Sir William Osler (Reproduced with permission from Wellcome Library, London)

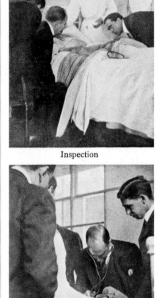
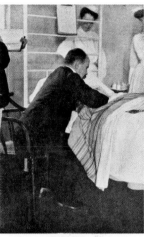
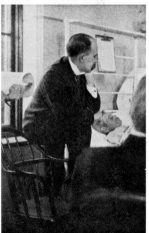

Inspection   Palpation

Auscultation   Contemplation

SNAPSHOTS OF OSLER AT THE BEDSIDE

From snapshots taken by T.W.Clarke

For the first 4 years at the John Hopkins, there were no medical students and Osler used these years to write *The Principles and Practice of Medicine*, first published in 1892.

In 1904, while visiting the UK, he was offered the Regius Chair of Medicine at Oxford. This was to succeed Burdon-Sanderson. Osler accepted and started his post in 1905.

Osler's name is associated with three medical conditions: Osler's nodes (tender, red swellings on the palms and fingers in bacterial endocarditis), Osler–Vaquez disease (polycythaemia rubra vera) and the Rendu–Osler–Weber disease (recurrent haemorrhages from multiple telengectasias in skin and mucous membranes).

Osler has written a lot about almost everything, and especially so about the relationship between the teacher and student, teacher and teacher, and teacher and patient. The quotation at the end of page 233 is from his book, *Counsels and Ideals from the Writings of Sir William Osler*, 1905.

Clinicopathological case study   circulatory failure

Clinical

A 65-year-old man complains of transient loss of vision in his right eye. He had two episodes in the previous month, each lasting for approximately 7–10 minutes. Two months ago, he also had transient slurring of his speech.

Pathology

Transient loss of vision or speech with full recovery is called a transient ischaemic attack. Generally it results from an embolus lodging in a small cerebral vessel and then being displaced or lysed. The commonest sites of origin are the heart or the carotid vessels.

Examination

Blood pressure 180/110.
Displaced apex beat and ejection systolic murmur.

He is hypertensive with an enlarged heart, i.e. left ventricular hypertrophy in response to increased workload.

Carotid bruits present.

The bruits indicate turbulent flow which is a result of stenosis and/or irregularities of the vessel wall due to atheroma.

No peripheral pulses palpable below the femorals.

Absent peripheral pulses indicate widespread arteriosclerotic disease.

Chest X-ray confirmed cardiomegaly but with no evidence of pulmonary oedema.

The presence of pulmonary oedema would have indicated cardiac failure.

An ECG showed atrial fibrillation and features of an old anterior infarction.

In atrial fibrillation, atria do not contract. The resultant stagnation of blood predisposes to thrombus formation.

An echocardiogram demonstrated thrombus within the left atrium.

Thrombus within the left atrium can be thrown into the systemic circulation. These can pass through the carotids to lodge in the cerebral vessels.

Carotid Doppler studies indicated moderate carotid artery stenosis.

Doppler studies detect turbulent flow. It is the electronic equivalent of the bruit.

Urine analysis: no glucose detected.

A simple test for diabetes. Diabetics are at high risk of atheroma and may also suffer from sudden temporary loss of consciousness.

Blood tests: serial cardiac markers, normal

Test for myocardial infarction.

Urea and creatinine: slightly raised

Mild renal impairment probably due to hypertension and atheroma

Management and progress

It was decided that he should be treated with antihypertensive agents to reduce his blood pressure and anticoagulants to reduce the risk of further thrombosis/embolism. However, within 24 hours, he developed a right-sided weakness with hemiplegia and a right extensor plantar response. He died without regaining consciousness.

The signs are of upper motor neurone damage involving the motor and sensory pathways with loss of consciousness. He has sustained a large left-sided cerebrovascular accident. The neural pathways cross, hence left-sided lesions give right-sided signs.

Postmortem findings:

Cardiovascular system – left ventricular hypertrophy. Atheroma in all three coronary arteries with an old anterior infarction. No evidence of recent infarct and no vegetations. A small amount of thrombus present in the left atrium. Extensive atheroma in aorta and carotids with narrowing of the mouth of the renal arteries.

Central nervous system – a large haematoma in the region of the left internal capsule. Extensive atheroma in the cerebral vessels.

Genito-urinary tract – small scarred kidneys showing ischaemic damage.

Clinically, the stroke could have been due to an embolus but, in his case, it was a result of rupture of a microaneurysm on the lenticulostriate branch of the middle cerebral, due to hypertension. These are called Charcot–Buchard aneurysms.

PART 4

CELL GROWTH AND ITS DISORDERS

Introduction: A brief history of cancer 241

Chapter 10: Benign growth disorders **243**

Clinical case: prostatic disease 243
Hyperplasia and hypertrophy 243
Atrophy 244
Metaplasia and dysplasia 246
Benign neoplasms 249

Chapter 11: Malignant neoplasms **251**

Clinical case: breast lump 251
Clinical features of malignant
tumours 251
Classification of tumours 259

Chapter 12: What causes cancer? **263**

Cancer as a disease of genetic
material 263
Risk factors for cancer 263
Summary 272

Chapter 13: Molecular genetics of
cancer **273**

Cytogenetics 273
Cancer-producing genes:
oncogenes 273
How can oncogenes promote
cell growth? 276
Mode of action of dominant
oncogenes 277

Tumour suppressor genes/
recessive oncogenes 279
DNA repair, apoptosis, telomeres,
telomerases and cancer 284
Which cell in the tissue gives
rise to cancer? 287
The multistep model for
carcinogenesis 287
Molecular methodology 289
Conclusion 290

Chapter 14: The behaviour of
tumours **291**

Tumour growth 291
How do tumours spread? 291
The role of the immune
system 296

Chapter 15: The clinical effects of
tumours **297**

Local effects 297
Endocrine effects 299
Paraneoplastic syndromes 300
General effects 301
Management of cancer 301
Conclusion 304
Clinicopathological case study:
cervical cancer 305

Does early death come
As a punishment?
Or
Does it come too late,
For those who are tortured
By incurable pain?
Is death really cruel?
Or
Is it merciful?

Gitanjali (1961–1977)

Gitanjali, as beautiful as the poem by Rabindranath Tagore, died at the age of 16 of cancer. To many people, cancer is a disease that appears suddenly, takes a tight grip, progresses relentlessly and causes a slow and painful death.

In 1731, Lorenz Heister, a German surgeon, wrote: 'The name *Scirrhus* is given to a painless tumour that occurs in all parts of the body, but especially in the glands, and is due to stagnation and drying of the blood in the hardened part. ... When a schirrus is not reabsorbed, cannot be arrested, or is not removed by time, it either spontaneously or from maltreatment becomes malignant, that is, painful and inflamed, and then we begin to call it *cancer* or *carcinoma*; at the same time the veins swell up and distend like the feet of a crab (but this does not happen in all cases), whence the disease gets its name; it is in fact, one of the worst, most horrible, and most painful of diseases.'

Is this pessimism really justified?

It is easy to forget that everything that comes to life dies: death is an integral part of life. There is a huge amount of large scale and impersonal death portrayed on television but few children in Western society ever see or discuss death at the individual and personal level. The obsession of society to seek all kinds of 'pleasure' has led to a world that is fearful of death (a final and definitive deprivation of pleasure) and hence the word 'pain' is seldom far from the word 'death'. Although about 20% of people will die of cancer, this is less than the number dying from cardiovascular disease (approximately 30%), but heart disease does not usually generate such intense dread.

Interesting? Perhaps death from cancer is seen as 'unfair' and therefore painful but death from a heart attack is seen as self-induced by over-eating and smoking and therefore 'deserved'?

A BRIEF HISTORY OF CANCER

Johannes Müller, a German microscopist, established that tumours were made of cells (1883). This laid the foundation for his pupil, Rudolf Virchow, who divided tumours into 'homologous' and 'heterologous'. The homologous group resulted from proliferation of cells already present and were generally benign, while the heterologous group showed a change in the character of the cell and were generally malignant. Virchow, however, failed to recognize the mechanism of metastasis which was later described by Billroth (1856) and von Recklinhausen (1883).

Many investigators have looked for causes of cancer. One of the most famous was Percival Pott who, in 1775, identified that scrotal cancer in chimney sweeps was related to chronic contact with soot. Occupational exposure to industrial tar and paraffin was recognized by von Volkmann in 1875 as causing cancers and many such associations have since been described. Recently, advances in molecular and cell biology techniques have facilitated the investigation of these associations at the level of genetic material. We are now in a position to attempt to answer some of the fundamental questions relating to the control of normal growth and differentiation and how these mechanisms go wrong in the process of neoplasia.

In this section, we shall consider the benign disorders of cell growth and the premalignant changes which are clues of early cancer and are important in screening programmes. We will go on to look at the symptoms which occur in cancer, how it is diagnosed and which features are important for prognosis and treatment. Then we will turn to the aetiology (causes of cancer) and the pathogenesis (natural history) of tumours, and finally, how they behave and what treatments are available. Perhaps at the end, you will be able to ask yourself again whether our social and cultural views about cancer, about death and about pain are justified.

CHAPTER 10

Cells have to adapt to any changes in nutrient supply or workload in order to survive and continue performing their cellular function, i.e to maintain homeostasis.

These adaptations take place at both the cellular and sub-cellular levels. We will discuss these adaptations with an emphasis on the changes that are important in pathology, and we will consider the clinical situations in which they are encountered. The changes that we will discuss are: hyperplasia, hypertrophy, atrophy, metaplasia, dysplasia and benign neoplasms.

CLINICAL CASE: PROSTATIC DISEASE

A 70-year-old man visited the urology clinic complaining of difficulty with micturition. He passed urine 15–20 times per day and several times during the night (nocturia). The stream of urine was poor and he found that on some occasions it dribbled. The urologist detected an enlarged prostate on rectal examination and the patient had part of his prostate removed to improve the flow.

Some of you may be wondering why an enlarged prostate obstructing urine flow through the urethra should result in increased urinary frequency. The reason (as indicated in Fig. 10.1) is that the enlarged median lobe protrudes into the bladder to produce a dam behind which some urine stagnates. This means that after micturition there is still urine in the bladder and the patient feels the urge to pass urine again. The stagnant urine is also prone to infection or stone formation. The poor urine flow is due to narrowing of the prostatic urethra and the 'ball valve' effect of the median lobe pressing forward on the urethral orifice.

HYPERPLASIA AND HYPERTROPHY

Hyperplasia is defined as an increase in the *number* of cells in an organ or tissue, while hypertrophy is an

Figure 10.1 Macroscopic specimen with prostatic hyperplasia and bladder showing numerous trabeculae due to urinary obstruction by a nodular enlarged prostate (see also Fig. 10.2)

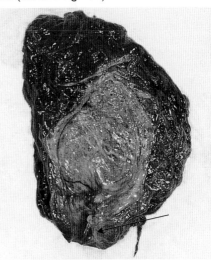

increase in *cell size*. Often the two co-exist in a tissue because some cell types are incapable of division and so must increase their size (hypertrophy) to cope with any extra work while other cells can proliferate to share their additional work (hyperplasia). In chapter 5 on healing and repair (page 125), we noted that cardiac and skeletal muscle and nerve cells have limited potential to replicate whereas epithelial cells and fibroblasts do so easily. Smooth muscle cells can respond by a combination of hyperplasia and hypertrophy. This means that in the prostate the glandular epithelium and the fibroblastic stroma will show hyperplasia and the smooth muscle is hypertrophic and hyperplastic. Why should the prostate enlarge with age, since its workload does not increase? Presumably there is an over-reaction to years of androgen stimulation but nobody really knows.

When the hypertrophy or hyperplasia is useful, i.e. it allows the organ to cope with extra work, it is called physiological. If the enlargement does not appear to serve a purpose, then it is termed pathological. Thus the prostatic changes would be pathological. Physiological hyperplasia and hypertrophy may be mediated through hormonal changes or growth factors. Pregnancy is an example of hormone-induced hyperplasia and hypertrophy that allows an organ the size of a pear to enlarge to accommodate a full term baby and prepares the breasts for lactation. The smooth muscle cells of the uterus enlarge (hypertrophy and hyperplasia) ready for the work of pushing the baby into the world (aptly named 'labour') and the number of glandular milk-producing cells in the breast increases (hyperplasia).

Figure 10.2 **Photomicrograph showing nodular hyperplasia of the prostate**

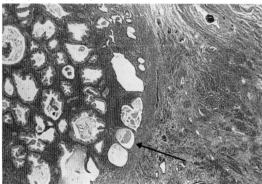

A fascinating example of physiological hyperplasia that occurs in the body is the regeneration of the liver following partial hepatectomy. There is a fascinating Greek myth about it. Prometheus, who was Atlas's brother, had incurred the wrath of the mighty Zeus.

In anger, Zeus had Prometheus chained naked to a pillar in the Caucasian mountains where an eagle tore at his liver all day, year in, year out; and there was no end to his pain. The reason was that the liver grew back each night! It is not recommended that you try this experiment. The evidence suggests that the remaining liver produces various growth factors and cytokines including, transforming growth factor-alpha (TGF-α), hepatocyte growth factor (HGF) and interleukin 6 (IL-6) which causes an increase in mitotic activity and hence an increase in the cell number. What is remarkable is that it knows when to stop! It is believed that growth inhibitors such as transforming growth factor-beta (TGF-β) and interleukin 1 (IL-1) are involved in this process. The ancient Greeks had remarkable insights into the body's capacity to regenerate.

ATROPHY

Atrophy is defined as a decrease in *cell size* and/or *cell number*. Extra cells are lost through the process of apoptosis

Figure 10.3 **The Ancient Greeks appreciated the body's capacity for liver regeneration. Prometheus was punished by Zeus for bringing fire to humanity. Every night for years his liver was torn at by an eagle**

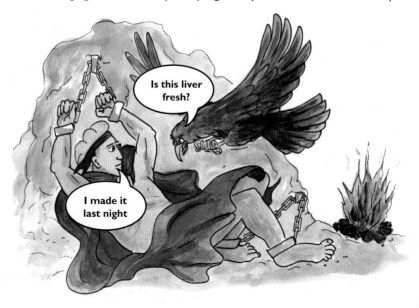

described in chapter 1. Strictly speaking, the reduction in *cell numbers* is called involution. Since this is part of normal development, it is termed physiological atrophy and the classic example is the involution of the thymus gland during development. It is distinguished from pathological atrophy which results from an abnormal state. An example of pathological atrophy is the severe muscle wasting that may follow an episode of poliomyelitis or the muscle wasting that is commonly observed in limbs immobilized in plaster following a fracture. See Fig. 10.4.

Key facts

Examples of hyperplasia and hypertrophy and their causative factors

- Hypertrophy of myocardium due to hypertension
- Skeletal muscular hypertrophy due to exercise
- Red-cell hyperplasia in bone marrow secondary to low atmospheric oxygen (living at high altitude)
- Uterine hyperplasia/hypertrophy secondary to hormonal changes of pregnancy
- Hyperplasia of epidermis and connective tissue due to release of growth factors to aid wound healing

Key facts

Causes of atrophy

Decreased functional demand
loss of hormone stimulation
decreased physical exercise
immobilization of limb following fracture

Loss of blood supply
injury to blood vessel
decreased flow – atheromatous occlusion

Loss of innervation
transection of nerve fibres
infective/inflammatory disorders, e.g. polio

Developmental
decrease in thymic size with age
atrophy of ductus arteriosus

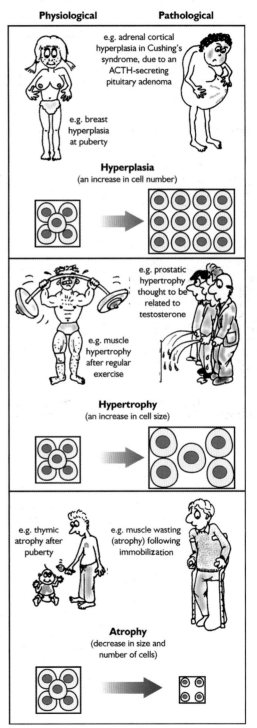

Figure 10.4 Hyperplasia, hypertrophy and atrophy may represent physiological responses to normal development or a pathological change in response to a disease process

Figure 10.5 In smokers, the normal ciliated columnar epithelium lining the bronchus undergoes metaplasia to stratified squamous epithelium. This confers greater protection against heat damage. Metaplasia is reversible if the stimulus is removed. Metaplasia is not a premalignant condition, but areas in which metaplasia occurs are at increased risk of developing dysplasia, which is premalignant. In this example, carcinogens in the cigarette smoke may induce mutations in the exposed, rapidly dividing epithelial cells (see also Fig. 10.6)

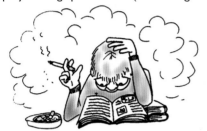

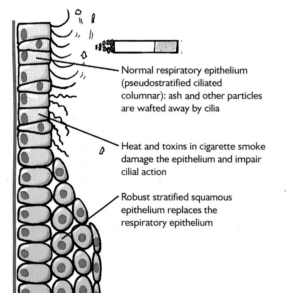

Normal respiratory epithelium (pseudostratified ciliated columnar): ash and other particles are wafted away by cilia

Heat and toxins in cigarette smoke damage the epithelium and impair cilial action

Robust stratified squamous epithelium replaces the respiratory epithelium

METAPLASIA AND DYSPLASIA

The uterine cervix serves as a useful model for this discussion of metaplasia and dysplasia. The changes in the cervix are now well documented because of national programmes designed to screen women of reproductive age to detect early changes associated with cancer. Screening involves scraping some cells from the junctional zone of the cervix using a spatula. These are generally spread onto a glass slide, fixed and stained by the

Figure 10.6 **Photomicrograph showing squamous metaplasia of endocervical glands**

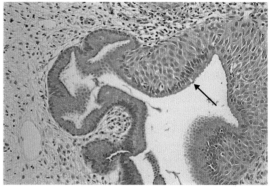

Papanicolaou technique. Liquid-phase cytology is also increasingly being used.

The cervix has a transitional zone between the squamous epithelium of the ectocervix and the columnar epithelium of the endocervix. If there is chronic inflammation of the cervix, the columnar epithelium may be replaced by squamous epithelium, so-called 'squamous metaplasia'. Other examples include 'intestinal metaplasia' in the stomach and 'Barrett's metaplasia' of the oesophagus where the squamous epithelium is replaced by gastric type tissue. Metaplasia is the *conversion of one type of differentiated tissue into another type of differentiated tissue*. This is most common in epithelial tissue although it can occur in other types of tissues such as mesenchymal tissues. Generally, it is a response to chronic irritation and is a form of adaptation which involves, for example, replacing a specialized glandular or respiratory epithelium with a more hardy squamous epithelium (Fig. 10.5). It is worth noting that the metaplasia probably occurs at the level of the tissue-specific stem cell as the metaplastic process leads to the production of a number of cell types characterizing that particular tissue. Hence the process occurs at the *tissue* level. The conversion of one *cell* into another is referred to as *transdifferentiation* rather than metaplasia. Currently little is known about the molecular mechanisms involved in this process; however, Cdx1 and 2 transcription-factor genes are believed to be important in intestinal metaplasia.

Metaplasia itself is generally an adaptive, benign and reversible process but its importance lies in the fact that the stimulants and irritants causing the metaplasia may persist and play a role in carcinogenesis (Fig. 10.7).

Figure 10.7 **Effects of stopping smoking at various ages on the cumulative risk (per cent) of death from lung cancer by age 75 (© Cancer Research Campaign 2001)**

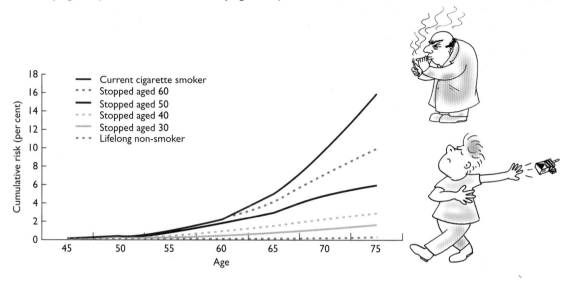

The exfoliated cervical cells in a smear may show dysplasia, which is more worrying because it is a step on the road to an invasive tumour. The term dysplasia was originally used to mean an abnormality of development. Unfortunately, it is a term that is used too loosely and this causes confusion. In pathology reports concerning the microscopy of tissues, dysplasia refers to a combination of abnormal cytological appearances and abnormal tissue architecture. Its importance lies in its precancerous association. However, the term is still used to describe some gross abnormalities of development encountered in neonatal pathology, such as renal dysplasia and broncho-pulmonary dysplasia, which have no precancerous association.

Dysplasia in the cervical squamous epithelium involves an increased cell size, nuclear pleomorphism (variation in size and shape), hyperchromatism (increased blueness due to abnormal chromatin), loss of orientation of the cells so that they are arranged rather haphazardly and abnormally sited mitotic activity (Figs 10.8 and 10.9).

Of course, these appearances are the same as those described in malignant change but they differ in *extent*. When the full thickness of the epithelium is involved, it can be called 'carcinoma *in situ*' while involvement of only the lower third is 'mild dysplasia'. Many pathologists and clinicians felt that it was inappropriate to have different names for the various stages and so the term 'cervical intra-epithelial neoplasia' (CIN) was introduced. CIN

I is the equivalent of mild dysplasia and describes abnormalities affecting the lower third of the epithelium, CIN II (replacing moderate dysplasia) is used for changes reaching the middle third, and CIN III (replacing severe dysplasia or carcinoma *in situ*) refers to full thickness involvement. Similar terminology can be used for changes in the squamous epithelium of the vulva (VIN) and larynx (LIN), although *glandular* epithelial changes (e.g. stomach or large bowel) are usually subdivided into mild, moderate or severe dysplasia. There is a move to simplify it further by dividing into low and high grade types. A potential problem with the terminology is that it implies a biological continuum from low grade (CIN I) to high grade lesions (CIN III), which may not be true. In some organ systems such as breast, it is clear that in most cases, high grade *in situ* carcinoma does not develop from low grade *in situ* carcinoma.

It should not be assumed that dysplasia is irreversible. It is believed that early stages of dysplasia may revert to normal if the stimulus is removed. However, severe dysplasia will often progress to cancer if left untreated and, for this reason, it is sometimes referred to as carcinoma *in situ*.

If severe dysplasia is cancer confined to the epithelium, what are moderate and mild dysplasia? This is a good question and without a 'correct' answer. In practice, severe dysplasia is treated as a favourable type of cancer, while milder degrees of dysplasia can be managed

Figure 10.8 Dysplasia is a precursor lesion to squamous cell carcinoma of the cervix and is invariably associated with wart virus (human papillomavirus) infection. (a) Medium-power photomicrograph of a cervix with warty change; this is 'koilocytosis', recognized microscopically as a halo effect around the nucleus (thick arrow), which appears spiky (thin arrow). (b) Dysplasia is classified as CIN I, II or III (cervical intraepithelial neoplasia), depending on the degree of nuclear atypia seen. Nuclear atypical changes predominate in the lower one-third of the epithelium in CIN I and throughout all layers in CIN III. CIN III carries a very much higher risk of progression to cancer than CIN I or II

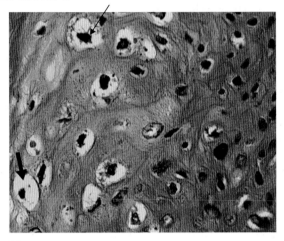

(a)

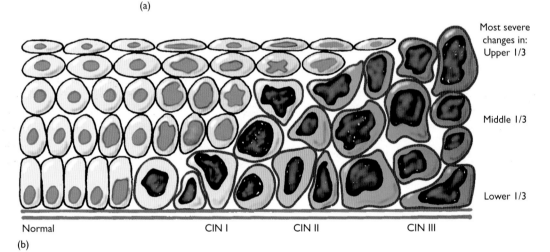

Most severe changes in:
Upper 1/3

Middle 1/3

Lower 1/3

Normal   CIN I   CIN II   CIN III

(b)

Figure 10.9 Dysplasia involving endocervical glands

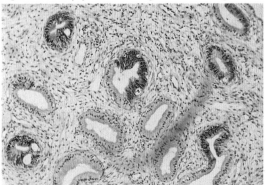

slightly less aggressively but followed to ensure that they do not progress to more severe disease.

The concept of dysplasia fits with our current multi-step theory of neoplasia (see page 287) in that it represents a stage between benign hyperplastic proliferation and overt cancer. The concept of dysplasia as a cancer in its early stages has also led to the institution of screening programmes for cervical and breast carcinoma. The logic behind this is that if dysplastic changes precede carcinoma by several months or years, and patients with dysplasia can be identified and treated, we can reduce the death toll from that cancer. Obviously, deaths from that cancer must be fairly common to make this worthwhile and we must be confident that the 'at risk' group are being screened sufficiently often to detect the early changes.

For example, if the progression from CIN II to invasive tumour took only one year, then it would be of limited value to screen patients every three years. Much of the interest in genetic and immunocytochemical markers of malignancy lies in the hope that they will be able to detect ever earlier precancerous changes to increase the potential benefits of such screening programmes.

There can be little doubt that the cervical screening programme has been effective in reducing mortality and there is some benefit from the breast programme but whether they are cost-effective remains a moot point. However, there is little doubt that it has led to an improvement in the quality of radiological, pathological and clinical services. This is an important health issue and worth thinking about and discussing with your colleagues. What would you do if you were the Minister of Health?

BENIGN NEOPLASMS

A neoplasm is defined as a new and abnormal growth and particularly one in which the cell division is uncontrolled and progressive. Neoplasms may be benign or malignant. We will deal with malignant neoplasms in the next chapter.

A benign neoplasm, such as an adenoma in the colon, is an uncontrolled focal proliferation of well-differentiated cells which does not invade or metastasize. Unfortunately, the term is sometimes used inaccurately and some tumours do not quite fulfill these criteria, but it will serve as a working definition. Although benign, these tumours can cause many clinical problems as discussed in the section on the local effects of tumours (page 1).

One of the commonest benign tumours necessitating removal is the leiomyoma (fibroid) of the uterine myometrium which may contribute to heavy and painful menstruation (Fig. 10.10). Benign melanocytic tumours of the skin are removed for cosmetic reasons or fear of malignant change (Fig. 10.11). Endocrine tumours are generally benign but can cause dramatic systemic problems through excessive production of hormones (Fig. 10.12; see also page 299), and some 'benign' intracranial tumours like meningiomas can kill the patient because the skull cannot stretch to accommodate the 'benign' expansion. Remember that something which is 'benign' to the pathologist may appear 'malignant' to the patient!

HYPERPLASIA AND HYPERTROPHY VERSUS BENIGN NEOPLASMS

The difference between a benign neoplasm and hypertrophy/hyperplasia is that the neoplasm, by definition, exhibits *uncontrolled* cell proliferation. This is unlike hyperplasia and hypertrophy where the growth, either due to increase in cell numbers or cell size, is an adaptive response to a stimulus and removal of this stimulus results in regression.

Figure 10.10 **Benign leiomyoma**

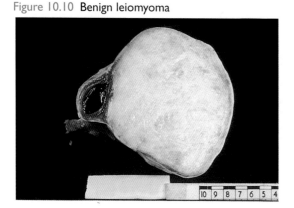

Figure 10.11 **Benign naevi**

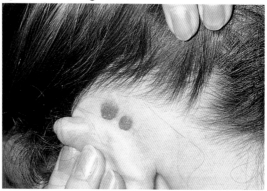

Figure 10.12 A comparison of the effects of hormone-secreting tumours on cortisol and ACTH (adrenocorticotrophic) levels in the blood and the way in which the dexamethasone test can help to distinguish between the causative lesions. Adenoma is a benign glandular tumour; small-cell lung carcinoma is a malignant tumour of probable neuroectodermal origin

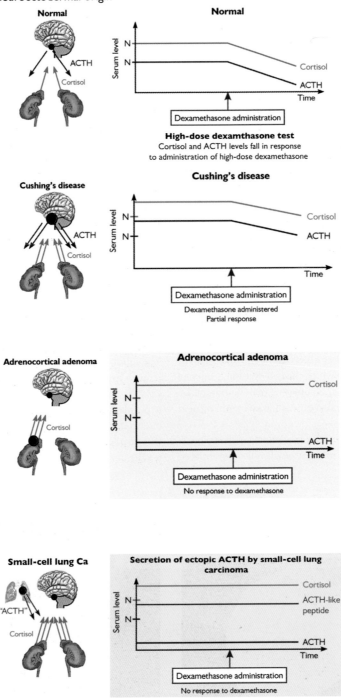

CHAPTER 11

MALIGNANT NEOPLASMS

CLINICAL CASE: BREAST LUMP

A 50-year-old woman presented to her family doctor with a lump in her left breast. She had noticed a recent enlargement in its size but the mass was not painful. She had no other medical problems but she had a positive family history, her mother having died of breast cancer 5 years previously. She had two daughters aged 27 and 25 years who were both well.

Her family doctor could feel a 2 cm diameter mass below the nipple in her left breast. This was hard, poorly defined and caused dimpling of the overlying skin. It was also fixed to the underlying tissues. The nipple and areola on that side had an eczematous appearance but the right breast and nipple were normal. He did not find any enlarged lymph nodes in either axilla or supraclavicular fossa and no abnormalities in the rest of the body. The family practitioner suspected that this was a malignant tumour and so referred her to hospital for further investigation.

But why did the family doctor consider that this mass was malignant?

CLINICAL FEATURES OF MALIGNANT TUMOURS

It should be stressed that it was not a single criterion but a combination of factors that allowed him to draw such a conclusion. In this case, the lump was ill defined, hard and involved adjacent tissues and skin. A characteristic feature of malignant tumours is that tongues of cancer cells infiltrate surrounding tissues, whereas benign tumours tend to grow with a smooth pushing edge.

Thus while benign lumps are generally mobile, malignant tumours are often fixed relative to the surrounding structures. Many malignant tumours induce a proliferation of benign fibroblasts which produce dense collagenous connective tissue. This reaction is termed desmoplasia and gives the tumour its hard texture.

The lesion's size was greater than most benign lesions, although this is a variable feature. More importantly, there was a recent rapid increase in size, which often indicates malignant growth. In this example, there was one other important clue for the doctor which is a peculiarity of some breast cancers. The 'eczema' that was noted over the nipple is referred to as Paget's disease of the nipple. This is due to carcinoma cells growing along the breast ducts towards the nipple and then into the epidermis of the skin (Fig. 11.1).

Two other factors, had they been present, would have influenced the doctor, these are pain and the presence of metastasis. Many tumours, both benign and malignant, are painless, but the presence of unremitting pain is suggestive of malignancy. The presence of metastatic disease is the definitive evidence that a tumour is malignant so it is important to understand possible routes of spread, in order that the most likely sites for metastasis can be examined especially carefully. In this woman's case, there was no pain or evidence of metastatic tumour spread, so the doctor suspected that

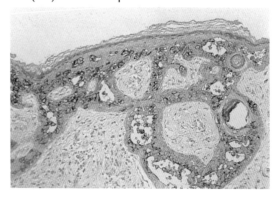

Figure 11.1 **Photomicrograph of nipple stained with epithelial membrane antigen (EMA) showing tumour cells (red) within the epidermis**

History   **Sir James Paget** (1814–1899)

James Paget was born in Yarmouth, Norfolk. He was apprenticed to a surgeon at the local hospital at the age of 16 and enrolled as a medical student at St Bartholomew's Hospital, London, at the age of 20 years. In 1837, a year after obtaining his MRCS, he was appointed curator of the museum at the hospital. Paget was an excellent clinical observer and an eloquent lecturer. He is best remembered for his descriptions of Paget's disease of bone (osteitis deformans) and Paget's disease of the nipple. He was elected FRS (1851) and Surgeon Extraordinary to Queen Victoria (1858). He was created a baronet in 1871.

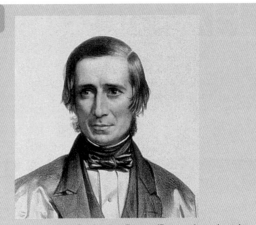

Figure 11.2 Sir James Paget (Reproduced with permission from Wellcome Library, London)

it was a localized malignant growth and the patient was referred to hospital.

EVALUATION IN HOSPITAL

Here a series of tests were performed to make a more precise diagnosis and to assess the extent of her disease; this included haematological and biochemical blood tests to look for anaemia and changes in liver function which might suggest metastases to bone marrow and liver, mammography (X-ray of the breast), a chest X-ray and bone scan to look for tumour spread. The mammography showed a 2 cm spiculated mass with linear calcification. The rest of her investigations were unremarkable.

The surgeon must make a definite diagnosis by obtaining some tissue from the breast lump. He has various options. He can:

- insert a needle attached to a syringe to suck out some cells for examination – fine needle aspiration (FNA) cytology (Fig. 11.3)
- insert a special biopsy needle which would ream out a core of tumour about 3 mm wide and 10–15 mm long (trucut biopsy)
- anaesthetize the patient and remove a part of it (excision biopsy)
- anaesthetize the patient and remove the whole lump (wide-local excision or mastectomy).

In this particular case the surgeon opted for FNA cytology (although in many institutions, this has been replaced by a core biopsy), which showed malignant cells.

Many centres use this type of 'triple approach' of clinical evaluation, radiology (in this case mammography) and FNA cytology in the initial evaluation of patients. Since all three investigations were positive, the surgeon went on to excise the lump and sample the axillary lymph nodes. In due course, the surgeon received the pathologist's report on these tissues and used that information to guide his management of the patient. The report is reproduced on the next page (see also Figs 11.4–11.7) and we shall discuss its relevance for patient management and some points it raises about the biology of tumours.

WHAT ARE THE MACROSCOPICAL FEATURES THAT DISTINGUISH MALIGNANT TUMOURS?

Let us consider this report in more detail. First, there is the gross appearance which records points similar to the criteria used clinically by the family practitioner and surgeon for distinguishing malignant from benign lumps. This includes the size, the infiltrating margin and the consistency of the tumour. Other features include the presence or absence of necrosis and haemorrhage. Most importantly, there is an assessment of excision margins since incomplete excision will result in rapid recurrence and increased opportunity for spread. The report of the microscopical appearances records the

Pathologist's report

Name:	Ida Hopps
Age:	50 years
Ward:	Thompson
Consultant:	I M Surgeon
Specimen:	Left mastectomy and axillary dissection
Date of operation:	12.11.07

Macroscopic appearance:

A simple left mastectomy specimen, weighing 160 g. It consists of skin, including nipple, which measures 170 × 90 mm and covers fatty tissue with maximum dimension of 80 mm. In the tissue beneath the nipple, there is a pale, firm, gritty mass measuring 25 × 20 × 20 mm which has an irregular, poorly defined margin. The closest excision margin (deep) is 15 mm from the mass. There is an area of erythema around the nipple. The axillary dissection measures 80 × 50 × 50 mm and 13 lymph nodes have been identified.

Microscopical appearance – synoptic report:

Invasive carcinoma

Type:	Ductal carcinoma
Size:	22 mm
Grade:	II
(Tubule score, 2; pleomorphism score, 3; mitoses score, 1)	
Lymphovascular permeation:	Not seen

In situ carcinoma

Type:	Ductal carcinoma *in situ* (DCIS)
Grade:	High
Type:	Solid and comedo
Calcification:	Present
Excisional margins	All clear, >10 mm

Lymph nodes

Site:	Axillary tissue
Number present:	10
Number involved:	0

Nipple   Paget's disease

Immunohistochemistry

Oestrogen receptor (ER):	Positive (3+ staining in 90 per cent of cells)
Progesterone receptor (PgR):	Positive (3+ staining in 90 per cent of cells)
HER2:	Negative (0)

Summary:

Left breast:	*In situ* and invasive ductal carcinoma Grade II, 22 mm (T2)
	Complete excision
	ER+, PR+, Her-2-
	Reported by Dr S. P. Ecimen

Figure 11.3 Investigation of a patient with a breast lump

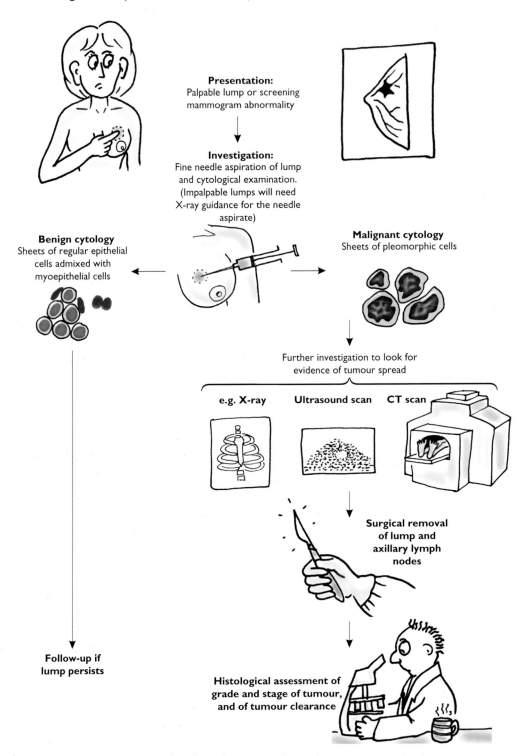

Presentation:
Palpable lump or screening mammogram abnormality

Investigation:
Fine needle aspiration of lump and cytological examination.
(Impalpable lumps will need X-ray guidance for the needle aspirate)

Benign cytology
Sheets of regular epithelial cells admixed with myoepithelial cells

Malignant cytology
Sheets of pleomorphic cells

Further investigation to look for evidence of tumour spread

e.g. **X-ray**   **Ultrasound scan**   **CT scan**

Surgical removal of lump and axillary lymph nodes

Follow-up if lump persists

Histological assessment of grade and stage of tumour, and of tumour clearance

pathologist's conclusion, i.e. that it is a primary malignant tumour of breast tissue. Let us consider how this conclusion has been reached.

WHAT ARE THE MICROSCOPICAL FEATURES THAT DISTINGUISH MALIGNANT TUMOURS?

Malignant tissues differ from benign tissues in that individual cells have an abnormal appearance and their arrangement is deranged. The disordered growth pattern is easy to appreciate provided that you know the normal histological appearance of that tissue.

Within the breast, the normal duct–lobular system is composed of an inner epithelial and an outer myoepithelial layer surrounded by basement membrane. A crucial factor, which is often essential for diagnosing carcinoma, is that cells should have breached the basement membrane, which marks the boundary between epithelial and sub-epithelial tissues. Within the breast, it is possible to identify disordered growth which is still confined within the ducts, an *in situ* carcinoma.

An atypical appearance of individual cells (cytological atypia) is a rather more subtle change. The malignant cells do not only differ from normal cells but also from each other; this is called pleomorphism.

Pleomorphism may involve both nucleus and cytoplasm. In practice, it often refers to the nucleus which may be many times the size of a normal nucleus and may show marked variability in *size* and *shape* – nuclear pleomorphism. It may also have an altered distribution of chromatin and is a darker colour in stained sections, so called hyperchromatism. These alterations reflect the increased amount and abnormalities of nuclear chromatin, which is common in tumours as they are frequently aneuploid.

Dictionary

Aneuploid: an abnormal number of chromosomes which is not an exact multiple of the haploid (23) number

Most normal cells have a small single nucleolus. In malignant cells, there may be many nucleoli of varying sizes or, alternatively, a large single nucleolus. The position of the nucleus within the cell is often abnormal, i.e. it exhibits a loss of polarity. Thus, the nucleus of, for example, a normal colonic cell is situated at the cell's

base with mucus in the cytoplasm nearer the surface whereas the nucleus is more central in a malignant cell. There is also an increase in mitotic activity due to the increase in cell proliferation and abnormal mitotic figures may also be identified. The general appearance of the cells is altered as there is an increase in nuclear–cytoplasmic ratio, either because the amount of cytoplasm is less or the nucleus is larger or a combination of the two.

The cytoplasmic changes vary depending on the tissue but generally involve a loss of specialized features; for example, absence or reduction in mucin content in a colonic adenocarcinoma. Ultimately, however, all of these features are only guidelines and the real test is whether the tumour behaves in a malignant fashion. Of course we cannot leave patients untreated just to see how the tumour behaves. Pathologists have learnt much about the behaviour of tumours from autopsy studies and, fortunately, tumours of similar appearance usually show similar behaviour in different patients.

Note that many of the features discussed here are the same as those used for the assessment of dysplasia (see page 247) and the distinction between grades of dysplasia and frank malignancy is based on both degree and extent of the changes.

WHAT FACTORS INFLUENCE PROGNOSIS?

Here we are concerned with factors which influence prognosis and can be assessed routinely by histopathologists. The important aspects are:

- the type of tumour
- the grade of tumour
- the stage of the disease
- tumour markers.

First it is essential to decide whether the tumour has arisen locally or whether it is a metastasis. Two points help make this distinction and these are whether there are precancerous changes or *in situ* carcinoma present and whether the lesion resembles tumours known to occur at that site.

In situ carcinoma is an alteration in the cytological appearance which is similar to that seen in malignant tumours but does not show any invasion through the basement membrane. If the tumour had been entirely *in situ* then it would have an extremely good prognosis because the lack of local invasion would mean that the

Figure 11.4 **Gross examination of mastectomy specimen**

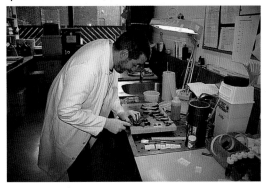

Figure 11.5 **Slice of lumpectomy specimen showing spiculated tumour close to the deep margin**

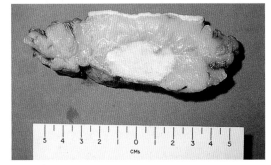

Figure 11.6 *In situ* **ductal carcinoma with central necrosis and microcalcification**

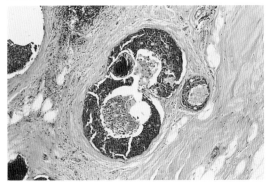

Figure 11.7 **Normal breast duct (right) with adjacent tissue showing infiltration by moderately differentiated ductal carcinoma**

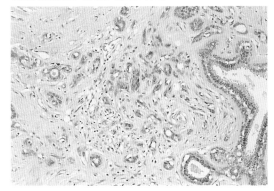

tumour had no ability to extend into lymphatic or blood vessels and no possibility of metastasis. Precancerous lesions are harder to define but are changes (e.g. atypical hyperplasia) which have been shown in large studies to be associated with the subsequent development of cancer and are believed to represent an early, but possibly reversible, stage of malignancy.

In most organs, there is one type of malignant tumour which is far more common than any other and this generally corresponds with the type of tissue which is proliferating in that normal organ. For example, the breast and colon have active glandular epithelium so the commonest malignant tumour at both sites is an adenocarcinoma composed of malignant glandular epithelium. The bladder is lined by transitional epithelium which gives rise to transitional cell carcinoma and the oesophagus has squamous epithelium and squamous carcinomas. Remembering the

normal histology can be a great help in predicting the commonest tumours for a particular site.

To return to our patient, she has an adenocarcinoma which has *in situ* and invasive components. The *in situ* carcinoma tells us that it is locally arising. Therefore, this is a primary tumour of the breast. Within the breast, there are a large number of different subtypes and it is worth remembering that not only is cancer many diseases, but individual organs also have many different types of cancer. Our woman has a ductal carcinoma which has a poorer prognosis than if she had a mucinous carcinoma (see Fig. 11.13).

Although the patient had an invasive carcinoma, the tumour was not seen in lymphatic or blood vessels. The most important prognostic feature is the *type* of tumour but after that the prognosis is influenced by the grade and stage. The grade of a tumour depends on its

Figure 11.8 Comparison of clinical, gross and microscopical features of benign and malignant tumours

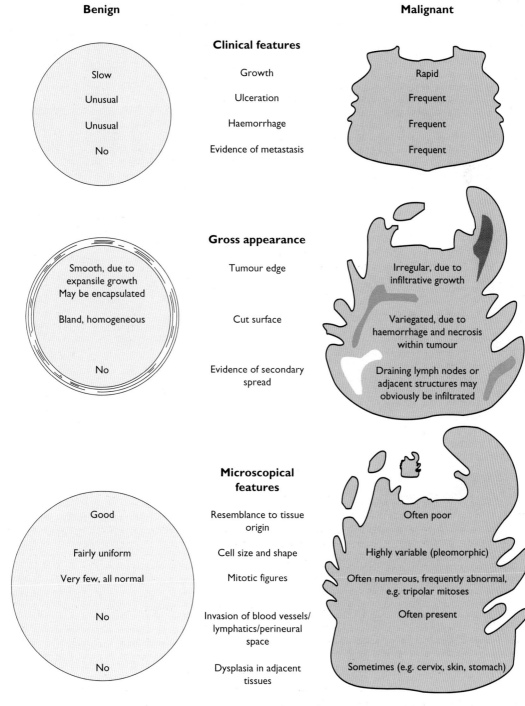

Benign

Malignant

Clinical features

Benign		Malignant
Slow	Growth	Rapid
Unusual	Ulceration	Frequent
Unusual	Haemorrhage	Frequent
No	Evidence of metastasis	Frequent

Gross appearance

Benign		Malignant
Smooth, due to expansile growth May be encapsulated	Tumour edge	Irregular, due to infiltrative growth
Bland, homogeneous	Cut surface	Variegated, due to haemorrhage and necrosis within tumour
No	Evidence of secondary spread	Draining lymph nodes or adjacent structures may obviously be infiltrated

Microscopical features

Benign		Malignant
Good	Resemblance to tissue origin	Often poor
Fairly uniform	Cell size and shape	Highly variable (pleomorphic)
Very few, all normal	Mitotic figures	Often numerous, frequently abnormal, e.g. tripolar mitoses
No	Invasion of blood vessels/ lymphatics/perineural space	Often present
No	Dysplasia in adjacent tissues	Sometimes (e.g. cervix, skin, stomach)

Figure 11.9 Cytological smear showing pleomorphic tumour cells admixed with smaller lymphoid cells

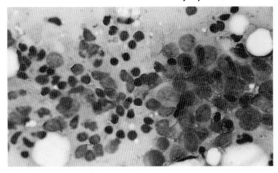

Figure 11.10 Normal terminal duct and lobule of breast

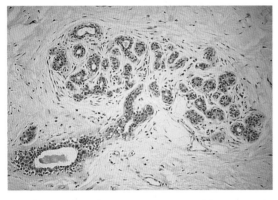

Figure 11.11 Breast carcinoma exhibiting pleomorphism, necrosis and mitotic activity

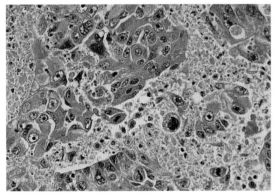

Figure 11.12 High-grade invasive ductal carcinoma

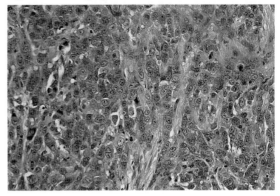

Figure 11.13 Invasive mucinous carcinoma of the breast

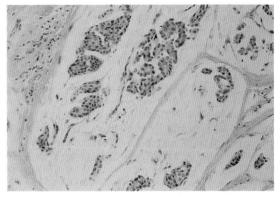

histological appearance while the stage of a tumour depends on its size and extent of spread. The histological grade is a crude measure of how closely the tumour resembles normal tissue combined with an estimate of its mitotic activity. There is a well-defined scoring system for breast tumours (see Table 11.1), based on tubule formation, nuclear pleomorphism and the mitotic count. This divides them into three grades, with grade 1 tumours having a better prognosis than grade 3 tumours. Many sites have no formal grading system and so the pathologist will merely record whether the tumour is well-differentiated, moderately differentiated or poorly differentiated, by assessing similar features but in a less objective way.

The stage of a tumour is a measure of the *extent of disease* and depends on pathological, radiological and clinical information. A TNM staging system is often used for breast carcinoma where T stands for size of primary tumour, N codes for regional node involvement and M for metastatic disease. Figure 11.15 illustrates the different pathological staging systems and links with the TNM classification.

This provides an easy shorthand for indicating the disease stage, which is helpful for deciding treatment and comparing the outcome of patients treated with new therapeutic regimens. Obviously, assessment of a

Table 11.1 Grading of breast cancer. Grading is based on the assessment of three criteria: tubule formation, nuclear pleomorphism and mitotic count. Each is scored from 1 to 3, as shown below

	Score
Tubule formation	
Majority of tumour >75 per cent	1
Moderate amount 10–75 per cent	2
Little or none <10 per cent	3
Nuclear pleomorphism	
Mild	1
Moderate	2
Severe	3
Mitotic count (count per 10 high-powered fields; varies with type of lens)	
0–5	1
6–10	2
>11	3
Total score	**Grade**
3–5	1
6–7	2
8–9	3

Figure 11.14

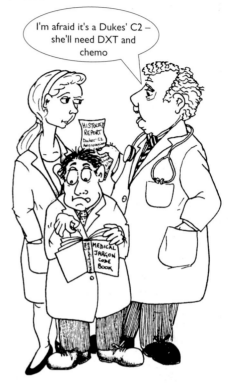

new treatment regimen must take account of the stage of a patient's disease to avoid spurious results.

The pathology report on our patient states that none of the lymph nodes contained tumour and the clinical investigation did not show metastases. Therefore, she would be categorized as T2 (size 2.2 cm), N0, M0 which translates as stage II disease. This short coded message tells the doctor that she is in a relatively good prognostic group.

Immunohistochemical markers for tumour associated gene(s) and gene products are sometimes carried out to help predict behaviour and decide on treatment options. Since the breast is an endocrine responsive organ and proliferates due to stimulation by oestrogen, breast cancers may express the oestrogen (ER) and progesterone receptors (PgR). Approximately 60–70 per cent of breast cancers will be ER and PgR positive and this is not only a better prognostic index but also predicts for response to anti-oestrogenic treatment (e.g. Tamoxifen). Her-2 is an oncogene (see page 278) that is over-expressed in a quarter of breast cancers and is usually seen in high-grade cancers and predicts for a poorer prognosis. A monoclonal antibody trastuzumab (Herceptin) has been developed against the Her-2 receptor and has been shown to be effective in the treatment of advanced breast cancer. It has recently been approved for use in adjuvant (at time of primary diagnosis) settings too. It is one of the first treatments in the category of 'targetted therapies', where specific molecular abnormalities seen in cancers are used as therapeutic targets. This is quite different to chemotherapy which represents general poisons to cancer (and normal) cells.

When the doctor talks to his patient about these results, she may well ask him a variety of questions about her prognosis; but before we attempt to answer those questions, we should digress to discuss the classification of tumours.

CLASSIFICATION OF TUMOURS

The pathological classification of tumours is illustrated in Fig. 11.16.

Figure 11.15 Staging of tumours

TNM system, e.g. Ca breast

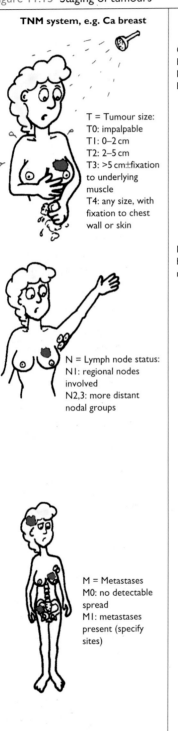

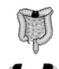

T = Tumour size:
T0: impalpable
T1: 0–2 cm
T2: 2–5 cm
T3: >5 cm±fixation to underlying muscle
T4: any size, with fixation to chest wall or skin

N = Lymph node status:
N1: regional nodes involved
N2,3: more distant nodal groups

M = Metastases
M0: no detectable spread
M1: metastases present (specify sites)

Dukes' staging of colorectal carcinoma

Comment: 5 year survival figures:
Dukes' A: 80–85 per cent
Dukes' B: 55–67 per cent
Dukes' C: 32–37 per cent

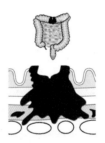

mucosa
m. mucosae
submucosa
m. propria
lymph nodes

Dukes' A: tumour confined within bowel wall; no spread through main muscle layer

Dukes' B: spread through m. propria into serosal fat, without lymph node involvement

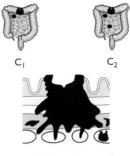

C_1 C_2

Dukes' C: tumour spread to lymph nodes.
C1: pericolic nodes involved
C2: involvement of higher mesenteric nodes

Cotswolds revision of Ann Arbor staging system for Hodgkin's lymphoma

Comment: the presence of 'B' symptoms, e.g. fever, drenching sweats, weight loss, adversely affects the prognosis, and is included in the stage, e.g. Stage IIA (no B symptoms), or Stage IIB.

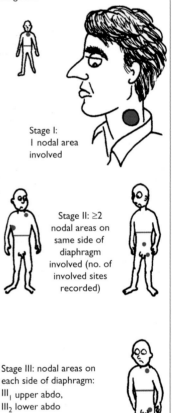

Stage I:
1 nodal area involved

Stage II: ≥2 nodal areas on same side of diaphragm involved (no. of involved sites recorded)

Stage III: nodal areas on each side of diaphragm:
III_1 upper abdo,
III_2 lower abdo

Stage IV:
visceral involvement

The spleen is part of the reticuloendothelial system. Splenic involvement does not carry the same staging implications as, for instance, bone marrow or liver

Figure 11.16 Pathological classification of tumours

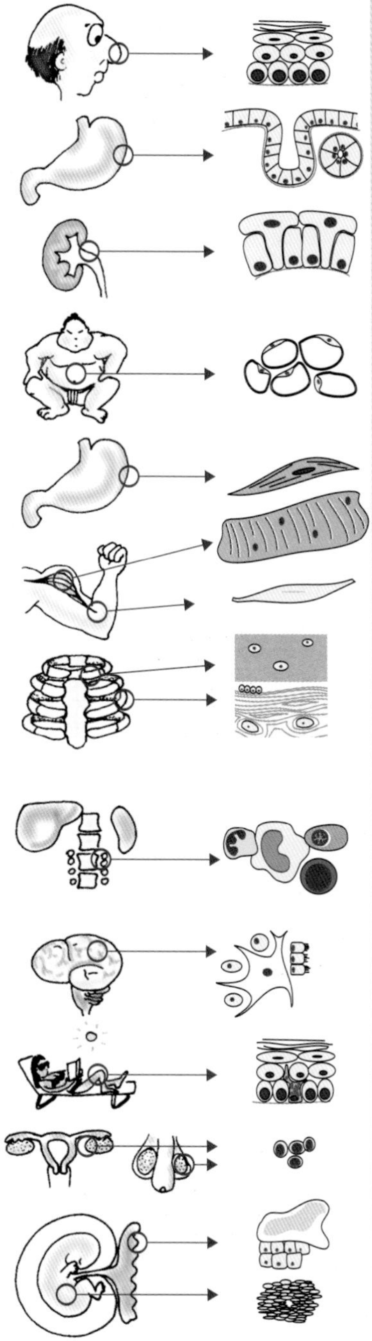

TISSUE TYPE	BENIGN	MALIGNANT
Epithelium		**Carcinoma**
Squamous, e.g. skin	Squamous papilloma	**Squamous** carcinoma
Glandular, e.g. gastrointestinal tract	Adenoma	**Adeno**carcinoma
Transitional, e.g. urothelium	Transitional cell papilloma	**Transitional cell** carcinoma
Connective tissue		**Sarcoma**
Fat	Lipoma	**Lipo**sarcoma
Muscle: i. Smooth muscle, e.g. wall of gastrointestinal tract	Leiomyoma	**Leiomyo**sarcoma
Muscle: ii. Striated muscle, i.e. voluntary muscle	Rhabdomyoma	**Rhabdomyo**sarcoma
Fibrous tissue, e.g. tendon	Fibroma	**Fibro**sarcoma
Cartilage	Chondroma	**Chondro**sarcoma
Bone	Osteoma	**Osteo**sarcoma
Special categories	(non-systematic nomenclature retained mainly for historical reasons)	
Bone marrow-derived cells:		
Myeloid cells		Myeloid leukaemia
Lymphoid cells		Lymphocytic leukaemias
		Lymphomas
Plasma cells	Plasmacytoma	Myeloma
Central nervous system, e.g. glial cells		Gliomas
Melanocyte	Benign melanocytic naevus	Melanoma
Germ cells	Benign teratoma	Malignant teratoma Seminoma/Dysgerminoma
Placenta	Hydatidiform mole	Choriocarcinoma
Embryonal cells		Embryonal cell tumours (may show differentiation towards tissue types, e.g. neuroblastoma)

You will recall that knowledge of the normal structures at a particular site can be of great help in predicting the commonest tumours. In most organs, there is one particular type of malignant tumour which is more common than any other and this generally corresponds with the type of tissue which is proliferating at that site. The stomach and colon have active glandular epithelium so the commonest malignant tumour at both sites is an adenocarcinoma, which is composed of malignant glandular epithelium. The bladder is lined by transitional epithelium which gives rise to transitional cell carcinoma and the skin has squamous epithelium and squamous carcinomas.

Since the tumour resembles part of the parent tissue, the classification is based on the assumed histogenesis, i.e. because a transitional cell carcinoma has some similarities with transitional epithelium, it is assumed to arise from it.

The broad classification divides tumours into those arising from epithelia (carcinomas), from connective tissue (sarcomas), from lymphoid tissue (lymphomas) and 'the rest', which includes specialized tissues such as the brain. Included in Fig. 11.16 are the benign counterparts arising from the same tissues.

At this point there needs to be a word of caution because, although this classification originated from ideas on histogenesis, it is now apparent that cells of one tissue type may 'differentiate' to resemble cells of another type (a process called metaplasia; see page 246). For example, bronchial glandular epithelium may become squamous due to the chronic irritation from smoking. A tumour arising in such a patient may hence appear squamous although the original epithelium at this site was glandular. The histogenetic approach to classification is destroyed in such circumstances.

Fortunately, we only have to classify tumours according to their type of differentiation and we eliminate the problem! Thus a tumour resembling squamous cells is a squamous cell carcinoma regardless of the original tissue type. You will discover that although rare, it is possible to get squamous carcinoma in the breast and adenocarcinoma in the bladder! Sometimes a tumour cell is very poorly differentiated so that, even to the trained histopathologist's eye, it does not resemble a particular type of normal cell. In this situation, special stains to demonstrate cytoplasmic or surface molecules can be helpful. Thus the presence of intracellular mucins would suggest an adenocarcinoma and immunohistochemical stains for different intermediate filaments or lymphoid antigens would help to distinguish between a wide variety of tumours. If it is not possible to demonstrate any differentiation, the tumour is referred to as anaplastic. Some of these substances are also released into the blood, which is useful both for diagnosis and for following the patient's response to treatment. For example, prostatic specific antigen (PSA) levels can be measured in the blood to help screen for prostatic adenocarcinoma, although levels are also raised in some non-malignant prostatic disorders because the antigen is present on both benign and malignant prostatic cells. The β subunit of human chorionic gonadotrophin (β-HCG) and alpha-fetoprotein (α-FP) are also useful markers in patients with germinal cell tumours.

Now we must turn to the patient's questions. What causes cancer? How will it behave? What treatments are available? Will there be a lot of pain?

If we are not to be stumped by the patient, we have to understand a little more about the natural history of cancer.

CANCER AS A DISEASE OF GENETIC MATERIAL

The view that cancer originates within single cells due to abnormalities within its DNA is now generally accepted. The evidence comes from five main sources:

- Some cancers have a heritable predisposition; examples include familial retinoblastoma and familial adenomatous polyposis.
- Many tumours exhibit chromosomal abnormalities and karyotypic studies have even identified specific changes in some tumours, e.g. 8:14 translocation in Burkitt's lymphoma.
- A number of rare inherited disorders involve an inability to repair damaged DNA. An example is xeroderma pigmentosa and these patients have an increased susceptibility to skin cancer following damage to DNA from ultra-violet light.
- Many chemical carcinogens are also mutagens, i.e. they have been shown to cause genetic mutations.
- DNA recombinant technology has demonstrated that DNA from tumour cells, when transferred into a normal cell, can convert them into tumour cells of the same type.

The isolation of genes with a direct role in tumour formation (oncogenes) has firmly established cancer as a disease of genetic material. However, unlike, for example, cystic fibrosis, where mutation in one gene causes the disease, no single gene defect has been shown to 'cause' cancer; cancer genes in general should be thought of as significant contributors to the development of malignancy rather than as 'causes' of cancer.

We will now consider the many predisposing and aetiological factors that lead to tumour formation. Although it appears that these factors must alter either the DNA structure or function in some way, the details of many of these processes remain unclear.

One of the patient's concerns will relate to what causes cancer and the risk factors that were important in his or her case.

RISK FACTORS FOR CANCER

AGE

The advent of antibiotics, improved sanitation and good nutrition has extended people's expected life span so that they can now achieve an age in which there is a high incidence of malignant tumours, particularly those of breast, colon, lung, prostate and bronchus. It is postulated that carcinogens may have a cumulative effect over time which may explain an increased incidence with age. The ability of carcinogens to induce genetic mutations is well known and the large number of cell divisions with increasing age may contribute to the neoplastic process. Cell division itself is a risk since each time the DNA is copied, there is a potential to introduce mistakes within the genome. There are elaborate DNA repair mechanisms in place to correct such errors but mutations in genes coding for proteins involved in DNA repair will allow such errors to pass on to the next generation of cells. All these factors together with the age-related metabolic or hormonal changes may combine to account for the increasing incidence of tumours with age. Tumours are of course not just confined to the elderly and some malignancies such as leukaemias are more common in children. In some childhood tumours (e.g. retinoblastoma) heredity plays a major part in the aetiology.

GENETIC FACTORS

In the case of breast carcinoma discussed in chapter 11, the doctor discovered that the patient's mother had died of breast carcinoma. The patient also had two daughters who at the time were both well. This history of malignant disease within close family members is of relevance as there are several tumour types where the risk of cancer in close family members is increased. How much the risk is increased in individual cases and with different tumours is not easy to specify but, in general, it is about two to three times the general population. Obviously, tumour development is not inevitable and many other factors such as environmental and dietary influences may modify the risk.

In some tumours, the genetic susceptibility is better understood and in two autosomal dominant conditions, familial polyposis coli and retinoblastoma, it involves loss of a tumour suppressor gene or anti-oncogene (see later). Familial polyposis coli (familial adenomatous polyposis) is a disorder in which individuals develop hundreds of polyps in the gastrointestinal tract. These polyps show varying degrees of dysplasia (page 247) and, although benign, should be regarded as premalignant because practically all of these patients will develop a colonic carcinoma if the colon is not removed by the age of 25 years. Retinoblastoma is a malignant tumour of the eye which is commonest in children. Twenty-five to 30 per cent of cases of retinoblastoma are hereditary and the rest are sporadic. Both the familial and sporadic cases arise due to two mutations in the retinoblastoma gene but the familial cases inherit one mutation through the germ line cells (see later).

GEOGRAPHY AND RACIAL FACTORS

Geographical factors merge with environmental factors, as a geographical factor is only an environmental factor which affects the population of a particular area. This may be a sunny climate, radioactive rock formations or a carcinogen in the water supply (Fig. 12.1).

Let us discuss the increased incidence of stomach cancer in Japan compared with North America. The tumour is seven times commoner in Japanese people living in Japan than in Americans living in the United States. Is this a racial difference or an effect of some climatic, geological or dietary factor which operates in Japan? To answer this we need to know the incidence in Japanese people who move to America and raise families. They will keep their racial (genetic) factors and may import their dietary factors but not their geographical factors. We find that the incidence drops in these immigrants and is halved in their first-generation offspring but is still higher than in white Americans; so we haven't achieved a definite answer to our question. Some reports suggest that the incidence drops further in future generations

Figure 12.1 Geographical variations in tumour incidence

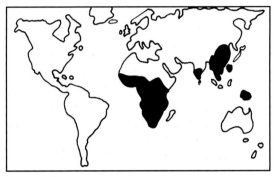

Hepatocellular carcinoma
Sub-Saharan black Africa
Far East

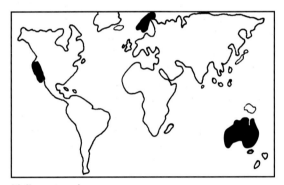

Malignant melanoma
Australia
Scandinavia
North America: Californian whites at highest risk

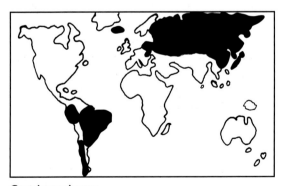

Gastric carcinoma
Japan, China
Brazil, Colombia, Chile
Iceland, Finland,
USSR, Poland, Hungary

until it equals the American rate. This would appear to rule out a racial (genetic) factor and may implicate a cultural dietary change. Similar arguments apply to the interesting observation of an increase in prostate cancer amongst the Japanese migrants to USA.

A much easier example is the incidence of melanomas in white-skinned Australians. Here there is a *racial predisposition*, because they do not have sufficient skin pigmentation to protect them from ultra-violet light, and the *geographical factor* of a sunny climate. If the Australian emigrates at birth to a cold grey country, then his risk of melanoma drops dramatically.

ENVIRONMENTAL AGENTS

Numerous environmental agents have been implicated in the causation of cancer. Everybody knows that there is a strong association between smoking and lung cancer. This problem may not only affect the smoker but also the 'innocent bystander' who inhales exhaled tobacco smoke (passive smoking).

Asbestos exposure increases the risk of developing lung carcinoma and malignant mesothelioma of the pleura and peritoneum. Exposure to β-napthylamine, which may occur in the rubber and dye industries, increases the risk of transitional cell tumours of the bladder. Exposure to vinyl chloride in the plastic industry enhances the development of liver angiosarcoma (malignant tumour of blood vessels).

One of the first examples of an environmental cancer was described in 1775 by Percival Pott, surgeon to St Bartholomew's Hospital. He had observed that chimney sweeps had a very high incidence of scrotal cancer, and correctly deduced that this was due to chronic contact with soot. In fact, Percival Pott achieved a double: he described an environmental carcinogen and an occupational cancer in one go! He is also remembered for his description of spinal tuberculosis, referred to as Pott's disease.

CARCINOGENIC AGENTS

So far we have discussed carcinogenesis under the broad headings of age, genetics, race, geography and environment. The next step is to consider what type of agent is operating (the aetiological agent) and to look at ideas on how the agent converts a normal cell to a malignant cell (pathogenesis).

It is worth remembering that, as in the case considered in chapter 11 of the woman with breast cancer, by the time a patient presents with a tumour, a large number of cellular events and many thousands of cell divisions have already taken place. Consequently, we are looking at a growth that has been in existence for quite some time, possibly 10–15 years. Identifying the responsible aetiological factors at this stage can be extremely difficult. There are three major groups of agents involved in carcinogenesis that we need to consider. These are:

- chemical carcinogens
- radiation
- viruses.

These groups should not be viewed in isolation. Chemicals may, for example, interact with ionizing radiation or with oncogenic viruses. Several different agents within any one group may also interact with each other. Further, all these extrinsic agents may interact with endogenous or constitutional factors in the host such as genetic susceptibility, immune status or hormonal status, emphasizing that the carcinogenic process is complex and multifactorial.

Chemical carcinogens

The figure below illustrates classical experiments of chemical carcinogenesis using mouse skin, which provide the basis for the multistep theory (page 287) and lead to the descriptions of the process of initiation and promotion. We now know that tumour development in humans is much more complex than depicted in Fig. 12.2.

Let us consider Fig. 12.2. If you apply a low dose of polycyclic aromatic hydrocarbon (initiator) to the shaved skin of the mouse and don't do any more, then no tumours will result. However, if you later apply another chemical, croton oil (promoter), to the same skin, local tumours will develop. The important points are that the initiator must be applied before the promoter and that the promoter must be applied repeatedly and at regular intervals. There may be a long time interval between initiation and promotion which suggests that initiation provokes an irreversible change in the DNA which is fixed by cell division. In contrast, the promoter acts in a dose-related, initially reversible fashion and appears to modify the expression of altered genes. Some chemicals (complete carcinogens) can act as both initiator and promoter whereas others (incomplete carcinogens) only fulfill one action.

Evidence that certain chemical are carcinogenic in humans is provided by epidemiological studies. Some chemical carcinogens occur naturally; for instance,

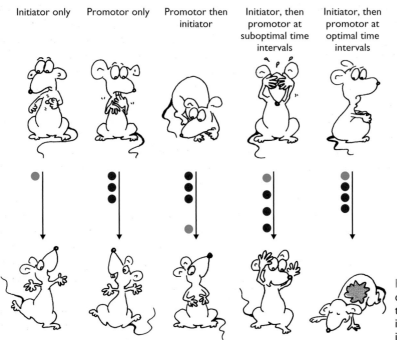

Figure 12.2 **Chemical carcinogenesis: the effects of tumour promoters and initiators. Key: green dot – initiator; red dot – promoter**

aflatoxin B_1 is a potent hepatocarcinogen which is a metabolite from the fungus *Aspergillus flavus*, a common contaminant of grain and other crops in the tropics. Several carcinogens occur as complex mixtures as in tobacco smoke. Chemical carcinogens typically take twenty or more years to exert their effects; hence there is a long latency period between first encounter with the chemical and the appearance of a tumour. The dose required to induce tumours varies widely. Carcinogens act on a number of fairly specific target tissues, broadly determined by the initial routes of exposure and by subsequent patterns of absorption, distribution and metabolism. β-Naphthylamine is an interesting example. It enters the body mainly via the respiratory system and is inactivated by conjugation with glucuronic acid. Following excretion in the urine, it is activated again due to the action of urinary glucuronidase which splits the conjugate releasing the active molecule. Its carcinogenic effects are hence confined to the urinary tract where it causes transitional cell tumours.

Chemical carcinogenesis is complex and occurs in several steps in which both genotoxic and non-genotoxic events contribute. Genotoxic carcinogens react with DNA. Various types of genetic damage will follow and, if the damage is not lethal to a cell, it will be transmitted to the daughter cells after cell division. The only protection the cell has is its array of DNA repair enzymes, which must reconstitute the DNA before the next cell division or else the abnormality will be 'stamped' in by being transmitted to the daughter cells. Most genotoxic carcinogens undergo metabolic changes and are converted from inactive procarcinogens to activated ultimate carcinogens which bind to DNA. Some genotoxic chemicals react directly with DNA without previous metabolic activation. The conditions which determine whether a potential genotoxic chemical is activated or detoxified are very complex, but two main groups of enzymes are involved: the family of cytochrome P-450-dependent mono-oxygenase isoenzymes, and various conjugating enzymes which catalyse the formation of water soluble glucuronides. The process by which activated genotoxic carcinogens bind to DNA is equally complex. Once an activated carcinogen is bound to DNA, a number of consequences follow, depending on the nature and extent of the DNA damage that has been sustained. If this damage is extensive and irreversible, the cell will die. If less severe, the damage can be restored by the process of error-free DNA repair. The third possibility, mentioned earlier, is that the cell will survive with damaged DNA which will then be passed on to the daughter cells following cell division.

Non-genotoxic carcinogens, by contrast, do not bind to DNA and do not directly damage it. They appear to act on cells in the target tissues mainly by directly stimulating cell division, or by causing cell damage and death (and thus indirectly stimulating cell division through the process of regeneration and repair). Other effects are less clearly understood, but the general mode of action of non-genotoxic chemicals can be thought of as causing disruption of normal cellular homeostasis. Some non-genotoxic chemicals, such as hormones, act through receptors on the surface of target cells.

One final point should be made. Some genotoxic chemicals exert both genotoxic and non-genotoxic effects in the target tissues. So although genotoxic and non-genotoxic effects are both required for tumour development, they do not necessarily depend on separate genotoxic and non-genotoxic agents.

Key facts

Examples of chemical carcinogens and the associated tumour types

Carcinogen	Tumour type
Aromatic amines, e.g. β-naphthylamine	Transitional cell carcinoma of lower urinary tract (principally of the bladder)
Polycyclic aromatic hydrocarbons, e.g. benzo(a)pyrene	Skin cancer, lung cancer
Vinyl chloride and Thorotrast	Angiosarcoma of liver
Arsenic	Skin cancers
Aflatoxin B_1	Liver cell carcinoma

Radiation

Ionizing radiation includes electromagnetic rays, such as ultra-violet light, X-rays and gamma rays, and particulate radiation, such as alpha particles, beta particles, neutrons and protons. All of these are carcinogenic.

As ionizing radiation passes through tissue, it interacts with atoms in its path to destabilize them. This disturbance in the electron shell of atoms may lead to chemical changes.

The precise mechanisms are still obscure. Radiation causes chromosomal breakage, translocations and mutations. Various protein molecules are also damaged and there are two principal theories to account for the observations. The direct theory states that ionizing radiation directly ionizes important molecules within the cell; while the indirect theory states that ionization first affects water within the cell, which leads to the production of oxygen free radicals which cause the damage. Whichever mechanism operates, the end result is that DNA is altered, analogous to the initiator effect in chemical carcinogenesis.

The carcinogenic effect of radiation is related to its ability to produce mutations and it is known that this depends on the type and strength of the radiation and the duration of exposure. Some tissues, such as bone marrow and thyroid, are particularly sensitive to the effects of radiation and children are more susceptible than adults.

Ultra-violet light is particularly important, as sun exposure causes vast numbers of melanomas, squamous cell carcinomas and basal cell carcinomas of the skin. Fortunately, squamous cell carcinomas and basal cell carcinomas generally can be cured by complete local excision, but melanomas metastasize early and kill. Many of the pioneers who studied radioactive materials and X-rays developed skin cancers, and miners of radioactive elements have a high incidence of lung cancers. The radiation from the atomic bombs dropped on Hiroshima and Nagasaki resulted in increased incidence of leukaemia, especially acute and chronic myeloid leukaemia, breast, lung and colonic cancers. In contrast, a dramatic increase in thyroid carcinomas has been described in children living in Ukraine and Belarus, who were exposed to fallout after the Chernobyl accident. Interestingly, no increase in the incidence of other types of childhood or adult solid cancers has been noted.

Viruses

A large number of viruses have been implicated in the causation of cancer (Table 12.1). We will discuss:

- Epstein–Barr virus (Figs 12.3–12.6)
- human papilloma virus (Figs 12.7 and 12.8)
- hepatitis B virus (Figs 12.9 and 12.10)
- human T-cell leukaemia virus-1
- Kaposi sarcoma-associated herpes virus (KSHV) (Fig. 12.11).

Table 12.1 Viruses and their associated cancers	
Virus	**Associated tumour**
Oncovirus	
HTLV-1	Adult T-cell leukaemia/ lymphoma
Hepadnavirus	
Hepatitis B	Liver cancer
Papovavirus	
Papilloma virus types:	
1, 2, 4, 7	Benign skin papillomas
6, 11	Genital warts
16, 18	Cervical cancer
10, 16	Laryngeal cancer
5	Skin cancer
Herpes virus	
Epstein–Barr (EBV)	Burkitt's lymphoma
	Nasopharyngeal carcinoma
	Immunoblastic lymphoma
Herpes simplex – 8	Kaposi's sarcoma
	Body cavity B-cell lymphoma
	Multiple myeloma

Figure 12.4 Photomicrograph showing classical 'starry sky' appearance of Burkitt's lymphoma due to apoptosis of tumour cells creating 'light holes' in a 'sky' of blue cells

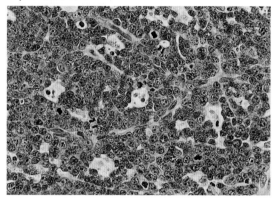

Figure 12.5 Reed–Sternberg cell in Hodgkin lymphoma, staining positively for Epstein–Barr virus. EBV has been found in the Reed–Sternberg cells in about one-third to one-half of all Hodgkin cases, though whether it truly has an aetiological role has not been conclusively established

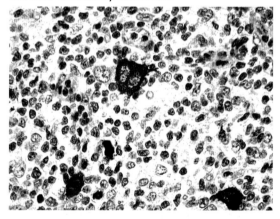

Figure 12.3 Young child with a large maxillary tumour distorting the face. This is a classical presentation of Burkitt's lymphoma

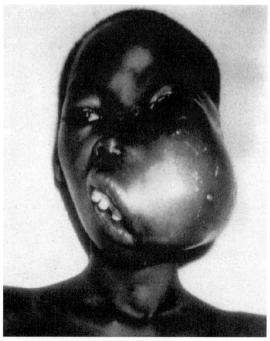

Epstein–Barr virus

There is a very strong association between EBV and the African variety of Burkitt's lymphoma, since over 98 per cent of the African cases show EBV genome in the tumour cells and all the patients have a raised level of antibodies to EBV membrane antigens. Fortunately, EBV does not inevitably cause cancer, as EBV is a common infection in developed countries, where it causes a flu-like illness called infectious mononucleosis or glandular fever. Burkitt's lymphoma can occur without EBV and few non-African Burkitt lymphomas (15–20 per cent) have the EBV genome. Therefore, EBV must be just one factor involved in the transformation of B lymphocytes to a B-cell malignancy.

It is interesting that the African regions where Burkitt's lymphoma is common are also regions where malaria is endemic. It would appear that malaria causes a degree of immuno-incompetence that allows the EBV-infected B cells to proliferate and, hence, gives them an increased risk of mutation. Burkitt's lymphoma exhibits a specific mutation resulting in the 8:14 translocation regardless of whether EBV is involved. This translocation moves the c-*myc* gene from its position on chromosome 8 to be adjacent to the immunoglobulin heavy chain gene on chromosome 14. c-*myc* codes for proteins which control cell proliferation and the effect of this translocation is to increase its transcription, possibly because that zone of chromosome 14 is an area of frequent transcriptional activity.

Another putative association of EBV is with Hodgkin's lymphoma, a heterogenous disorder of B cells in which the tumour cells are often a small component of the proliferation. The classical cells are called the Reed–Sternberg cells.

Human papilloma virus

Human papilloma virus (HPV) is a papova virus which has long been known to be associated with skin papillomas (warts). Its role in causing cancer was recognized during the study of a very rare disease, epidermodysplasia

Figure 12.7 Inflamed cervical epithelium with multinucleated giant cell due to herpes simplex virus infection. The role of HSV in cervical cancer is still debated; human papilloma virus (HPV) is of far greater importance.

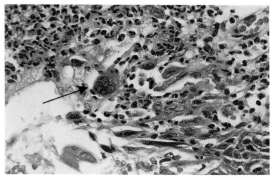

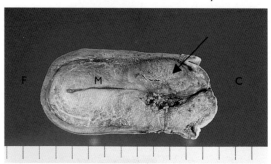

Figure 12.8 Invasive cervical carcinoma (arrow). Each division is 10 mm. C, cervix; F, fundus; M, myometrium

History   Thomas Hodgkin 1798–1866

Thomas Hodgkin was a devout Quaker who was generally unsuccessful in practice because he was very reluctant to accept fees. In his early years, his major interest was pathology and he was curator of the pathology museum at Guy's Hospital and later lecturer in pathology for 10 years; but resigned after being passed over for the job of assistant physician, much to the disappointment of his students. In later years, he devoted his time to philanthropic causes, travelled widely and died from dysentery in Jaffa.

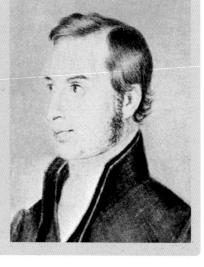

Figure 12.6 Thomas Hodgkin

Figure 12.9 **Viral hepatitis showing an apoptotic liver cell (arrow) surrounded by inflammatory cells**

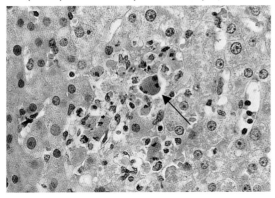

Figure 12.10 **Hepatocellular carcinoma arising in a cirrhotic liver**

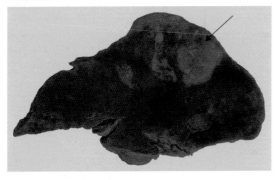

verruciformis, in which patients have defective cell-mediated immunity and numerous skin papillomas. These papillomas may transform into squamous cell carcinomas which frequently contain the genome of HPV 5, 8 or 14. HPV is not a single virus but a group of around 85 genetically distinct viruses. Interestingly, some types appear to produce benign tumours while others predispose to malignancy. Thus HPV 16 and 18 (the most common amongst many others) are implicated in squamous cell carcinoma of the uterine cervix while HPV 6 and 11 are common in benign cervical lesions (Figs 12.7 and 12.8).

HPV can be transmitted by sexual intercourse and it is noted that there is a high incidence of carcinoma of the cervix in those who begin sexual activity at an early age and in those who are promiscuous. The question is: why doesn't our immune system eradicate the virus? Many people have skin warts on their hands and feet (verrucae) as children but appear to develop immunity so that the warts are less common in later life. HPV genome comprises a number of genes, two of which are believed to be important in malignancy. The protein products of the E6 and E7 genes bind to p53 and retinoblastoma protein respectively inactivating their function in regulating the cell cycle (see page 282).

Now that we know the viral types involved in some cancers, it opens the door for developing vaccines. Immunization for the prevention of hepatitis B and its associated hepatocellular carcinoma is already in progress and proving successful. Two vaccines for the prevention of cervical cancer are on the market, Cervarix, targeting HPV 16 and 18, and Gardasil which targets HPV 16, 18, 6 and 11. These are likely to have a major impact on the disease but have to be given before the first sexual intercourse as the time course for progression is more than 10 years.

Hepatitis B virus

Hepatitis B virus (HBV) is associated with the production of a chronic hepatitis, cirrhosis and carcinoma of the liver.

In sub-Saharan Africa and south-east Asia, where infection with HBV is endemic, the infection is transmitted vertically from mother to child during pregnancy. These children, therefore, have chronic HBV infection and a high incidence of hepatocellular carcinoma at a relatively young age (20–40 years).

The importance of HBV in hepatocellular carcinoma (HCC) is apparent from this sort of epidemiological work and also from molecular biological investigation looking for integrated HBV DNA sequences. These have been identified in the hepatocytes of some patients with chronic HBV infection and some HCC tumour cells. It appears that integration of the viral genome precedes malignant transformation by several years but, to date, no known oncogenic sequences have been identified. The HBV genome does contain a transactivating gene, termed X, which codes for a product that alters the level of transcription of other genes, including the genes in the hepatocytes. An additional mechanism that has been postulated is that HBV infection also leads to liver cell injury and regeneration due to the effect of cytotoxic T cells. It is possible that both the direct (DNA effect due to X) and indirect mechanism (proliferation in response to immune mediated injury) are important in the aetiology of HCC.

Liver cell carcinomas are also associated with alcoholic liver disease, androgenic steroids and aflatoxins. Aflatoxins are toxic metabolites of a fungus, *Aspergillus flavus*, which can contaminate food in the tropics. Aflatoxin B is thought to contribute to the high incidence

Figure 12.11 **A larynx with Kaposi's sarcoma composed of slit-like channels filled with red blood cells**

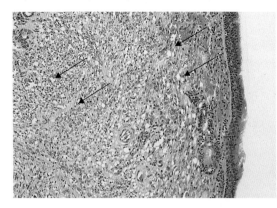

of liver cancer in parts of south east Asia and Africa. Possibly these agents act by causing damage which leads to regenerative activity and, hence, the production of proliferative nodules that are susceptible to further cellular alterations by HBV.

Human T-cell leukaemia virus-1 (HTLV-1)

Human T-cell leukaemia virus-1 (HTLV-1) is important because it is the only example (so far!) of a retrovirus causing a human cancer. It is implicated in adult T-cell leukaemia/lymphoma (ATLL) which is a rare tumour of the lymphoid system. HTLV-1 infection is commonest in southern Japan, South America and parts of Africa and precedes the development of malignancy by decades. It has a transactivating gene, *tat*, that increases IL-2 receptor expression in infected T cells, which promotes their growth. The study of retroviruses has advanced our knowledge of the role of genes in tumour biology by allowing the identification of specific transforming genes. This is discussed in greater detail below. However, to date, they have not been shown to be important in common human tumours.

Kaposi sarcoma-associated herpes virus

Kaposi's sarcoma is an important vascular neoplasm which has come to prominence in HIV-infected patients. Since early 1980 it has been frequently associated with patients who have AIDS. It is an endemic lesion in central Africa, predominantly in healthy men but also in women and children. Evidence is accumulating that this odd vascular tumour is due to a novel herpes virus. This virus has been termed Kaposi's sarcoma-associated herpesvirus (KSHV) or human-herpes virus 8 (HHV-8). There is

strong evidence demonstrating that this virus is linked to several other neoplasms, such as body cavity B-cell lymphoma, multiple myeloma, benign lymphoproliferative disease, angiosarcoma of the face, angiolymphoid hyperplasia with eosinophilia, and multicentric Castleman disease. Although the data are unclear, there is a suggestion that HHV-8 may play a role in some enigmatic inflammatory diseases, such as sarcoidosis. The study of HHV-8 has been very fruitful in revealing new aspects of viral carcinogenesis. The genome of this virus encodes proteins that take part in molecular mimicry of cell cycle regulatory and signalling proteins (see section on molecular genetics).

Retroviruses

The study of viruses has helped enormously in unraveling the relevance of genes in human cancer. Of particular use are the retroviruses, which normally contain just three genes, two coding for structural proteins (*gag* and *env*) and one (*pol*) for the enzyme, reverse transcriptase, that produces DNA from RNA. The addition of a fourth gene can often give the virus acute transforming properties, i.e. infection with the altered virus can produce tumours under experimental conditions, so called transfection experiments. These viruses acted as tools to enable scientists to identify the genetic sequences that could transform cell lines. Many of the viral oncogene sequences were recognized as variants of cellular genes that the retrovirus had acquired from the human genome. This focused attention on the human cells' proto-oncogenes and led to an understanding of the mutations and translocations that can lead to their activation.

Oncogenic RNA viruses

Oncogenic RNA viruses are all retroviruses, i.e. they contain reverse transcriptase, and they can be divided into acute transforming viruses, slow transforming viruses and transactivating viruses. The acute transforming viruses produce tumours within a few weeks in infected animals and often are capable of transforming cell cultures. The slow transforming viruses take months to produce tumours, which are frequently forms of chronic leukaemia. These two groups of viruses alter the infected cell in different ways. The acute transforming viruses are usually incapable of normal replication because they have lost some genes related to replication but gained genes which confer their transforming capabilities. These additional genes are variants of their host's genes; genes that are called proto-oncogenes when in the host, and viral oncogenes when in the virus. The proto-oncogene is a normal cell gene that is normally involved in growth or differentiation. The viral oncogene is not identical to the proto-oncogene, although there is quite extensive sequence homology. The viral oncogene is structurally altered which, in some way, deregulates cell growth. Alternatively, at the time of inclusion into the viral genome, the proto-oncogene may be inserted near a potent viral promoter, resulting in increased expression. In some cases, acute transforming viruses and normal retroviruses co-infect cells so that the non-transforming retrovirus can provide the replication information that the transforming virus lacks.

Slow transforming retroviruses do not contain oncogenes, have the normal three gene structure to their genome and are capable of replication. They alter the host cell's behaviour by inserting near to a cellular proto-oncogene, so that they either cause increased activity of the cellular gene or, possibly, induce a structural change in the gene. This is called insertional mutagenesis.

Transactivating viruses do not contain oncogenes but, in addition to the *gag, pol* and *env* genes, they have a fourth region which confers transforming properties. The human T cell leukaemia virus is in this group and its extra genes (*tat*) code for a variety of proteins, one of which activates the host's IL-2 and IL-2 R genes resulting in uncontrolled cell proliferation.

Oncogenic DNA viruses

Oncogenic DNA viruses contain genes which act early in infected cells to increase expression of a wide variety of genes. The purpose of this is to activate later viral genes concerned with replication and assembly. However, it can also have the effect of inducing excessive expression of host cell genes responsible for growth regulation. For example, the 'early genes' of the virus can produce proteins (e.g. T proteins of polyoma and SV40 viruses) that localize in the nucleus and alter the regulation of DNA synthesis. In some cases, this is through binding to the p53 protein so that its half life is increased and DNA synthesis remains activated. Some 'growth enhancing' actions may actually result from inhibiting normal 'growth inhibiting' proteins.

There is an 'old wives' saying: 'Where God puts disease, he also puts a cure'. Viruses undoubtedly cause infectious disease and can be one step on the road to cancer. However, they may also provide a possible cure

for disease as they may be ideal vehicle for altering the genetic code within human cells. Ultimately, it would be best if patients with single-gene disorders could have their defective gene replaced by the correct gene. In theory, this is possible by using a retrovirus to introduce the gene, although in practice there are many problems to conquer. The most useful practical application of our rapidly expanding knowledge of the genes is in the manufacture of specific proteins.

SUMMARY

Although we started the chapter with the statement that cancer is a disease of genetic material, it should be evident that it is also a multifactorial disorder. This might appear initially as a paradox; but remember that in any given person, the combination of a genetic makeup, the environment in which the person lives and the factors to which he/she is exposed, the longevity of the person and 'chance' will combine to produce the genetic changes (mutations) that may ultimately lead to cancer. One could argue that at least in some circumstances, the cancer is a direct payback of an evolutionary advantage of the past. It is not difficult to envisage a genetic make-up that gives such an advantage; a good example could be decreased pigmentation in races living in the cloudy and colder northern hemisphere which would help in obtaining adequate amounts of vitamin D from sunshine. This advantage from the genetic make-up could become a distinct disadvantage if put into the context of chance mutations, increased exposure to sunlight due to sunbathing on numerous holidays on tropical beaches and a long enough life for the mutations to result in a cancer – a melanoma.

Key facts

Major aetiological factors involved in tumour formation

- Age
- Genetic factors
- Geographical and racial factors
- Environmental agents
- Carcinogens: chemicals, radiation, viruses
- Immunity

It is now well over a hundred years since Gregor Mendel first carried out his experiments with peas and almost exactly a century since Mendel's laws were 're-discovered'. It is also just over a century since David von Hansemann (1890) described abnormal mitotic figures in cancer cells, and since Theodore Boveri proposed that alterations in the chromosomes were the basis of cancer formation. Remarkably, it was half a century later that the Philadelphia chromosome (discussed below) was identified.

There is little doubt that Theodore Boveri is one of the giants of twentieth century cancer genetics. His classical experiments on fertilization of sea urchin eggs with two sperms demonstrated the phenomenon of abnormal chromosomal segregation and he was quick to realize that this abnormal chromosomal number may account for the unrestricted growth of tumours. In fact, he made a number of pertinent remarks relating to regulation of the cell cycle, the presence of oncogenes and tumour suppressor genes and genetic instability in tumours. To put it into context, Boveri made his observations between 1902 and 1904, the Philadelphia chromosome was identified in the 1960s, Knudson's two-hit hypothesis and the identification of the first dominant oncogene in the 1970s, the cloning of the first tumour suppressor gene, retinoblastoma gene (RB), in the 1980s, discovery of mismatch repair defects in tumours and cloning of BRCA1/2 in the 1990s, and the publication of the first draft of the human genome in 2000. What an incredible century!

CYTOGENETICS

Not surprisingly, following Boveri's publications, some of the earliest indications for genetic alterations came from classical karyotypic analysis. This type of study reveals gross abnormalities at the chromosomal level. Classical examples of tumours showing such gross chromosomal abnormalities include chronic myeloid leukaemia and Burkitt's lymphoma. We have already considered Burkitt's lymphoma in the section on viruses (page 268). We will briefly consider chronic myeloid leukaemia here.

The Philadelphia (Ph1) chromosome is present in 90 per cent of cases of chronic myeloid leukaemia and can be used as a diagnostic marker. It is produced by a reciprocal and balanced translocation between chromosomes 22 and 9. The breakpoint on chromosome 9 occurs at the locus of the *abl* proto-oncogene and the breakpoint on chromosome 22 is in the region termed the breakpoint cluster region (bcr). Some recent work suggests that the *bcr* genes code for a protein kinase that could have oncogenic potential. The *abl* proto-oncogene has sequence homology with the tyrosine kinase family of oncogenes but it is only after translocation to chromosome 22 that it produces a mutant protein with tyrosine kinase activity. This particular tyrosine kinase activity is located in the nucleus where it is believed to influence transcription of DNA. Further examples of tumours and the cytogenetic abnormalities are shown in Table 13.1.

CANCER-PRODUCING GENES: ONCOGENES

The term 'oncogene' refers to any mutated gene that contributes to neoplastic transformation in the cell. Two major types of oncogenes have been identified: *dominant oncogenes* and *tumour suppressor genes (anti-oncogenes)*. A third category of genes are also known to be important, so-called 'stability' genes or genes involved in DNA repair.

Some oncogenes involved in carcinogenesis are mutated versions of normal cellular genes (called proto-oncogenes, p-*onc*). The function of these normal genes is enhanced by the mutations and hence they are referred to as 'activating' or 'gain in function' mutations. These genes are also known as 'dominant' oncogenes since

Table 13.1 Chromosomal alterations in human tumours

Tumour type	Chromosomal aberration	Possible action	Gene(s)
Haemopoietic tumours: translocation			
Chronic myeloid leukaemia	t(9;22)(q34;q11)	Alteration of nuclear tyrosine kinase	ABL
Burkitt's lymphoma	t(8,14)(q24;q32) t(2;8)(p12;q24) t(8;22)(q24;q11)	Cell cycle regulation	c-myc-IgH Igk,c-myc
Acute myeloid leukaemia	t(8;21)(q22;q22)		ETO
Mantle cell lymphoma	t(11;14)(q13;q32)		Bcl-1-IgH
Follicular lymphoma	t(14;18)(q32;q21)		IgH-bcl-2
Solid tumours: translocation			
Ewing's sarcoma/PNET*	t(11;22)(q24;q12) t(21;22)(q22;q12) t(11;22)(q13;q12)		EWS-FL1 EWS-ERG EWS-WT1
Synovial sarcoma	T(X;18) (p11.23,q11.2) T(X;18) (p11.21,q11.2)		SYT-SSX1 SYT-SSX2
Malignant melanoma	t(1;19)(q12;p13) t(1;6)(q11;q11) t(1;14)(q21;q32)		? ? ?
Salivary adenoma	t(3,8)(p21;q12)		CTNNB1
Renal adenocarcinoma	t(X;1)(p11;q21) t(9;15)(p11;q11)		TFE3 ?
Solid tumours: deletions			
Retinoblastoma	del13q14	Loss of oncosuppression	RB
Wilms' tumour	del11p13 del11p15 del17q12–21	Loss of oncosuppression	WT-1 ? FWT1
Bladder, transitional cell carcinoma	del11p13		?
Lung cancer, small-cell type	del17p13	Loss of oncosuppression	TP53
Colorectal adenocarcinoma	del17p13 del 5q21	Loss of oncosuppression Loss of oncosuppression	TP53 APC
Breast cancer	del17p13 del17q21 del13q12–13 del16q22.1	Loss of oncosuppression Loss of oncosuppression Loss of oncosuppression Loss of oncosuppression	TP53 BRCA1 BRCA2
Solid tumours: amplification			
Neuroblastoma		Cell cycle control	N_MYC
Breast cancer		Increased growth factor activity	CERBB2

mutation of one allele is sufficient to exert an effect, despite the presence of normal gene product from the remaining allele. It is over 30 years since such genes were discovered. This category of genes are now referred in the literature as just 'oncogenes'.

Dictionary

Allele: Alternative form of the gene found at the same locus in homologous chromosomes

In contrast, tumour suppressor genes (TSGs) are normal genes whose function is inactivated by mutations and hence these are known as 'inactivating' or 'loss of function' mutations. The genes are also known as 'recessive' oncogenes since inactivation of both alleles is required to have an effect at the cellular level. Evidence for the existence of such genes has been largely circumstantial and was based on classical genetics, cytogenetics and molecular genetics. You should beware that the terms 'dominant' and 'recessive' refer to action at the genetic level; confusion sometimes occurs since the terminology has been borrowed from classical Mendelian genetic inheritance patterns.

The stability or DNA repair genes include mismatch repair (*MMR*) genes as well as the breast cancer predisposition genes *BRCA1* and *BRCA2*. *MMR* genes repair subtle mistakes in the genome which occur during normal cell division or due to exposure to carcinogens. *BRCA1* on the other hand is also involved in chrosomal stability during mitotic recombinations and segregation. These genes are fundamental to the cell as mutations in these genes allows alterations in the DNA to go unrepaired, and hence mutations in other genes occur at a higher rate. You can imagine that if these increased mutations occur in cell-cycle related genes or genes involved in aopotosis, genetic changes will be consolidated as the cell will be allowed to proceed and complete a round of division despite defective DNA.

Where do oncogenes come from? There are both exogenous and endogenous sources. The exogenous sources include viral oncogenes (v-*onc*) which may be introduced into cells by tumour viruses. Endogenous genes are called cellular oncogenes (c-*onc*) and these are genes that are normally present in the cell but have been altered to produce the oncogene. As mentioned above, the normal gene from which the oncogene is derived is called the proto-oncogene.

The viral or exogenous oncogenes can be divided into two types: those that show similarity to normal cellular genes and those that are completely different. This is important because viral oncogenes that resemble cellular genes are actually derived from the cell's genes. This is quite amazing when you think about it! A virus infects a cell and incorporates some of the cellular genes into its own genome. These genes, finding themselves in a new piece of DNA or RNA, become altered in their properties and are then viral oncogenes. When the virus infects another cell, it can introduce the viral oncogene (a process called transduction), which leads to altered growth of the infected cell. Retroviruses, which consist of RNA that becomes incorporated into the host DNA through the action of the enzyme, reverse transcriptase, can readily 'pick up' some host DNA and so can carry viral oncogenes derived from cellular oncogenes. Oncogenic DNA viruses generally possess gene sequences that are uniquely viral and have no homology with cellular oncogenes.

Key facts

Main differences between dominant oncogenes and tumour suppressor genes

	Dominant oncogenes	Tumour suppressor genes
Number of alleles in normal cells	Two	Two
Number of alleles mutated to exert effect	One	Two
Effect of mutation on the function of the protein product	Enhanced	Reduced
Germline (inherited) mutations identified, i.e. important in genetic predisposition	Rare-*RET*, *KIT*	Many-*TP53*, *RB* etc.
Adjectives to describe mutations	Activating, gain in function, dominant	Inactivating, loss of function, recessive

Figure 13.1 Point mutation

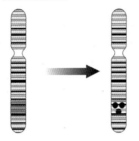

e.g. ras oncogene family in Ca colon

Figure 13.2 Translocation

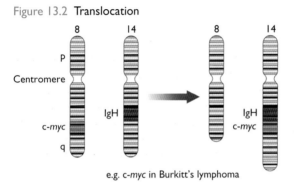

e.g. c-myc in Burkitt's lymphoma

Figure 13.3 Gene amplification

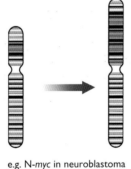

e.g. N-myc in neuroblastoma

HOW CAN ONCOGENES PROMOTE CELL GROWTH?

There are a number of ways by which the function of oncogenes can be altered and this includes (1) point mutations, (2) amplification, (3) gene rearrangement/translocation, (4) deletion of part or whole of chromosome and (5) altered expression. Since most of the mechanisms described apply to both type of oncogenes, they are considered here together; however, there are

Figure 13.4 Deletion

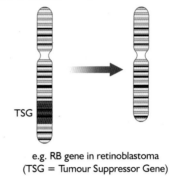

e.g. RB gene in retinoblastoma
(TSG = Tumour Suppressor Gene)

differences in the pattern of alterations between dominant oncogenes and tumour suppressor genes. In contrast to dominant oncogenes which are mutated in a consistent manner either by point mutation (e.g. *ras*), translocation (e.g. *abl*) or gene amplification (e.g. N-*myc*), mutations in tumour suppressor genes tend to be diverse both in type and position within the gene (e.g. *TP53*).

POINT MUTATIONS

This results in the substitution of one base pair by another, e.g. substitution of G:C by A:T. The effect of the point mutation depends on its position and includes alteration of the protein structure by change in the amino acid composition and insertion of a stop codon with premature termination of the protein. The clearest example of point mutations in human tumours are found in the *ras* family (Fig. 13.1). Mutations at codons 12, 13 and 61 of H-, K- and N-*ras* contribute to oncogenesis in many of the main types of human tumours. *ras* mutations are encountered in both benign and malignant neoplasms. *Kit* gene encodes a transmembrane tyrosine kinase receptor that is consistently expressed in hematopoietic stem cells, mast cells, melanocytes, germ cells, and interstitial cells of Cajal (ICC). Activating germline mutations of *kit* gene are associated with ICC hyperplasia, familial gastrointestinal stromal tumours (GISTs), cutaneous mastocytosis, and cutaneous hyperpigmentation. Depending on the site where the mutation has occurred, patients will present a combination of all or some of the above lesions.

GENE REARRANGEMENTS/TRANSLOCATIONS

This refers to the production of a hybrid chromosome due to joining of part of one chromosome with another

(Fig. 13.2). The rearrangement of DNA sequences can lead to creation of an altered gene (and product) either as a result of structural change or due to change in the control of transcription. Examples include 8:14 (or 8:22, 2:8) translocation in Burkitt's lymphoma and the 9:22 translocation in chronic myeloid leukaemia (CML).

AMPLIFICATION

The normal genome contains two copies of each gene (the two alleles). In amplification, one copy is multiplied numerous times and may result in increased mRNA and hence increased protein product (Fig. 13.3). At the level of the chromosome, these areas of amplification are seen as double minutes (DM) or homogeneously staining regions (HSRs). DM are extrachromosomal chromatin bodies without centromeres that segregate randomly during mitosis. HSRs are expanded chromosomal regions which are linked to the centromere and therefore segregate in the normal way. Most classes of oncogenes have been shown to be amplified in human malignancy. Examples include N-*myc* in neuroblastoma and *HER2* in breast cancer. Only some of these amplifications have been demonstrated to have pathological significance. N-*myc* amplification is correlated with advanced stage and recurrence of neuroblastoma and *HER2* amplification in breast cancer correlates with poor prognosis. It should be noted however that in many tumours, over-expression of mRNA and protein are seen in the absence of gene amplification.

DELETIONS

This ranges from the loss of single base pairs to loss of entire chromosomes. The small intragenic deletions have similar effects (abnormal protein, stop codons) to point mutations. Larger deletions will of course inactivate many genes at a time. See Fig. 13.4.

ALTERED EXPRESSION

The inactivation of a gene via deletions or intragenic mutations is now a familiar story. It has recently become apparent that some putative tumour suppressor genes do not exhibit these common phenomena in certain tumours. Instead changes in the methylation patterns of the promoter region of the gene or even alterations in the chromatin pattern regulated by histone deacetylases lead to an altered expression of some genes (i.e. alteration in the transcription of the mRNA and translation of the protein). This occurs without any mutational event in the gene; hence if the gene was sequenced, no changes would be detected. Some good examples are the inactivation of *p16* gene on chromosome 9p21, the inactivation of *BRCA1* gene in sporadic breast carcinomas, and the inactivation of the second allele in some rare types of gastric carcinomas (isolated or signet ring cell gastric carcinoma). It is worth bearing in mind that in tumorigenesis, methylation and acetylation play roles in the downregulation of the expression of tumour suppressor genes.

MODE OF ACTION OF DOMINANT ONCOGENES

Normal cell growth is believed to be influenced by growth factors binding to receptors on the surface of the cell. This produces a stimulus through a 'signal transduction pathway(s)' which influences the cell's nucleus to produce instructions for proliferation. Within the nucleus itself, there are also molecules that regulate transcription and those that regulate the cell cycle during cell division. Therefore, cell growth could be stimulated due to:

- increased growth factor production
- increase in growth factor receptors on the cell's surface
- abnormal growth factor receptors
- abnormal signalling through the cascade of signal transduction pathways in the cytoplasm
- abnormalities in the nuclear acting molecules
- alterations to the control of the cell cycle.

Oncogenes have been identified which act through each of these mechanisms.

GROWTH FACTORS AND GROWTH FACTOR RECEPTORS

Growth factors are polypeptides that act locally to stimulate proliferation and, sometimes, differentiation. If tumour cells produce substances that act as growth factors, then they will be continually self-stimulating (autocrine stimulation). Several classes of growth factors have been classified according to sequence homology and biological activity. The categories include epidermal growth factor family (EGF and TGF-α), the fibroblast growth factor family (acidic and basic FGF, hst and int-2), platelet derived growth factor (PDGF), colony stimulating factors (CSFs), interleukins and the insulin-like growth factors (IGFs). Growth factors act by

Figure 13.5 **Growth factor receptors and signalling pathways: points of interaction of cellular oncogenes**

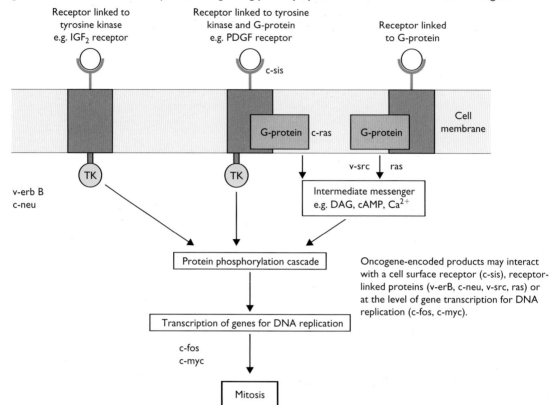

Oncogene-encoded products may interact with a cell surface receptor (c-sis), receptor-linked proteins (v-erB, c-neu, v-src, ras) or at the level of gene transcription for DNA replication (c-fos, c-myc).

binding to a receptor residing in the plasma membrane. The binding leads to activation of the receptor and signal transduction to the interior of the cell (Fig. 13.5).

When the normal cell surface receptors are activated by growth factors, the receptors usually dimerize, leading to phosphorylation of the tyrosine residues and an increase in their tyrosine kinase activity (Fig. 13.6). When the genes coding for these receptors are abnormal, there is persistent activity without receptor binding. The growth factor receptors can be activated in this way by a number of mechanisms including gene amplification, re-arrangement and over-expression. For example, the *HER2* gene is amplified in about 25 per cent of breast cancers and also in a variety of other cancers such as lung. Breast cancers, which over-express the *HER2* receptor, are more aggressive and have a poor prognosis. Recently, a humanized monoclonal antibody against *HER2* has been developed and is used to treat patients with breast cancer. In other situations, the receptor may not be over-expressed but may instead have altered kinase activity as with *HER1* (epidermal

growth factor receptor, EGFR). Some tyrosine kinases are not attached to a receptor but are anchored to the plasma membrane and participate in signalling. The *c-src* oncogene alters the activity of one of these non-receptor tyrosine kinases.

SIGNAL TRANSDUCTION PROTEINS: GTP-BINDING PROTEINS

Three mammalian *ras* genes – H-*ras*-1, K-*ras*-2 and N-*ras* – have been identified. They form one of the most important families of oncogenes identified to date. *ras* genes usually acquire transforming activity as a result of point mutation within their coding regions. These activating point mutations are restricted to certain sites, notably codons 12, 13 and 61. The p21 product of both *ras* proto-oncogene and transforming genes are located in the inner surface of the cell membrane. They bind guanosine nucleotides (GDP and GTP) and possess intrinsic GTPase activity. These biochemical properties resemble those of the G proteins which are associated with the cell membrane and are implicated in the modulation of signal transduction. It is becoming clear that ras proteins function as critical relay switches that regulate signalling pathways between the cell surface receptors and the nucleus.

Overall, point mutation in the *ras* gene is the commonest dominant oncogene abnormality in human tumours. It appears to play a major role in colon, pancreatic and thyroid cancers as well as in myeloid leukaemia.

NUCLEAR ONCOPROTEINS

These oncoproteins share the feature of nuclear localization and proven or suspected ability to bind to specific DNA sequences.

An important family of such genes involved in human malignancy is *myc*. This was originally identified as the oncogene carried by several acutely transforming retroviruses. The *myc* family consists of c-*myc*, N-*myc*, L-*myc*, R-*myc*, P-*myc* and B-*myc*. They have been isolated on the basis of homology to v-*myc* or one of the *myc* proto-oncogenes. c-*myc* is expressed in many tissues and correlates with cell proliferation. Activation due to gene amplification occurs in breast cancer and small-cell lung cancer (SCLC). In B- and T-cell lymphomas, translocation to an immunoglobulin (Ig) or T-cell receptor locus is seen.

The end result of all the signalling pathways is the transition of the cell through the cell cycle. Here another important family of molecules is critical. These are the cyclins and cyclin-dependent kinases (CDKs). The cyclins activate the CDKs by phosphorylation and these activated kinases are critically important in allowing the various stages of the cell cycle to progress smoothly (see Fig. 13.11). Control of the cell cycle also involves the products of tumour suppressor genes such as retinoblastoma (see later).

TUMOUR SUPPRESSOR GENES/RECESSIVE ONCOGENES

Although 'activated' or 'dominant' oncogenes held centre stage 25 years ago, it is interesting that there was evidence for yet another type of gene long before that. The successful identification of genes whose proteins are physiological inhibitors of growth stemmed from two main types of studies: (1) somatic cell hybrids, and (2) genetic studies of inherited cancer syndromes. Furthermore, cytogenetic studies had already shown that many tumours exhibit loss of DNA involving almost all chromosomal arms.

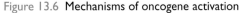

Figure 13.6 Mechanisms of oncogene activation

↑Growth factor
c-sis

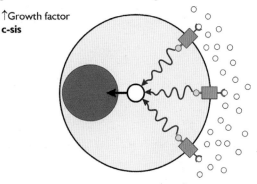

Permanent activation of receptor
v-erb B

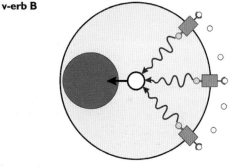

↑Growth factor receptor
c-neu

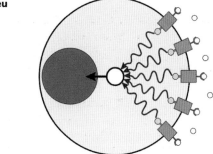

Abnormal signal transduction
c-K-ras

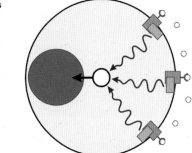

Figure 13.7 **Section through the eye showing retinal detachment due to underlying tumour**

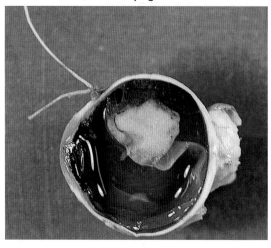

Figure 13.8 **Photomicrograph showing characteristic rosettes of retinoblastoma**

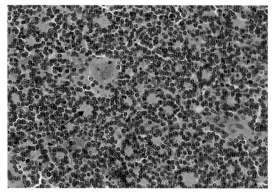

In somatic cell hybrids, the normal cell is fused with a transformed ('malignant') cell to form a hybrid cell. The main action of fusion was to produce a non-transformed state. This phenomenon of tumour suppression suggested that the normal cell must replace a defective function in the cancer cell. The first tumour suppressor to be identified was by the study of a rare familial disease, retinoblastoma (Figs 13.7 and 13.8).

Retinoblastoma, a tumour arising from the embryonal neural retina, has a worldwide incidence of 1:20 000. The tumour is of interest because it has both a sporadic and familial forms, with approximately 25–30 per cent of the tumours being heritable. These cases tend to present earlier and develop bilateral disease. In contrast, the sporadic cases have unilateral tumours. Advancement in surgery and radiotherapy led to improved survival and it became clear that 50 per cent of the offspring of patients with bilateral tumours were themselves at risk of the disease. Evaluation of family pedigrees clearly shows the inherited form as Mendelian dominant.

In 1971, Knudson proposed his 'two-hit' hypothesis (Fig. 13.9). He pointed out that if cancer arises due to a series of somatic events, then it is possible that sometimes, one of these changes is inherited in the germline and hence is present in every cell of the body. All the cells are therefore already one step along the pathway of carcinogenesis and this forms the basis for the dominantly inherited (Mendelian) cancer susceptibility. In addition, a further mutation occurring somatically during life in the same gene would knock out the function of the gene. Hence, while the susceptibility is dominant, the action at the cell level is recessive. This therefore predicted for a class of genes which had to be inactivated or to have 'loss of function' in order to provide the malignant phenotype. Knudson examined data relating to the age of first appearance of the tumour in both familial and the sporadic cases and showed that it followed the expected statistical model based on this hypothesis.

Cytogenetic studies had revealed that a few of the familial tumours showed germline deletions of chromosome 13 and careful karyotyping revealed deletions of 13q14. The retinoblastoma gene (*RB1*) was cloned in 1986. It was the first tumour suppressor gene to be isolated. With the cloning of the gene, it could be confirmed that familial retinoblastoma is indeed due to an inactivating mutation. Further evidence for oncosuppression comes from fusion experiments. Insertion of the 4.7 kb complementary DNA sequence (cDNA) into retinoblastoma and osteosarcoma cell lines lead to reversion of the tumorigenic phenotype and introduction of these cells into nude mice failed to produce tumours. Interestingly, mutations of the retinoblastoma gene and expression of the protein product have also been seen in almost every tissue despite the restricted oncogenic effects. Mutations are also found in other types of tumours such as breast carcinoma, although breast cancer does not form part of any syndrome in association with retinoblastoma.

THE MODE OF ACTION OF TUMOUR SUPPRESSOR GENES

Interestingly, although the mode of action of genes that are inhibitory for growth might follow the same pathways

Figure 13.9 Two-hit model of retinoblastoma. Black arrow indicates inactivating mutation

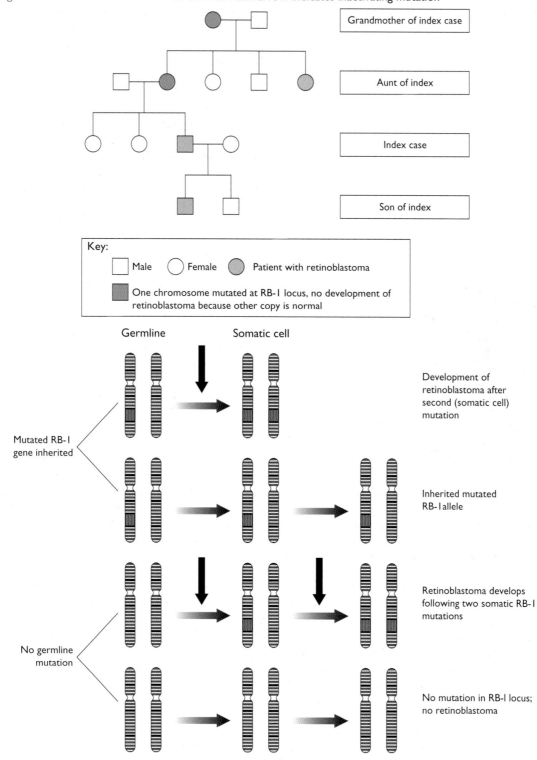

as those that promote growth, there is much less information on this topic than for dominant oncogenes.

Perhaps the best examples of molecules that act at the cell surface include the cadherins, which are cell–cell adhesion molecules. E-cadherin (an epithelial cell–cell adhesion molecule) is abnormal in a special type of breast cancer – lobular carcinoma. Mutations in the E-cadherin gene are also responsible for predisposition to inherited gastric cancer of diffuse type in a percentage of patients.

Another good example is the binding of transforming growth factor beta (TGF-β) to its receptor which leads to the transcription of genes that inhibit growth. The TGF-β signalling pathway is abnormal in colonic and pancreatic cancers.

A good example of a protein that regulates cell signalling is the APC (adenomatous polyposis coli) protein. This gene, which predisposes to familial adenomatous polyposis (FAP), is an important player in the development of colonic carcinoma (Fig. 13.10). The APC protein plays an important role in the signalling pathway that involves a molecule called β-catenin. This protein acts in the nucleus to increase the activity of growth promoting genes. APC causes degradation of β-catenin, hence removing the proliferative signal. It is easy to see then that mutations in APC gene will lead to increased levels of β-catenin and hence increased proliferating signal.

Not surprisingly, most information relating to the function of tumour suppressor genes comes from the study of RB and p53. These molecules have an effect on nuclear transcription and the regulation of the cell cycle. The regulation of the cell cycle is complex and illustrated in Fig. 13.11.

Briefly, when the cells are in the resting or quiescent stage, the retinoblastoma protein is hypophosphorylated. In this state, RB is able to bind to a transcription factor E2F and hence prevent the activation of genes that play a role in pushing the cell through division. Various growth factors including the EGF family (discussed above) activate the proteins of the cyclin family. The cyclins D/CDK 4, 6 and cyclin E/CDK2 complexes phosphorylate the RB protein, leading to release of the E2F molecule which is then free to bind to DNA and activate transcription of genes involved in cell division. This process is balanced by signals which inhibit the process, with p16 playing an important role.

Unlike RB, p53 protein does not play a role in maintaining a check on the normal cell cycle. However, damage caused to the DNA by irradiation or by chemicals

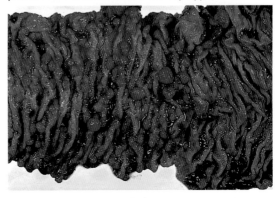

Figure 13.10 Large bowel with numerous polyps in patient with familial adenomatous polyposis

Figure 13.11 The cell cycle is largely governed by the actions of cyclins and cyclin-dependent kinases (CDK), some of which are manufactured during the cycle, others are recycled. Phosphorylation of the retinoblastoma protein (product of the RB-1 gene) enables the transition from G1 to the synthesis phase by releasing E2F protein, which activates DNA synthesis genes. p53 protein operates a quality control system at this checkpoint: if DNA damage or mutation is identified the defect is either repaired by DNA-repair enzymes or the cell is consigned to apoptosis. G2 is the pre-mitotic phase, during which preparation is made for mitosis. The resultant cells either re-enter the cycle, terminally differentiate and leave the cell cycle, or enter a resting phase, G0

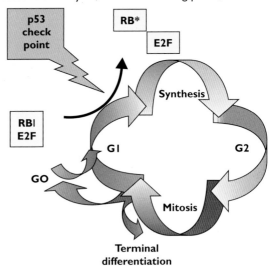

brings p53 into play. Levels of p53 protein rises following DNA damage and this leads to two main effects: it leads to cell cycle arrest by the transcription of an inhibitor of CDK, p21, or if the damage is too severe, to cell death via activation of apoptosis. The cell cycle arrest is necessary and important as it allows the cell time to repair the damage before completion of cell division. It is not too difficult to see that if cells that undergo cell division to produce daughter cells do so without repairing the defect then, in essence, the damage is consolidated (Fig. 13.12). This is one of the features of tumour cells. No surprise then that p53 has been called 'the guardian of the genome'.

Many TSGs have now been identified and although the exact mechanism of action is not clear in every case, the biology is slowly being unravelled. Some examples of TSGs that have a familial predisposition are shown in Table 13.2.

Figure 13.12 Clonal evolution

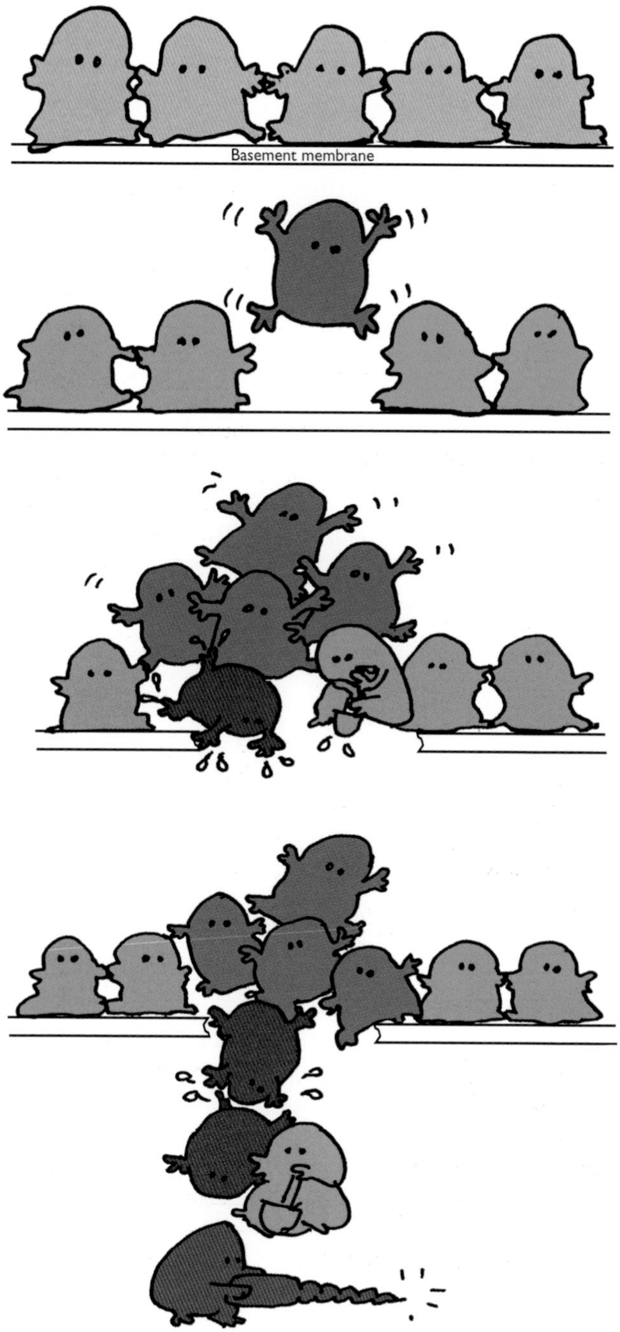

Normal epithelial cells, with cell–cell junctions and normal regulation of proliferation

Mutation in one cell confers freedom from normal growth control mechanisms. It proliferates without restraint

During proliferation, new mutations occur, some of which confer an increased growth advantage and an ability to spread through basement membrane

Further mutations occur. Thus, although the tumour has originated from a single mutated cell (i.e. it is clonal), it is clear that the final population is mixed, each new population evolving to the advantage of the tumour. This is clonal evolution

Table 13.2 Tumours and familial predisposition

Syndrome	Principal tumour types	Genetic locus/gene
Familial polyposis coli	Colorectal carcinoma	5q21 (APC)
MEN I	Pituitary, parathyroid thyroid, adrenal cortex, islet cell tumour	11q13
MEN IIa	Medullary carcinoma of thyroid, phaeochromocytoma, parathyroid tumours	10q11 (RET)
MEN IIb	Medullary carcinoma of thyroid, phaeochromocytoma, mucosal neuromas	10q11 (RET)
Von Hipple–Lindau	Haemangioblastoma of cerebellum and retina, renal cell carcinoma, phaeochromocytoma	3p25 (VHL)
Tuberous sclerosis 16p13.3 (TSC2)	Angiomyolipoma	9q34 (TSC1)
Familial retinoblastoma	Bilateral retinoblastoma, osteosarcoma	13q14 (RB)
Neurofibromatosis type I	Neurofibromas, neurofibrosarcoma, glioma, meningioma, phaeochromocytoma	17q11 (NF1)
Neurofibromatosis type II	Bilateral acoustic schwamnnomas, multiple meningiomas	22q (NF2)
Li–Fraumeni	Breast cancer, sarcoma	17p13 (TP53)
Breast–ovarian	Breast cancer, ovarian cancer	17q21 (BRCA1)
Breast	Breast cancer, ovarian cancer, prostate cancer	13q12–13 (BRCA2)
Hereditary non-polyposis colorectal cancer (HNPCC)	Colorectal carcinoma	2p (MSH2) 3p (MLH1) 7p (PMS2)
Familial gastrointestinal stromal tumours (GIST)	Multiple GIST, hyperplasia of intestinal cells of Cajal, mastocytosis, hyperpigmentation	4q12 (c-Kit)
Wilms' tumour (WAGR syndrome)	Wilms' tumour, aniridia, genitourinary abnormalities, mental retardation	11p13.3 (WT1)
Familial cylindromatosis	Cylindromas (skin)	16q (CYLD)
Peutz–Jeghers syndrome	Intestinal polyps, ovarian and pancreatic tumours	19p13.3 (STK11/LKB1)
Cowden's syndrome	Hamartoma polyps of gastrointestinal tract, gliomas, endometrial cancer, breast cancer	10q22–23 (PTEN)

MEN, multiple endocrine neoplasia.

DNA REPAIR, APOPTOSIS, TELOMERES, TELOMERASES AND CANCER

DNA REPAIR

If the human genome is not to fall apart as a result of exogenous (environmental chemicals, radiation) and endogenous (DNA replication) damage, it has to have efficient DNA repair and ability to execute programmed cell death (see below). There are many different types of DNA repair mechanisms within the cell and undoubtedly the knowledge will become more complicated and refined with time. Since some of the important genes involved in cancer are already being assigned to have a role in particular types of repair mechanisms, they will be listed here but it is not the intention that you should be able to regurgitate the different mechanisms in detail.

The mechanisms include homologous recombinational repair (HRR), non-homologous end-joining (NHEJ), nucleotide excisional repair (NER), base excisional repair (BER) and mismatch repair (MMR). HRR, as its name suggests, relies on the homologous chromosome to provide the template for repairing the defective strand; it is therefore an accurate and error-free way of dealing with damage. In contrast, NHEJ is prone to error as no complementary strand is available to provide a template for accurate replication. The recently identified breast cancer predisposition genes, *BRCA1/2,* are involved in DNA repair through HRR. In their absence following mutations in the genes, DNA repair is still possible but it now occurs through the error-prone pathway of NHEJ, hence making the cell more susceptible to further genetic changes and hence cancer formation.

The other major pathway that has been identified to play a role in tumour formation is MMR. Genomic instability plays an important role in the development of tumours in patients with hereditary non-polyposis colorectal cancer (HNPCC). Most HNPCC patients have mutations in the human counterparts of the bacterial mismatch repair genes *mutS* and *mutL*. Mutations in these genes leads to an inability to repair DNA mismatch (mistakes that happen during DNA replication) and hence contribute to neoplastic transformation by allowing mutations to be transmitted to daughter cells. Microsatellites are repeat units generally found within the non-coding part of the genome. They are highly polymorphic (the two alleles differ in size) and hence they provide a useful tool for the investigation of mutations within the genome. Patients with HNPCC show widespread alterations in these microsatellites and are therefore said to exhibit microsatellite instability (or a mutator phenotype). The implication of finding microsatellite instability is that the mismatch repair genes must be inactivated otherwise the mismatch repair gene proteins would have corrected the mutations identified in the microsatellites. Hence analysis of microsatellite instability provides indirect evidence for mismatch repair gene abnormality and patients with high levels of instability can have direct genetic testing to look for the mutations in the mismatch repair genes.

APOPTOSIS AND CANCER

Following genetic damage, the cell may have an opportunity to repair the defect via the pathways described above. Occasionally, the damage is so severe that the cell is unable to do this and a set of signals is initiated which lead to programmed cell death. This is an important protective mechanism as a cell with severe genetic damage is no threat if it is dead! It is only when it manages to go through the cell division cycle with its damage and pass the alterations onto the daughter cells that problems are likely to occur.

Apart from showing increased proliferation, cancer cells also fail to undergo apoptosis and hence have an increased life span compared to normal cells. The inability of cancer cells to commit suicide is an important contributory factor to tumour growth both at the primary site and at the sites of metastatic spread.

Many genes involved in the control of apoptosis have now been identified. The first to be identified was *bcl-2*. This gene is a member of a large family of genes, some of which are pro-apoptotic (*bax, bad*) while others are anti-apoptotic (*bcl-2, bcl-xL*). The mechanisms controlling apoptosis are complex. In response to DNA damage, a whole series of cascades is set up, the balance of which determines whether the cell is sent into a death programme (Fig. 13.13). In the presence of an overall death outcome, the *bcl-2* family of proteins operates via activation of a series of proteolytic enzymes called 'caspases' which chop up the DNA into fragments.

Two other genes which are also prominent in the apoptotic pathway are *p53* (discussed above) and c-*myc* oncogene.

TELOMERES, TELOMERASE AND CANCER

Telomeres are a series of short tandem nucleotide repeat sequences of six base pairs (TTAGGG) that are found at the end of chromosomes. They cap the chromosomes and protect the ends from degradation during DNA replication that occurs as part of cell growth and differentiation. They also work as a molecular counting mechanism (an intracellular clock), because with each round of DNA replication, the telomeres shorten until the cell reaches a 'crisis' (also known as the Hayflick limit). At this point the chromosomal ends become dysfunctional, end-to-end joining occurs and the cell is sent into apoptosis via a p53 mediated pathway.

An enzyme called telomerase plays a role in the maintenance of the telomeres by preventing the erosion of telomeres that occurs during replication. This enzyme is a ribonucleoprotein reverse transcriptase that is composed of two components, hTERC (the RNA subunit that acts as the template for addition of new telomeric repeats), and hTERT (the catalytic protein component). Its expression is tightly regulated

Figure 13.13 DNA damage can take several forms, some shown here. Several enzymes patrol the cell's DNA to detect DNA distortion or mismatch and effect DNA repair. Once a cell has divided, any mutation will be perpetuated if the daughter cell is capable of further division. This may lead to tumour development

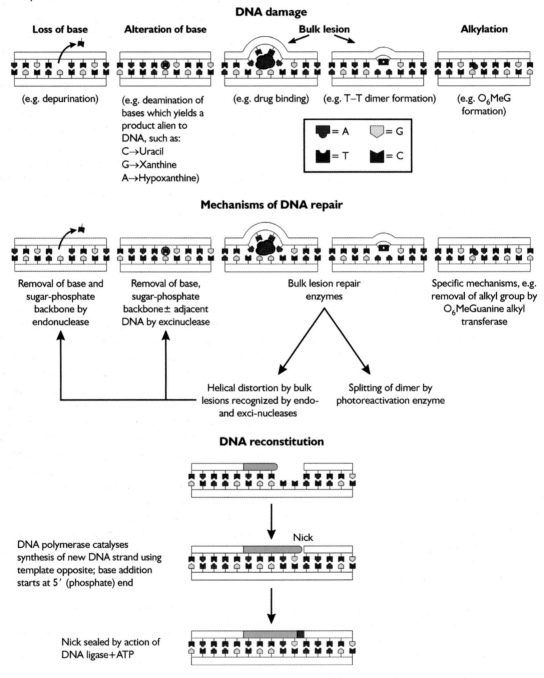

during development and, after this period, in humans, it is expressed in quantities sufficient to prevent telomere erosion in male germ cells, lymphocytes and stem cell populations, including basal keratinocytes. The state when the cell cannot divide anymore is called 'cellular senescence'.

It is becoming clear that in order to create a cancer cell, two barriers must be overcome: cellular senescence and crisis, which limits replicative potential. This hypothesis seems to be valid for both benign and malignant tumours, at least in '*in vitro*' experiments. It is not difficult to postulate that cancer cells have learnt how to circumvent the erosion of telomeres. This is indeed the case and unlike normal, non-germ cells, most cancer cells have detectable and increased telomerase activity or develop an alternative mechanism for telomere lengthening (ALT), which is thought to involve recombination mechanisms and results in abnormal telomeres.

Several lines of evidence have supported the major role of telomerase in oncogenesis. When normal cells reach the 'crisis' (complete erosion of telomeres), lack of telomerase leads to major chromosomal abnormalities (aneuploidy and chromosomal fusions). Other connections between telomerase and other oncogenes and tumour suppressor genes are currently under intense investigation.

WHICH CELL IN THE TISSUE GIVES RISE TO CANCER?

The traditional view has been that a cell, capable of replication, undergoes a mutation in a gene which allows it to have a growth advantage. This mutated cell produces a small clonal expansion. Subsequent mutations over a long time period leads to further clonal expansions which then become the reservoir for further mutations and expansions. This idea follows the traditional Darwinian model of evolution.

There has been an increasing interest in stem cell biology over the last two decades and a role for stem cells in the development of cancers has been proposed. Normal stems cells, by definition, must be able to undergo self renewal (produce an identical copy of itself) and be able to produce daughter/progenitor cells. Progenitor cells retain some characteristics of stem cells initially but lose these features as they differentiate into the different tissue types with subsequent cell divisions.

One of the problems with the traditional model is the knowledge that cancers take a long time to initiate and progress, and this contrasts with the relatively short lifespan of mature, differentiated cells. It has been proposed that stem cells, which are long lived and hence predisposed to the slow accumulation of genetic changes, may be the tumour initiating cells. Although a huge amount of effort is currently invested in studying normal and cancer associated stem cells, it is unclear at present whether cancers do indeed arise from normal stem cells or whether some cancer cells develop the ability to have stem-like characteristics as a result of transformation. This is a field in transit and worth keeping an eye on as it will change the way we think about primary and metastic disease and how we manage it in the future.

THE MULTISTEP MODEL OF CARCINOGENESIS

In the course of examining malignant tissues, histopathologists frequently encounter lesions that show transitions with appearances intermediate between normal morphology and frank malignancy. Occasionally, such lesions are closely associated with the invasive cancer (Fig. 13.14). This led to the suggestion that many of these lesions may be precursors of the invasive carcinoma. With the identification of dominant oncogenes and tumour suppressor genes, genes involved in DNA repair and apoptosis, it became possible to investigate tumours and putative precursor lesions using molecular techniques. The study of colorectal carcinoma with its well-defined pre-invasive lesion, the adenoma, has paved the way for this type of investigation (Fig. 13.15). The results demonstrate that both activating and inactivating events are involved and it is the co-ordinated

Figure 13.14 **Multistep model for colorectal carcinoma**

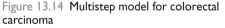

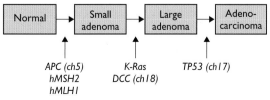

Figure 13.15 **The colonic adenoma–carcinoma sequence**

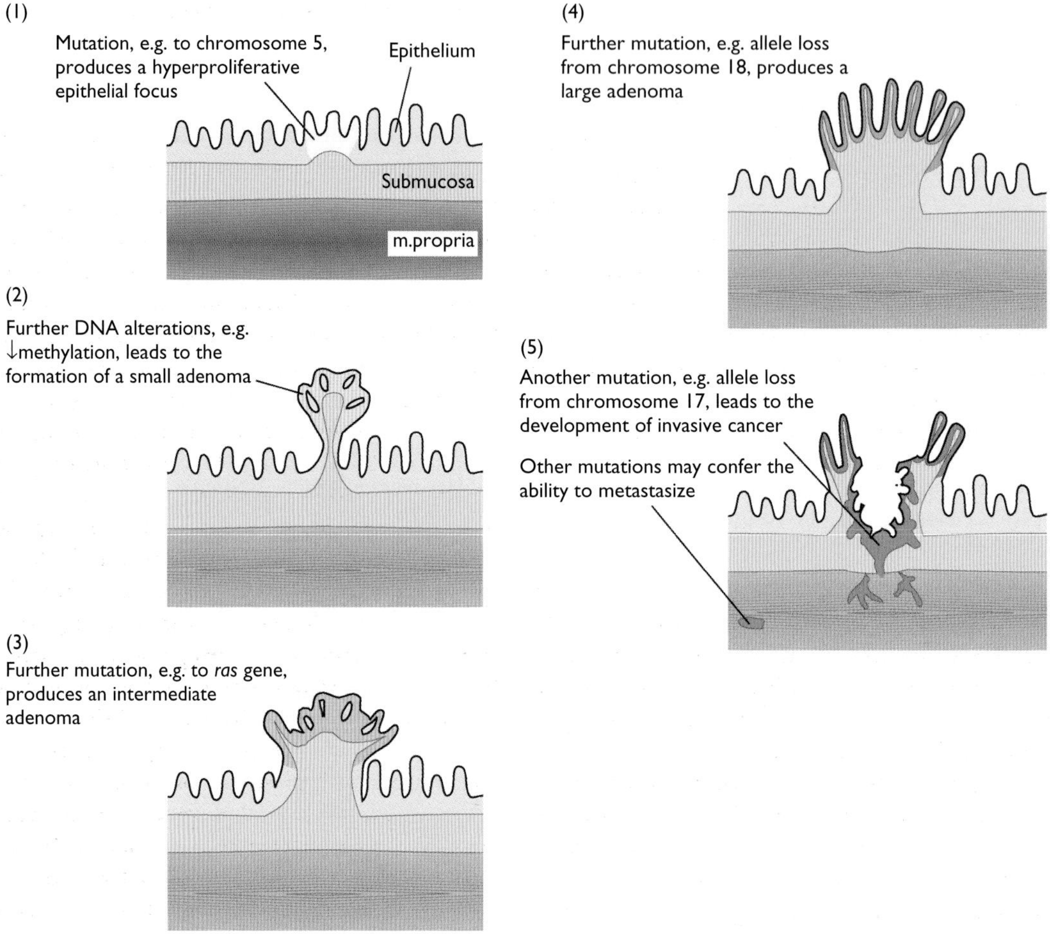

(1)

Mutation, e.g. to chromosome 5, produces a hyperproliferative epithelial focus

Epithelium

Submucosa

m.propria

(2)

Further DNA alterations, e.g. ↓methylation, leads to the formation of a small adenoma

(3)

Further mutation, e.g. to *ras* gene, produces an intermediate adenoma

(4)

Further mutation, e.g. allele loss from chromosome 18, produces a large adenoma

(5)

Another mutation, e.g. allele loss from chromosome 17, leads to the development of invasive cancer

Other mutations may confer the ability to metastasize

involvement of many of these types of alterations that are important in colon tumour formation. Furthermore, it is not just the timing of the events but the sequential accumulation of genetic damage that is also important in tumour formation. This idea that it is not one event but a sequence of genetic alterations that produces tumours is referred to as the 'multistep theory of neoplasia'.

The idea of the multistep model has been extended to almost every tumour type and there is good evidence that cancers in general develop in this way. The idea behind this type of model has also been fundamental in recommending screening programmes for cancer, the argument being that if you pick up a 'tumour' either when it is very small or still in its early stages of development, you can cure it. While the idea is a good one, it has also opened up a whole lot of problems. The screening programmes are identifying lesions at a very early stage in development and the classification and natural history of many such lesions is at present unknown. Once a lesion has been removed, the patient inevitably wants to know what it is and what its implications are. Since this is not always possible to predict with accuracy, it can cause much distress, for the clinician as well as the patient.

There has been a hope that new molecular techniques will help to understand the biology of cancer and in particular the early lesions. So what are these techniques and how are they helping with patient management?

MOLECULAR METHODOLOGY

LOSS OF HETEROZYGOSITY

In 1971, Knudson proposed his 'two-hit' hypothesis for the presence of tumour suppressor genes (TSGs). The recognition that the second mutation that leads to inactivation of the gene is usually in the form of a large deletion led to the development of the technique of loss of heterozygosity (LOH) by Cavenee and colleagues. The technique relies on the observation that markers (microsatellites) that are heterozygous and near the TSG would become homo- or hemizygous in the tumour compared to normal tissue. This was confirmed in the case of retinoblastoma where markers close to the gene were seen to exhibit LOH in both sporadic and familial cancers.

Since the introduction of the technique by Cavenee, there have been numerous studies looking at LOH in many cancer types. Although patterns of LOH have been reported in some series as being of prognostic significance, this information has not yet translated into routine practice. LOH has also been used extensively to investigate precancerous lesions in the hope that patterns of LOH would help to stratify lesions into 'benign' and 'malignant'. It has been apparent that many lesions traditionally thought of as 'benign' are monoclonal and that there is considerable overlap in LOH between these lesions and those accepted as 'malignant', i.e. ductal carcinoma *in situ* (DCIS). Hence at present, there are no robust profiles using LOH that help to definitively distinguish such lesions in clinical practice.

COMPARATIVE GENOMIC HYBRIDIZATION

CGH is a fluorescent *in situ* hybridization technique capable of determining changes in DNA copy number between differentially labelled test (e.g. tumour) and reference (e.g. normal) samples. Unlike LOH analysis which gives information at a very specific locus on a chromosomal arm, CGH analysis provides information from the entire genome. This has the advantage that a single experiment can give an idea about the many changes on all the different chromosomes, data that would require hundreds of experiments using LOH analysis. Traditionally, CGH has been done using competitive hybridization to normal metaphase chromosomes, hence resolution is poor, and is only capable of detecting high-level amplifications of around 2 Mb, and deletions of the order of 10 Mb (these represent large areas of the chromosomes wih many genes). Hence, there is a compromise between global information and identifying very specific location of the change. A large number of investigators have used CGH analysis to understand the changes in DNA copy number in invasive cancer as well as precancerous lesions. As yet, specific profiles that are of prognostic significance or predict for response to therapy have not been developed for routine use, but clearly there is a hope that such a profile may be developed in time. More recently, this

Figure 13.16 These images demonstrate small-cell carcinoma of the lung, a neuroectodermally derived tumour, common in smokers. It is renowned for its ability to metastasize widely before producing clinical symptoms and is therefore almost always fatal. New molecular techniques may assist in understanding the mechanisms by which such tumours develop, in creating early tumour detection systems and engineering tumour-specific treatments. Left: CXR, right hilar and anterior mediastinal mass (blue arrow); small-cell lung cancer. Right: CXR, right apical and paramediastinal mass (red arrow) invading the mediastinum; non-small-cell lung cancer (NSLC)

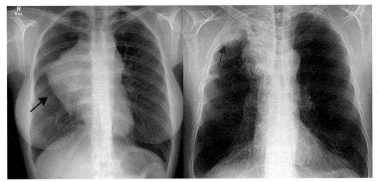

method has been adapted to produce an array CGH analysis (see below), where a large number of genetic loci are spotted onto a glass slide and hybridization is done to these loci rather than to metaphase chromosome. This has improved the resolution of the technique.

EXPRESSION ARRAYS

As well as cataloguing the amplifications, deletions and complex rearrangements at the genomic (DNA) level, analysis of changes in the profiles of gene expression (mRNA) may give clues to the underlying molecular events in tumorigenesis. The method consists of thousands of sequences of complementary DNA (cDNA, derived from reverse transcribing the RNA) robotically arrayed onto a glass slide. The samples to be examined are labelled with different colour fluorochromes, mixed and co-hybridized to the arrays in a competitive manner, and the resulting fluorescence values reveal the relative levels of each RNA transcript in the test sample compared to the reference sample (e.g. tumour versus normal or between two different normal cell types). Mathematical algorithms are used by bioinformaticians to probe differences in expression patterns between sample sets. Expression profiles generated by cDNA arrays can reveal similarities and differences that are not necessarily evident from traditional approaches, such as morphological or immunohistochemical analysis.

The power of this technique has been elegantly demonstrated in a number of studies published since 2000. The first demonstrated that within the morphologically homogeneous category of large B-cell lymphoma, two subtypes exist with differing patterns of gene expression. Subsequent papers have looked at other tumour types such as breast, lung and ovarian cancers and also identified sub-classes of tumour not easily identified using routine microscopy.

PROTEIN ARRAYS

Protein molecules, rather than DNA or RNA, carry out most cellular functions. The direct measurement of protein levels and activity within the cell may be the best determinant of overall cell function. Techniques are being developed to quantify the levels of all the proteins within a cell and compare protein levels between different cell types. Proteomic analysis, consisting of

two-dimensional gel electrophoresis (2-D PAGE) and tandem mass spectrometry, has been used to map protein profiles in normal and tumour cells. As would be expected, the studies have highlighted differences in protein profiles between subsets of normal cells and between normal cells and tumour cells. It is unlikely that the 'proteome' is stable over time as the cell requirements are constantly changing as it adapts to its environment. Any proteomic data is therefore likely to represent only a snapshot of the 'proteome'.

The development of proteomic arrays (using antibodies) are in development. At present, the technique is labour intensive and requires large amounts of purified samples. It is therefore not yet appropriate for use in clinical practice. However, use of this technology will undoubtedly lead to the identification of new cancer-associated proteins.

CONCLUSION

Pathological assessment of tissues has remained the linchpin of diagnostic practice for over a hundred years. It has become the core science of clinical medical practice, providing data for clinical management and a framework for future correlation of new markers and new therapies. With the current explosion of technology and data, it is important for pathologists and other clinical specialists to embrace and incorporate these changes into their training and practice. Molecular biologists will also benefit from a closer interaction with pathologists.

That brings us to the end of this section on the cellular events involved in producing the cancer cell. Of course, we have a long way to go before we have a full understanding, but our knowledge is advancing at an exciting pace, and a whole new language of tumour terminology is emerging. For the scientist, the battle is the biology, for the clinicians and students trying to understand and apply the new knowledge, it is often the terminology!

The next question we need to address and one that will be in the forefront of the patient's mind is: How will a given tumour behave?

CHAPTER 14

The behaviour of a tumour can be considered under a number of headings covering how fast it will grow, whether it is likely to metastasize, which sites are affected and what symptoms and complications the patient is likely to suffer.

TUMOUR GROWTH

It is often assumed that tumours grow faster than normal tissues because they expand to compress the surrounding structures. However, this does not mean that the cells are dividing more often, but that there is an imbalance between production and loss. The time taken for tumour cell division varies between 20 and 60 hours, with leukaemias having shorter cell cycles than solid tumours but, in general, tumour cells take *longer* than their normal counterparts. Cells can be in a resting phase or in growth phase, i.e. in one of the stages of mitosis. Some normal tissues have a high turnover of cells, such as the intestine, where around 16 per cent of the cells will be in the growth fraction. In contrast, most tumours have only 2–8 per cent of their cells actively dividing. This is important therapeutically because the cells in the growth phase are most readily damaged by chemotherapy and so tumours with a large growth fraction (e.g. leukaemias, lymphomas and lung anaplastic small cell carcinoma) will respond better than tumours with few cells proliferating (e.g. colon and breast).

Can we predict how fast a tumour is growing? To some extent, yes. The number of mitotic figures present per unit area in a light microscopical section is a crude measure of how active the proliferation is within a tumour. A tumour with a large number of cells in mitosis is likely to behave aggressively and this is why a mitotic count is one of the criteria for grading tumours (see page 258). However, the number of cells seen to be in mitosis is not only influenced by the growth fraction and the cell cycle time but also by whether they get 'stuck', i.e. the tumour cell can enter mitosis but, possibly because of an irregularity in chromosome number or in the internal organization of the mitotic spindle, may fail to complete the mitosis. Thus, on the examination of a tissue section, the tumour appears to be highly proliferative but it is really 'stuck'. Tumour growth will also be influenced by factors like the blood supply and, possibly, the host's immune response (page 295).

It would also be wrong to assume that every cell in a tumour behaves similarly. The daughter cells of a dividing cell are identical genetically to the parent cell and are said to be a clone (clonal expansion). However, tumour cells are also prone to develop genetic instability which results in some cells developing further abnormalities and hence resulting in the formation of multiple sub-clones. These may have certain survival advantages; for example, they may have enhanced angiogenic, invasive or metastatic capabilities. This is referred to as tumour heterogeneity and it is important to consider when planning treatments because it means that some tumour cells may respond differently to particular chemotherapeutic agents. This is rather analogous to bacterial resistance to antibiotics. Just as a combination of antibiotics is most effective against an unknown organism, so a mixture of treatment modalities is often used against a tumour.

HOW DO TUMOURS SPREAD?

Just over a hundred years ago, Stephen Paget (no, not the man who described Paget's disease, that was Sir James Paget) collected post mortem records of 735 patients who had died of breast cancer and he found that the majority of the metastases were in the liver and brain. He concluded therefore that certain tumours were predisposed to metastasize to certain tissues. He wrote, 'When a plant goes to seed, its seeds are carried in all directions; but they can only live and grow if they fall on congenial soil.' Not surprisingly, it came to be known as the 'seed and soil' theory.

James Ewing, 40 years later, suggested that tumours went to particular organs not because of the seed and soil effect, but rather because of the routes of the blood supply to the primary organ. Using his hypothesis, organs directly in line away from the primary site would be targets for metastatic disease.

We know now that they are both partially correct. Tumours of the colon do indeed go to the liver which is next in line through the portal circulation, but then so do many other tumours much farther away, such as melanomas arising in the eye. We also know that organs such as the heart and skeletal muscle, despite being exposed to large volumes of blood, rarely develop metastases. In broad terms, tumour spread through lymphatics will produce metastases in the anatomically related lymph nodes whilst spread through the blood is influenced more by 'seed and soil' considerations although anatomy is still of some importance.

The main routes of spread are via:

- lymphatics
- veins
- transcoelomic cavities
- cerebrospinal fluid
- arteries (Fig. 14.1).

Figure 14.1 **Routes of tumour spread**

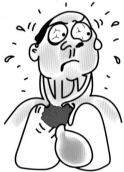

Direct: e.g. Mediastinal tumour surrounding and compressing the superior vena cava. This causes venous engorgement of the head, neck and arms, to produce headache and proptosis (bulging eyes due to cavernous sinus distension)

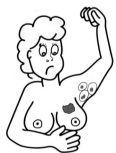

Via lymphatics: e.g. Carcinoma of breast first spreads to the local axillary lymph nodes

Carcinomas generally first spread via lymphatics

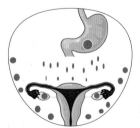

Transcoelomic: e.g. Gastric carcinoma cells seeding through the peritoneal cavity. Krukenberg gave his name to metastatic gastric carcinoma involving the ovaries

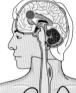

CNS spread: Primary central nervous system tumours will metastasize to brain or spinal cord, but appear to be confined by the blood–brain barrier and the dural membranes

Field change: e.g. Transitional cell carcinoma. Urothelial tumours may synchronously arise at several sites, e.g. renal pelvis, ureter and bladder. This is not tumour spread, but a 'crop' of separate primary tumours, thought to arise due to a 'field effect', in which several sites are exposed to the same urinary carcinogens

Via the bloodstream: e.g. Osteosarcomas metastasize to the lungs, or gastrointestinal carcinomas spread to the liver via the portal vein. Sarcomas generally spread via the bloodstream

Figure 14.2 Chest X-ray showing multiple 'cannon ball' metastases

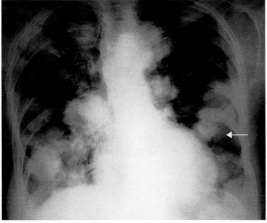

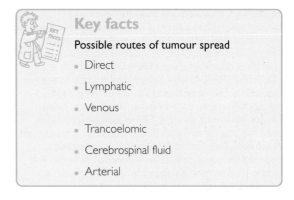

tumours may even grow along a vein, causing its obstruction, for instance renal cell carcinoma in the renal vein. Arteries are not often penetrated by tumours but, in the later stages of metastatic spread, tumour nodules can start to develop almost anywhere and it is likely that this happens after pulmonary metastases enter the pulmonary vein and are then distributed through the systemic arterial system. It is easy to understand how tumours which reach the pleural or peritoneal cavities can drop into the fluid and be disseminated throughout that coelomic cavity. Similarly, the CSF (cerebrospinal fluid) provides an easy route of spread for cerebral tumours, which do not generally metastasize outside the central nervous system.

One cubic centimetre of tumour can shed millions of cells into the circulation each day; so why are metastases not inevitable? Let us consider the steps required to produce a metastasis.

First, the tumour has to grow at the primary site and infiltrate the surrounding connective tissue, which may necessitate breaking through a basement membrane and the connective tissues nearby. It may also have to overcome inhibitor substances to the enzymes it produces to break down these connective tissue proteins. Then it can reach the lymphatic and blood vascular channels, which are an important route for dissemination. It has to find a way of attaching to the endothelium and subsequently enter the channels. The vessel wall is traversed and the tumour cells must detach to float in the blood or lymph and hope to evade any immune cells which might destroy them. Next they must lodge in the capillaries at their destination, attach to the endothelium again and penetrate the vessel wall to enter the perivascular connective tissue where they finally proliferate to produce a tumour deposit. Even here, the local environment is important in dictating whether the cells will grow or not.

Figure 14.3 Photomicrograph of lymphatic invasion by breast cancer

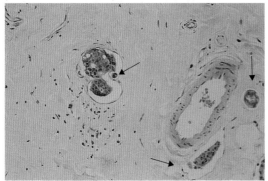

Lymphatic spread is common in carcinomas (tumours of epithelia) and the nodes which are involved first are the nodes which drain the tumour site (Fig. 14.3). Thus knowledge of the lymphatic anatomy is useful for predicting where the tumour will spread and is the basis for many of the staging protocols (page 260). However, lymph nodes near tumours can enlarge as part of an immune reaction that particularly results in expansion of the macrophage compartment (sinus histiocytosis). This means that the doctor must try to distinguish between soft, mobile nodes, which are likely to be reactive, and the hard, fixed nodes which contain metastatic tumour.

Venous spread will take tumours of the gastrointestinal tract to the liver and tumours from a variety of sites to the lungs. It is also the favoured route of spread for sarcomas (tumours of connective tissue). Some

Figure 14.4 Whole-body positron emission tomography (PET) scan in a 20-year-old patient with metastatic melanoma. (PET is a nuclear medicine imaging technique.) The radioactive compound used is [18F]fluorodeoxyglucose (18F-FDG) which is a glucose analogue taken up by metabolically active tissue. The PET scan detects areas of very high metabolic activity such as brain, muscle and brown fat, but also most cancers. PET is being increasingly used for staging malignancies, and assessing treatment responses. This scan shows multiple metastatic deposits including subcutaneous deposits in the left breast (red arrow), a deposit in the femur (black arrow), a pelvic uterine metastasis (green arrow) and multiple hilar, mediastinal and mesenteric lymph node deposits (brown arrow)

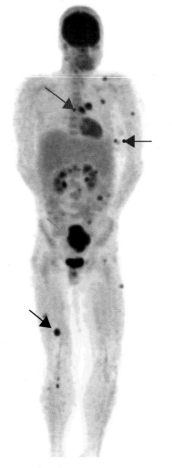

What stands between the primary tumour and the vessel? First, there is a variety of extracellular matrix components to break through for which the tumour may produce a number of enzymes. Loose connective tissue is not much of a barrier but dense fibrous areas, such as tendons and joint capsules and cartilage, can resist tumour spread. In addition, the tumour cells might acquire the ability to be more motile within this environment by developing a mesenchymal phenotype; this process is referred to as epithelial–mesenchymal transition (EMT). A number of stimuli are thought to be important in acquiring EMT; these include TGF-β, loss of E-cadherin and oncogenic signalling through the PI3 kinase pathway. The growth and dissemination of the tumour at this site is also limited without the process of angiogenesis and lymphangiogenesis. This increased vascularity is achieved by formation of new vessels (neoangiogenesis), by recruiting exisiting vasculature or by mimicry (where tumour cells form channels resembling vascular spaces).

Next is the basement membrane so that the tumour has to be able to secrete a type IV collagenase. Tumours often have collagenases to dissolve collagen but are less able to digest elastic tissue. This may be one of the reasons why arterial walls, which contain a lot of elastic, are less readily penetrated than venous walls. Alternatively, it may be because arterial walls are thicker and contain protease inhibitors. Once in the vessel lumen, tumour cells are prey to immune surveillance by the body's lymphocytes and monocytes. Some experimental data suggests that most of these cells die; however, this is controversial and it is not clear at present what proportion of cells survive and extravasate at distant sites. Of course, apart from the immune mechanisms, the tumour cells must also resist the huge sheer forces that will be present in the circulation. Finally, the tumour must attach to the endothelium at its destination which may involve specific adhesion molecules (addressins) that 'home' the metastatic tumour to a particular site, analogous to the 'homing' of lymphocytes (page 140). It is not entirely clear what dictates the site of metastatic disease. Some genes appear to predict metastases in general while others appear to be associated with site-specific disease. Much remains to be done to understand this process in detail.

Most of our discussions about tumour cell biology have concentrated on how genetic changes enhance cell proliferation. However, we should now look at how a proliferating tumour cell differs from a proliferating normal cell. Early experiments involving *in vitro* cell cultures demonstrated that normal cells would grow to form monolayers and then stop. This was referred to as contact inhibition. If some cells from this culture were

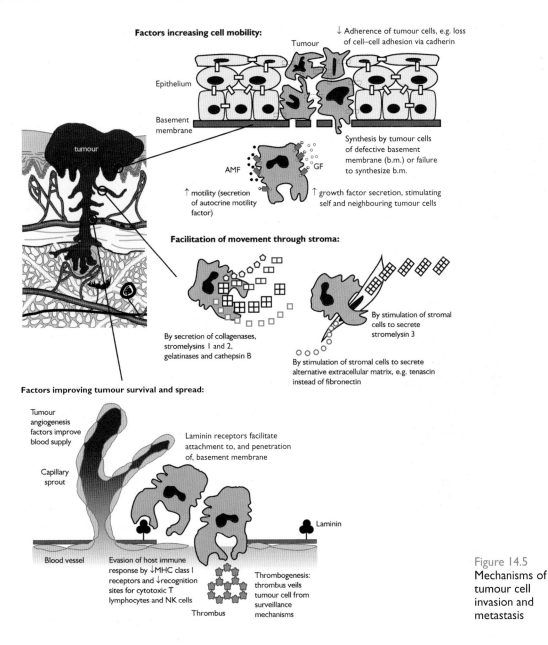

Factors increasing cell mobility:

↓ Adherence of tumour cells, e.g. loss of cell–cell adhesion via cadherin

Tumour

Epithelium

Basement membrane

Synthesis by tumour cells of defective basement membrane (b.m.) or failure to synthesize b.m.

AMF

GF

↑ motility (secretion of autocrine motility factor)

↑ growth factor secretion, stimulating self and neighbouring tumour cells

tumour

Facilitation of movement through stroma:

By secretion of collagenases, stromelysins 1 and 2, gelatinases and cathepsin B

By stimulation of stromal cells to secrete stromelysin 3

By stimulation of stromal cells to secrete alternative extracellular matrix, e.g. tenascin instead of fibronectin

Factors improving tumour survival and spread:

Tumour angiogenesis factors improve blood supply

Laminin receptors facilitate attachment to, and penetration of, basement membrane

Capillary sprout

Laminin

Blood vessel

Evasion of host immune response by ↓MHC class I receptors and ↓recognition sites for cytotoxic T lymphocytes and NK cells

Thrombogenesis: thrombus veils tumour cell from surveillance mechanisms

Thrombus

Figure 14.5
Mechanisms of tumour cell invasion and metastasis

transferred to a new culture vessel (passaged), they would begin to grow again in the same way; however, normal cells would only survive about 30–50 serial passages. Cultures of proliferating tumour cells differed in that they lost contact inhibition and so could grow as disorganized multilayers and they were also immortal, i.e. although each individual cell did not last forever, the clone of cells could be passaged indefinitely. Now it is known that tumour cells may show decreased expression of E-cadherin, which normally acts as an adhesion molecule between epithelial cells, and that their increased motility may be influenced by an autocrine motility factor which some transformed culture cells release. Tumour cells can also influence the production of stroma so that tenascin may predominate which does not bind readily to tumour cells. This sort of information suggests that it is not only changes in the tumour cells which produces local invasion and metastasis but that interactions between tumour cells, normal cells and stroma are also important.

THE ROLE OF THE IMMUNE SYSTEM

We are all aware of the role played by the immune system in defending us against infections, so it is not surprising that questions have been raised as to whether it has any role in protection against cancer. It was Paul Ehrlich, in 1909, who postulated that without the immune system constantly removing the 'aberrant germs', human beings would inevitably die of cancer. Many attempts were made to establish the role of the immune system in cancer and initial experiments, which transplanted tumours from one animal to another, appeared to support the concept. It was later realized that the destruction of these transplanted tumours was not due to immunity but to transplant rejection. Now, inbred mice can be used experimentally, thus avoiding the factor of transplant rejection. In certain tumours it has been shown that, if the tumour is removed from a mouse and the animal rechallenged with the tumour, the tumour is rejected. This supports the idea that immunity is involved in tumour rejection, but life is not quite so simple as we shall see.

You will recall that the cells of the immune system have to be able to distinguish between 'self' and 'non-self', by identifying specific antigens on the cell surface. Malignant tumours are derived from 'self', so if the immune system is to defend against tumours, the malignant cells must acquire antigens that differentiate them from normal cells. These are termed tumour-specific antigens (TSAs) and the whole subject has been highly controversial. In man, such tumour associated antigens are beginning to be defined and include differentiation antigens (e.g. CD19 and CD29), growth factor receptors such as epidermal growth factor receptor (EGFR) and intracellular proteins such as the MAGE family of proteins which are highly expressed in melanoma. These antigens have been identified by isolating tumour reactive T cells from patients with malignancies.

While tumours clearly do elicit immune responses, the degree of response does not appear to be sufficient to hold the progression of the malignancy in most cases. It is conceivable that as tumours progress, clones of cells without the antigens proliferate and escape immune destruction. A whole new area of cancer vaccine is developing rapidly and initial trials appear encouraging. Vaccination with ganglioside GM2 in melanoma appears to increase survival; vaccines against cervical cancer and liver cancer are already on the market, but time will tell whether the effects of immunization live up to the promise suggested by initial trials.

There is also evidence from animal experiments that surface antigens are altered in some tumours induced by viruses or chemicals. Viral-induced tumours in animals can display a new surface antigen (T) which is believed to be a viral peptide associated with major histocompatibility complex (MHC). This provokes a specific cytotoxic T-cell response and all tumours induced by a particular virus display the same antigen, regardless of the cell of origin. The obvious potential application for this lies in immunizing against tumours.

Chemically induced tumours in animals (e.g. by benzopyrene) may also display new surface antigens which induce a specific immune response, but these antigens are very varied, with primary tumours in the same animal exhibiting antigenic differences, so there is no cross-resistance through immunization.

Of course, the immune response need not be antigen-specific. Besides B and T lymphocytes, the body has at its disposal natural killer cells (NK cells) and macrophages. NK cells have the capacity to destroy cells without prior sensitization as well as the ability to participate in antibody-dependent cellular cytotoxicity (ADCC). Macrophages are also involved, either due to non-specific activation or in collaboration with T lymphocytes, and can participate via ADCC or by the release of cytotoxic factors, such as tumour necrosis factor (TNF), hydrogen peroxide and a cytolytic protease.

CHAPTER 15

THE CLINICAL EFFECTS OF TUMOURS

LOCAL EFFECTS

The local effects depend on the site of the tumour, the type of tumour and its growth pattern. Some complications, such as haemorrhage, are more common in malignant tumours because of their ability to invade underlying tissues and their vessels, but it must be remembered that even a microscopically benign tumour (e.g. a meningioma on the surface of the brain) can kill the patient due to its local effects.

Local effects can complicate both benign and malignant tumours. They include:

- compression
- obstruction
- ulceration
- haemorrhage
- rupture
- perforation
- infarction.

COMPRESSION AND OBSTRUCTION

A patient with any intracranial tumour (e.g. meningioma, astrocytoma, oligodendroglioma) may present with headaches, nausea and vomiting, because the mass growing within the closed cavity of the cranium raises the intracranial pressure. If the tumour is not removed and the pressure continues to rise, the patient will die from pressure effects on the vital respiratory centres.

A more localized example of the effect of compression is when the pituitary gland enlarges in the small cup-shaped space of the sella turcica. Local pressure will cause erosion of the bony sella and compression of the optic chiasma that sits directly above. The patient will then present with visual disturbance, classically a bitemporal hemianopia (Fig. 15.1).

Compression and obstruction have been included in the same section because there is often an overlap.

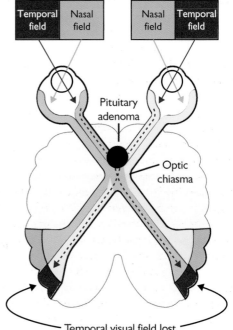

Figure 15.1 **Benign tumours may have profound effects. Here, a small pituitary adenoma produced blindness in both temporal visual fields by compressing optic nerve fibres at the optic chiasma**

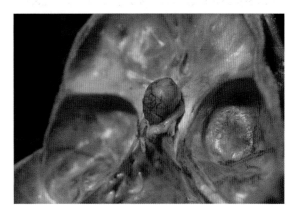

Figure 15.2 **X-ray showing constriction of lower oesophagus by oesophageal carcinoma**

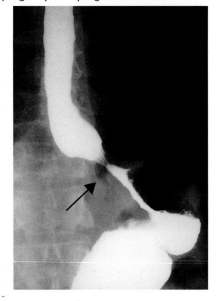

Figure 15.4 **Photomicrograph showing rectal ulceration due to adenocarcinoma**

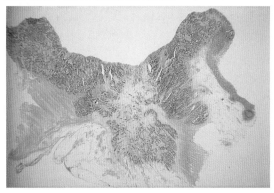

Figure 15.5 **Haemorrhage within intracerebral tumour**

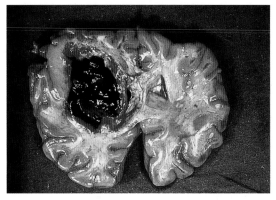

Figure 15.3 **Compression of cardiac ventricles by metastatic lung carcinoma infiltrating the pericardium**

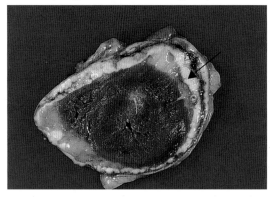

ULCERATION AND HAEMORRHAGE

An ulcer is defined as a macroscopically apparent loss of surface epithelium and may be benign or malignant. Ulceration of the skin will lead to a crust of dried fibrin and cells covering the area and is unlikely to produce severe haemorrhage. However, ulceration in the gastrointestinal tract, particularly the stomach and duodenum, may result in life-threatening haemorrhage or perforation. Here the absence of epithelium means the loss of an important defence mechanism which normally protects the underlying tissue from acid and enzymes. Once the submucosa is exposed to these agents, large vessel walls can be digested resulting in massive bleeding. See Figs 15.4 and 15.5.

RUPTURE OR PERFORATION

Rupture or perforation typically affects tumours of the gastrointestinal tract and will occur if the intraluminal

Compression can directly damage normal tissue, as described in the pituitary, or it may cause obstruction. This occurs, for instance, when a tracheal tumour obstructs a normal oesophagus or vice versa. In the brain, compression of the brainstem structures may obstruct the flow of cerebrospinal fluid, and a large prostate (benign or malignant) may compress the prostatic urethra. Alternatively, a tumour can grow into the lumen of the gut or into an airway so that it produces obstruction directly. See Figs 15.2 and 15.3.

Figure 15.6 Colonic carcinoma with perforation indicated by probe

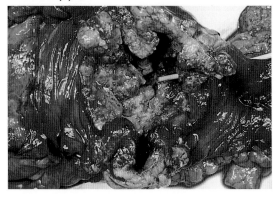

Figure 15.7 Extensive infarction in tumour, leaving small islands of viable cells (arrows)

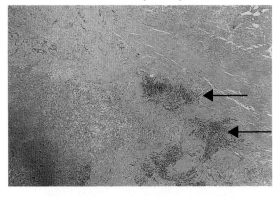

pressure exceeds the strength of the wall or if the wall is eroded or weakened by tumour, ischaemia or enzymic action, etc. (Fig. 15.6). Obviously, there is a risk of dilatation and rupture when part of the gut becomes obstructed as the gut contents cannot follow their normal route. Rupture may also occur in closed organs, such as the ovary, because the tumour has stretched the capsule, often because of accumulation of fluid or mucin as well as the proliferation of neoplastic cells.

INFARCTION

Many malignant tumours will show necrosis and infarction in their central region, which is believed to result from inadequate blood supply (Fig. 15.7). In experimental models, a tumour can only expand to a diameter of 1–2 mm before it must stimulate new blood vessel formation and, in human tumours, zones of necrosis may be encountered approximately 1–2 mm from a blood vessel. Therefore, it appears that this is the maximum distance for diffusion of nutrients. Tumours attempt to solve this by secreting angiogenic factors which stimulate capillaries to grow into the neoplasm.

Local anatomy influences the likelihood of infarction related to large vessel obstruction. The bowel, ovaries and testes are particularly liable to torsion, i.e. twisting on their vascular pedicle which occludes the vessels.

Although we often separate the complications of tumours under the headings of local tumour and metastatic tumour, a metastasis can produce any of the local effects mentioned above. In particular, lymph nodes containing metastases can cause obstruction at crucial sites, such as the porta hepatis or the hilum of the lung.

ENDOCRINE EFFECTS

Well-differentiated tumours do not only look like their tissue of origin but can also act like them. Thus tumours of endocrine organs can produce hormones which act on the same tissues as their physiological counterparts but are not under normal feedback control.

Cushing's syndrome provides an interesting example of where different endocrine tumours can produce the same clinical problems. In Cushing's syndrome, the patient suffers from osteoporosis, muscle wasting, thinning of the skin with purple striae and easy bruising, truncal obesity and impaired glucose tolerance. All this is the result of excess glucocorticoids. The same picture can be produced by prolonged administration of steroids to treat diseases (e.g. chronic asthma).

The adrenal produces corticosteroids when stimulated by adrenocorticotrophic hormone (ACTH) from the pituitary. The corticosteroids then provide negative feedback to the pituitary and ACTH levels drop. Cushing's disease can result from an adenoma in the pituitary gland, which produces ACTH, or a cortical tumour in the adrenal cortex, which secretes corticosteroids. Normal feedback does not operate as the adenoma cells behave autonomously. However, if very high doses of steroid (dexamethasone suppression test) are given, then the pituitary adenoma will reduce its ACTH production and endogenous steroid levels will fall, but excess steroid due to an adrenal adenoma will not be suppressed.

Some non-endocrine tumours can produce substances which have the same effects as hormones, so-called inappropriate production. One of the commonest

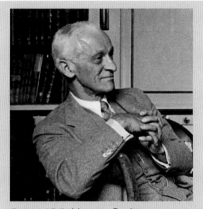
results is Cushing's syndrome when ACTH is produced by oat cell (anaplastic small cell) carcinoma of the bronchus, carcinoid tumours, thymomas or medullary carcinoma of the thyroid. This inappropriate and autonomous production does not suppress with high doses of dexamethasone.

PARANEOPLASTIC SYNDROMES

This refers to symptoms in cancer patients that are not readily explained by local or metastatic disease. Endocrine effects are generally included as a paraneoplastic syndrome if the production is inappropriate (as above) but not if the tumour arises from a tissue that normally produces that hormone.

Hypercalcaemia is a common, clinically important and complex problem with malignant tumours. In a patient with widespread metastases in bone, it may be explained as a local destructive effect of the tumour on bone which releases calcium. However, hypercalcaemia can also occur without metastatic bony deposits and, in some cases, it appears that a parathyroid hormone like peptide or TGF-β is secreted by the primary tumour and this is most likely with bronchial squamous cell carcinoma and adult T-cell leukaemia/lymphoma.

Clubbing of the fingers and hypertrophic osteoarthropathy are also common with lung carcinoma but can occur in non-neoplastic conditions including cyanotic heart disease and liver disease (Fig.15.9). It is

Figure 15.9 The drumstick appearance of finger clubbing is associated with hypoxia (e.g. lung cancer, cystic fibrosis, chronic pulmonary disease) and cirrhosis of the liver. Most patients with clubbing have increased blood flow through the fingers, possibly mediated by autonomic nerves (vagal transection can relieve symptoms). Such shunts may enable platelets to lodge in capillary beds and the interaction between platelets and endothelial cells, by releasing PDGF, may lead to overgrowth of bone and connective tissue. There is characteristic tufting of the distal phalanges on X-ray. Other joints may also be affected

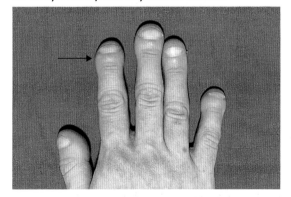

not clear how it develops, nor why sectioning the vagus nerve can lead to its disappearance! Equally mysterious are the skin disorders, peripheral neuropathy and cerebellar degeneration which may also occur in association with malignant tumours, particularly lung and bronchial carcinomas.

GENERAL EFFECTS

The general effects of tumours are not classed as paraneoplastic syndromes, although they are extremely common and must not be forgotten. These include general malaise, weight loss and lethargy, which are due to a combination of metabolic and hormonal influences exacerbated by any malnutrition or infection. This results in the clinical picture known as 'cachexia' (Fig. 15.10). An important chemical factor that may play a role in cachexia is cachexin, which is also known as tumour necrosis factor (TNF). This molecule is not produced by the tumour cells, but by activated macrophages. Anaemia is also common and can contribute to the general malaise. This may be a direct effect of metastatic deposits in bone marrow or an indirect effect of mediators which suppress haemopoiesis.

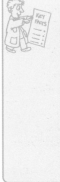

Key facts

Paraneoplastic manifestations of tumours

Endocrine effects
Cushing's syndrome
Inappropriate ADH secretion
Hypercalcaemia
Clubbing
Hypertrophic osteoarthropathy
Peripheral neuropathy
Cerebellar degeneration
Skin rashes

MANAGEMENT OF CANCER

We will discuss this under individual headings; however, many patients receive a combination of management strategies.

SCREENING PROGRAMMES

The concept of the multistep model of carcinogenesis has led to the idea that mortality from the tumour may be reduced if it is identified at an earlier stage or when it is still precancerous. Screening programmes have been instituted for cervical and breast cancer and there is considerable debate as to whether other tumour types such as prostate and colon should be included. In some countries, screening for colorectal cancer using faecal occult blood testing has been implemented. The

Figure 15.10 Cancer-related muscle wasting (cachexia). Similar appearances can be seen with some chronic diseases, e.g. tuberculosis or AIDS. Cachexia differs from starvation in that lean mass – skeletal muscle, especially of the shoulder girdle and head – is lost as well as adipose tissue, thus there is both proteolysis and lipolysis. Cytokines such as TNF, IL-1, IL-6 and IFN-γ are thought to drive the liver to produce high levels of acute-phase proteins, depleting amino acid reserves. Dietary measures alone are not effective. EPA in fish oils (an omega 3 fatty acid) interferes with PIF (proteolysis inducing factor, which releases protein from skeletal muscle), found in the urine of 80 per cent of cachectic patients. EPA does not affect lipolysis

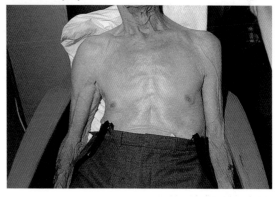

screening programmes have undoubtedly reduced mortality although not as dramatically as had been envisaged, but it has also highlighted deficiencies in our knowledge of classification and natural history of the early lesions, making management of patients with these 'pre-cancers' problematic. In order to circumvent this problem, management decisions are now made in multidisciplinary teams (comprising surgeons, oncologists, pathologists, radiologists etc.), bringing all the expertise to bear in deciding the final strategy.

LOCAL EXCISION

Local treatment is aimed either at achieving a cure or providing specific symptomatic relief. Cancers, such as squamous and basal cell carcinomas of the skin and cancers arising within polyps in the colon, can be cured by local excision. In tumours of the bowel, local excision may relieve an obstruction and provide good long-term remission of symptoms or even cure.

RADIOTHERAPY

Radiotherapy can be given from an external source or by implanting a small radioactive source into the

Figure 15.11 The ten most common cancers diagnosed in the UK, 1999. Excludes non-melanoma skin cancer (Copyright and courtesy of Cancer Research UK, 2005; http://info.cancerresearchuk.org/cancerstats/incidence/commoncancers/)

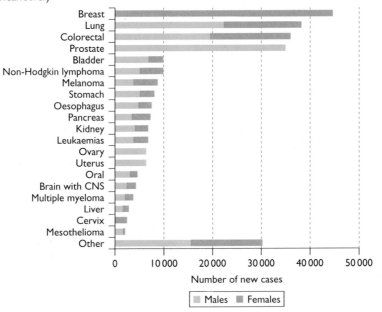

Figure 15.12 The ten most common causes of death from cancer in the UK, 2000 (Copyright and courtesy of Cancer Research UK, 2005; http://info.cancerresearchuk.org/cancerstats/mortaility/cancerdeaths/)

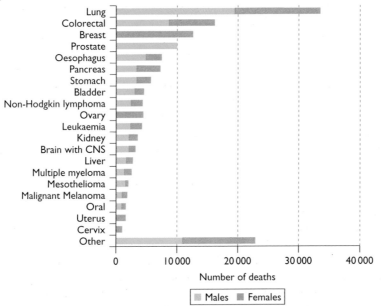

tissues. Delivery schedules vary from centre to centre but the general idea is to divide, or fractionate, the doses in order to get the maximum kill of tumour cells with the minimum damage to normal tissues. Implanted radioactive sources are very useful for providing high-dose local radiation and are particularly useful in cancers of the head and neck where there are many vital structures close together.

CHEMOTHERAPY

Chemotherapy is a relatively crude but potentially effective form of treatment. In patients suffering from haematological malignancies (e.g. leukaemia) or disseminated disease, surgery and radiation are not realistic options. You cannot excise a leukaemia and you cannot irradiate metastases which are widespread in the body!

In the 1950s, alkylating agents (e.g. busulfan) and anti-metabolites (e.g. methotrexate) were introduced and proved useful in the management of disseminated cancers. The main problem with such agents is that all of the body's normal tissues are also exposed to the drug and so the challenge is to deliver enough drug to kill the tumour without killing the patient! It has also become apparent that chemotherapy is much more effective in combination with other agents than as single agent.

ENDOCRINE-RELATED TREATMENT

This often involves giving a drug that inhibits tumour growth by removing an endocrine stimulus. For example, many breast carcinomas have receptors for oestrogen which stimulate tumour growth. A drug such as tamoxifen (an anti-oestrogen) will block these receptors and reduce progression of the disease. An alternative approach would be to remove the ovaries which produce oestrogen, much as the testes can be removed in men with prostatic adenocarcinomas to reduce the stimulus for tumour growth from androgens.

IMMUNOTHERAPY

DNA recombinant technology has enabled the production of cytokines in sufficient quantities for therapeutic use. The interferons (IFN) and tumour necrosis factors (TNF) are of particular interest. IFN-α and IFN-β have been used to treat a variety of tumours with some good effect, although it appears that they may best be used in combination with other treatments. Renal carcinomas, melanomas and myelomas have shown a 10–15 per cent

response, various lymphomas show a 40 per cent response and hairy cell leukaemia and mycosis fungoides have an 80–90 per cent response rate. TNF-α has been used in the treatment of melanoma although, to date, the response has been disappointing. Lymphokine activated killer (LAK) cells are a subset of NK cells which have been used in combination with interleukin-2 to treat renal carcinomas and some melanomas and colorectal cancers.

As mentioned previously, attempts at specific tumour antigens are in progress and initial trials of vaccination seem encouraging. There is also considerable interest in raising monoclonal antibodies to tumour cells. The hope is that it might be possible to attach drugs to these antibodies so that they would be delivered specifically to the tumour cell; the concept of the 'magic bullet'. A lot of questions remain unanswered but the field of immunization and targeted treatment is bound to create excitement over the next decade.

MOLECULAR MECHANISM-BASED THERAPIES (TARGETED THERAPIES)

With our increasing understanding of the mechanisms of disease, therapies directed at specific molecular pathways are rapidly emerging. These include monoclonal, antibodies and enzyme inhibitors directed at specific genetic changes.

HER-2 is a tyrosine kinase-associated receptor; the gene is located on 17q. It is amplified in 10–34 per cent of human breast carcinomas. A humanized monoclonal antibody directed against HER2 oncogene, trastuzumab (Herceptin), has been used to treat women with metastatic breast carcinomas who have HER-2 amplification. Recently it has also been approved in the adjuvant setting (at time of primary diagnosis).

Since the beginning of the 1990s, much effort has been put into the discovery of molecules that would be able to block specific kinases. The first drug that showed promising results was STI-571 (Gleevec), which was tailored to specifically inhibit the ABL-BRC tyrosine kinase fusion gene product. ABL-BCR results from a balanced translocation between chromosomes 9 and 22, and is found in more than 95 per cent of chronic myeloid leukemias (CMLs). Patients treated with this drug showed remarkable improvement. Not unexpectedly, STI-571 is not specific for this kinase and has been shown to inhibit other oncogenic tyrosine kinases, such as c-KIT and PDGFR. STI-571 seems to have a remarkable effect on neoplasms arising as a result of mutations of these genes and in particular in patients with gastrointestinal stromal tumours (GISTs) (with c-KIT activating mutations). The epidermal growth factor receptor (EGFR) is also a potential target. Gefitinib (ZD1839, Iressa™) has been on trial for esophageal and colorectal cancer (CRC) and cetuximab (IMC-C225, Erbitux™), a monoclonal EGFR antibody, has been approved for the therapy of colorectal cancer.

Vascular endothelial growth factor (VEGF) and its receptor (VEGFR) are involved in tumour angiogenesis. Bevacizumab (Avastin™), a monoclonal antibody against VEGF, is being used in conjunction with conventional chemotherapy for a variety of cancers. The era of targetted therapy and the 'Holy Grail' of individualized treatments are certainly pushing ahead with speed.

GENE THERAPY

Gene therapy emerged as an alternative to conventional cancer treatments as it become possible to transfer genetic material into a cell to transiently or permanently alter its biology (i.e. to induce cell cycle arrest/apoptosis). This may be achieved by using modified virus encoding specific DNA sequences (viral vector systems). The introduction of genes that encode tumour-suppressor proteins is known as therapeutic gene transfer. There are a number of drawbacks to this type of treatment and include the specificity of the virus for neoplastic cells, the side effects of the presence of the 'new gene' in normal cells and the reaction of the host immune system. The use of gene therapy for treatment had a setback when a young patient died as a result. Research continues in order to learn more about safe delivery of the vector into cancer cells and learning how to combat the different cell populations within a cancer. If the stem cell hypothesis is correct, cancers will contain slowly replicating stem cells, rapidly replicating transit-amplifying cells, as well as a variety of differentiated cells. Conventional chemotherapy may kill the dividing cells but may not have any impact on the stem cells, and use of additional gene therapy to target specific cells such as the stem cell population may be a way forward.

PALLIATIVE TREATMENT

The treatment of cancer has a wider role than merely providing a cure and cancer physicians are not interested in simply achieving a response to the administered treatment. Palliative treatment does not just refer to treatment that is given to patients in order to make them comfortable prior to death. It is and should be part of the oncological support given to all cancer patients and not only includes medication for the control of pain and nausea but also chemotherapy and radiotherapy for the relief of local symptoms and stabilization of disease. This is helped by the fact that we now have a larger panel of oral drugs, allowing patients to be managed in their own homes. The term 'continuing care' is sometimes used for this multidisciplinary approach starting with diagnosis and extending to the patient's death. The important point is that our knowledge of all modalities of treatment including pain control have advanced considerably in recent years and the pessimistic view that, if one has cancer one must pass one's last hours either conscious, but in agony, or pain-free but unconscious is no longer justified.

CONCLUSION

Science, like most aspects of life, has its fashions. Much of this section has concentrated on our evolving understanding of the role of the genetic code in producing cancer. Current fashion lies very much with large scale sequencing of all cancer genes and with expression profiling to identify subsets with differing prognosis and response to treatment. Stem cells are also a hot topic and there is a tendency to classify everything on the basis of hypothetical heirachies of cell lineage. There is little doubt that the ability to produce differentiated tissue from stem cells to help repair, such as in cerebrovascular accidents, myocardial infarcts and traumatic neural injuries will be a biotechnological miracle in the coming years. Whether stem cells have such a high profile in cancer biology remains to be seen.

Clinicopathological case study — cervical cancer

Clinical

A 38-year-old woman came to the surgery for a cervical smear.

She was single and had been living with her boyfriend for the last 6 months. She divorced her husband 2 years ago and since then had had a number of casual relationships. Her first sexual contact was at the age of 16.

Four years ago her smear showed warty change, and the last one, 1 year ago, again showed extensive warty change with possible dyskaryosis. The hospital had asked for a repeat smear as the epithelial cells were obscured by inflammatory debris.

She initially ignored the recall due to social problems.

The result of the repeat smear showed warty change and severe dyskaryosis and she was referred for a colposcopic biopsy.

The cervical biopsy confirmed the above findings and she was booked in to have a cervical cone biopsy.

The results of the cone biopsy came as a shock. The report read that she had extensive squamous metaplasia with wart virus change together with severe dysplasia between 3 o'clock and 5 o'clock and a focus of invasive squamous cell carcinoma which was completely excised. Invasive tumour did not involve deep tissues or invade blood vessels. The dysplastic epithelium extended to the endocervical excision margin and was therefore not completely excised.

Pathology

Carcinoma of the cervix is an important cause of death and the cervical screening programme has been instituted to try and reduce this toll. The idea is that, if the disease can be picked up at an early stage, it should be possible to cure it.

The risk factors for cervical cancer include:

smoking, early onset of sexual intercourse, multiple sexual partners, a sexual partner with a history of promiscuity and infection with the human papilloma virus (HPV).

Her history reveals that she had a number of risk factors including wart virus change on her previous cervical smears.

The normal routine recall for cervical smears is 3 years, but early recall is instituted for suspicious or abnormal smears.

Severe dyskaryosis is the cytological equivalent to severe dysplasia on histological examination.

Dysplasia is a premalignant condition in which there are cytological features of malignancy, i.e. increased nuclear:cytoplasmic ratio, nuclear pleomorphism, hyperchromatism, loss of maturation and mitotic activity. Dysplasia can be graded into mild, moderate or severe. Severe dysplasia implies a full-thickness abnormality and the feature distinguishing this from carcinoma is the presence of invasion through the basement membrane.

Metaplasia, on the other hand, is entirely benign. It is a form of adaptation to injury, where one type of epithelium is replaced by another. In the cervix, the glandular epithelium, after repeated bouts of inflammation, changes to a more resistant squamous epithelium.

The cone biopsy is a way of performing a local excision of the cervix; the tissue removed is in the form of a cone. A suture is usually put at 12 o'clock to orientate the specimen. The role of the pathologist is to map the abnormal areas, to assess the abnormality in terms of severity and to comment on completeness of excision.

The report was discussed with the patient and she was advised to have radiotherapy and a hysterectomy

The examination of the hysterectomy specimen showed residual foci of severe dysplasia but no invasive carcinoma. The excision was complete and she was discharged after an uneventful recovery.

This patient was 38, and still capable of having children. The decision to have a hysterectomy can be a difficult one, although she had very little choice.

The hysterectomy specimen did not reveal any more areas of carcinoma and the single focus of carcinoma was completely excised, so she should be cured. Often the ovaries are not removed, to prevent menopausal symptoms.

So what is a disease? The definition provided at the outset regarding a loss of homeostasis is, we believe, a good one. What we hope is apparent though is that the mechanisms involved in maintaining the balance are incredibly intricate and complex. This is the paradox of life, complexity and simplicity existing together. To maintain homeostasis – balance – seems a simple thing to do. We hardly notice the constant adaptations that the body undergoes moment to moment as we move about our daily lives, the change in body temperature, heart rate and the flexing or relaxation of muscles as we change posture. Yet the processes that allow such a seamless transition from moment to moment are both complex and beautiful.

Imagine a cell with its 30 000 to 40 000 genes. These genes are transcribed into messages, which are then read and translated into proteins, which are modified to make yet more proteins, which in turn regulate the genes and messages. The pattern of gene expression is different from cell to cell depending on its function and its role at that time. Imagine this whole network like a three-dimensional tube/metro system buzzing within the cell, constantly adapting to fulfil its function. Now imagine this cell as one of a hundred forming a tissue and one of thousands forming an organ and one of billions forming the body. Can you imagine a billion tube/metro networks all working together in a coordinated manner?

We have to admit that we can't! It is totally mind-boggling and yet, this is exactly what must be happening every second, every minute of the day for the tissues, organs and body to maintain the homeostasis that allows us to function as part of a bigger 'organism' that we call life. This is not such a crazy concept; we know that our own homeostasis is not just to do with our own genes and proteins but also with the interaction of our bodies with the environment in which it finds itself. Cancer may be a 'genetic disorder' but we are all aware that the genes provide a 'predisposition', which given the right lifestyle and interaction with the environment leads to cancer. Not everyone with an inherited mutation develops cancer, but they are at increased risk which becomes manifest given the right circumstances.

The beginning of the twentieth century marked the change in the way physicists looked at the world. The quantum theory and the theory of relativity has questioned what we mean by 'reality' and the wave–particle duality continues to show us just how simple (we all think we understand it) and complex light really is. Lest you think that this 'new' physics has nothing to do with you, the quantum physics that is used to describe light is also the same physics that applies to all atoms including those in our DNA.

The end of the twentieth century saw the emergence of a revolution in biology, the sequencing of the human genome and the ability to look at thousands of genes and their expression profiles in one experiment. This will undoubtedly change the way we look at disease and we are already in this new century into an era of targeted therapy. The technological advances are also going to change the way we diagnose disease, with magnetic resonance imaging (MRI) looking at how we think and respond to stimuli and nanotechnology providing us with tools for near-patient testing and drug delivery. Perhaps that is the key; disease, like education and life itself, should be viewed as a process rather than a defined thing with a beginning and an end.

> *I saw a child carrying a light.*
> *I asked him where he had brought it from.*
> *He put it out, and said:*
> *'Now, you tell me where it is gone.'*
> *Hasan of Basra*

Page numbers followed by (f) refer to pages on which figures appear; page numbers followed by (t) refer to pages on which tables appear.

ABL-BCR tyrosine kinase fusion gene product   303
abl proto-oncogene   273
abortive viral infections   39
abscesses
    dental   115
    lung   113
Acanthamoeba   39(t)
accessory cells   140–2
ACE inhibitors, on arteriolosclerosis   207
acetylation, on tumour suppressor gene action   277
acid and alcohol fast bacilli   118
acidosis
    hypothermia   32
    intracellular   9
acquired immune deficiency syndrome *see* AIDS; human immunodeficiency virus
ACTH, hormone-secreting tumours and   250(f), 299, 300
active immunity   159
active immunization   160–1
acute coronary syndrome   212–13
acute-phase proteins   110–13
acute-phase reactions   109–14
acute rejection, transplanted organs   158
acute respiratory distress syndrome *see* adult respiratory distress syndrome
acute transforming viruses   271–2
acute tubular necrosis (ATN)   228
adaptive immunity   81, 139, 143–55
Addison's disease   46
addressins   98, 140
adenocarcinoma   256, 262, 298(f)
adenomas
    adrenocortical   250(f)
    colon   249
    precancerous   287–8
adenomatous polyposis coli protein   282
adhesion, platelets   172
adhesion molecules   96–8
adjuvants, vaccines   160
adrenal gland
    adenoma   250(f)
    see also steroid hormones
adrenaline, for anaphylactic shock   46
adrenocorticotrophic hormone, hormone-secreting tumours and   250(f), 299, 300
adult polycystic kidney disease   59
adult respiratory distress syndrome (ARDS)   228, 229(f), 230(f)

adult T-cell leukaemia/lymphoma (ATLL)   271
aflatoxin   266, 270–1
age/ageing   27–8
    atherosclerosis   193
    tumours   263
agglutination, antigens   148
AIDS
    apoptosis   24
    CD4$^+$ T-lymphocytes   154
    Kaposi's sarcoma   271
    tuberculosis and   118
    see also human immunodeficiency virus
air-borne infection   79
air emboli   186
alcohol   49, 136(f), 137–8
    on cholesterol ester transfer protein gene   202
    fatty change from   14, 15
    hypothermia   32
alkylating agents   25
alleles   57, 275
allelic exclusion, immunoglobulin genes   152
allergic reactions   44–6
alpha-1-antitrypsin   102, 103(f)
alpha-fetoprotein   64, 72
alternative pathway, complement system   108
alveolar macrophages   80, 113
alveolitis, extrinsic allergic   48(f), 49
amniocentesis   64
amniotic fluid emboli   186
amplification
    oncogenes   276(f), 277
    polymerase chain reaction   69
amyloidosis   138
anaemia   220–7
    coeliac disease   53
    microangiopathic haemolytic   187
    tumours   301
anaphase lag   60, 61(f)
anaphylactic hypersensitivity   44–6
anaphylactic shock   45–6
anaplastic tumours   262
aneuploidy   66, 255
aneurysms   165, 166, 207–10
    cardiac   218
    thrombosis   175
    see also microaneurysms
angina   214

angiogenesis
  tumours 299
  wound healing 130
angiography, coronary, CT 219
angiotensin II, hypertension 205
angiotensin-converting enzyme inhibitors, on arteriolosclerosis 207
anisocytosis 220
ankylosing spondylitis 63
Ann Arbor staging, Hodgkin's lymphoma 260(f)
antibiotics
  for cancer treatment 26
  on gut flora 80
  resistance to 83–5
    tuberculosis 85–7, 121
  sites of action 38(f)
antibodies 144–52, 159
  cancer treatment 303
  see also immune complex mediated hypersensitivity
antibody-dependent cytotoxic hypersensitivity 46, 47(f), 148, 154
anticoagulants 219
antigen(s) 148
  agglutination 148
  autoimmune diseases 157(t)
  changing 81, 82(t)
  exogenous 48–9
  sequestered 155
  tumour-specific 296
antigen-presenting cells 145(f)
  MHC class II molecules on 150
  see also dendritic cells
antimetabolites 25–6
anti-oestrogens 303
antiplatelet agents 219
anti-proteases 102
alpha-1-antitrypsin 102, 103(f)
antiviral agents, resistance of viruses to 87–8
anus, infection defence 80
aorta
  aneurysms 207(f), 208
  atherosclerosis 191
  dissection 208, 209
  fatty streaks 193
aortic incompetence 210
APC protein 282
aplastic marrow 220
apoprotein, deficiency 14
apoptosis 19–22, 23(f), 24–5, 26
  tumours and 24–5, 285
apoptotic bodies 22
arachidonic acid derivatives 102, 104(f)
array technology 290

arrhythmias 12–13, 216–18
arteries
  thrombosis 169, 175, 180
  see also atheroma; vascular supply
arteriolosclerosis 190, 206–7
arteriosclerosis 190
Arthus, Nicholas 48
Arthus reaction 48–9
asbestos 265
aspartate aminotransferase 13
Aspergillus 43(f)
aspirin
  on fever 110
  on platelets 172
Assman focus 120
asystole 218
atelectasis, ARDS 229(f)
Atg genes 22
atheroma 174, 189–203
  aneurysms 208
  embolism from 185
  myocardial infarction 214, 215
  plaques
    classification 192
    development 196–8
    fissuring 193, 214
    stability 192, 214, 232
  risk factors 193–5
  strokes 232–3
athlete's foot 43
atomic bombs 30(f), 267
atopic allergies 44–6
ATP binding cassette transporter A1 200
atrial fibrillation 236
atrioventricular node (A–V node) 13
atrophy 244–5
Augmentin 87
Australia, melanoma 265
autocrine motility factors 295
autocrine stimulation, tumour cells 277
autoimmune diseases 22, 46, 116, 155–8
autolytic change 18
autophagy 19–21, 22–4, 25(f), 27(t)
  in tumours 26
autopsies
  perinatal, thymus 21
  reports 8
autoregulation
  blood pressure 209
  brain 231
avascular necrosis, femoral head 70(f)
axons, healing 133

AZT (zidovudine) 87–8
azurophilic granules 102

Bacillus Calmette–Guérin (BCG)
  vaccine 121
Bacillus cereus 35
bacteria
  endotoxins 33–4
  exotoxins 34–8
  gram-negative 34(t), 35(f)
  gram-positive 34(t), 35(f)
  killing in inflammation 101–9
  liquefactive necrosis from 16
  organisms classified 34(t)
bactericidal permeability increasing protein 101
bacteriophages 84, 85(f)
Barrett's metaplasia, oesophagus 246
basophils, inflammation 91(t)
B cell receptor complex (BCR) 144
B cells *see* B-lymphocytes
BCG vaccine 121
bcl-2 gene 285
bcr genes 273
beclin1 gene, breast carcinoma 26
bed sores 135(f)
Belarus, tumours 267
'bends' 186
benign hypertension 204
benign prostatic hyperplasia 243, 244(f)
benign tumours 249, 250(f)
beriberi 51(t)
berry aneurysms 207
beta-naphthylamine 265, 266
bevacizumab 304
biomedical concept of disease 3
biopsy
  breast lumps 252
  cervix 305
blood-borne infection 79
blood flow
  atheromatous plaques 191
  thrombosis and 175
  see also circulatory disorders; vascular supply
blood loss *see* anaemia; shock
blood supply *see* vascular supply
blood transfusion reactions 46
blood volume, hypothermia 32
B-lymphocytes 143(f)
  humoral immunity 144–6
  IgD 148
  inflammation 91(t), 140, 142
  intestinal 147–8
body mass index 51

bone
  deformities, anaemias causing 224
  fractures 125, 126
  healing 128, 131–3, 135
    abnormal 135
bone marrow
  aplastic 220
  cells 93(f)
  emboli from 185
  hyperplastic 220
  hypoplastic 220
botulinum toxin 36, 38(f)
Boveri, Theodore 273
bovine spongiform encephalopathy 43
bovine tuberculosis 117
Boyden chamber 99
bradycardia 218
bradykinin 107
brain
  aneurysms 207–8
  damage from shock 228–9
  emboli 185
  haemorrhage 230, 232(f)
  healing 133
  herniation 231, 234(f)
  infarcts 17(f), 228–37
  space-occupying lesions 231, 297–8
  tumours 297–8
  see also nervous system
BRCA1 and *BRCA2* genes 275
breakpoint cluster region 273
breast
  calcification 18
  carcinoma 251–9
    beclin1 gene 26
    E-cadherin 282
    family history 263–4
    predisposition genes *see* *BRCA1* and *BRCA2* genes
    tamoxifen 303
  fat necrosis 17
  pregnancy 22
bronchi
  blood supply 184–5
  metaplasia, smoking 246(f)
bronchopneumonia 114
bundle branch block 13
Burkitt's lymphoma 268–9
  chromosomal translocations 269, 276(f)
bypass surgery, coronary 219

cachectin *see* tumour necrosis factor
cachexia 301
cachexin *see* tumour necrosis factor

cadherins 98(t), 282
  E-cadherin 282, 295
caisson disease 186
calcification 19(f)
  necrosis 18, 19(f)
  pancreatitis 17
  tuberculosis 120, 137
calcium, role in necrosis 9–12
calmodulin 12
calories, deficiency 51(t)
cancer *see* carcinoma; tumours
capillaries
  inflammation 92, 96
  permeability 170
  see also endothelium; granulation tissue
carbon tetrachloride 14
carcinogenic agents 265–72
carcinoma 256
  breast 251–9
    see also breast, carcinoma
  cervix 305–6
    see also cervix, carcinoma
  colorectal
    Dukes' staging 260(f)
    hereditary non-polyposis CRC 285
    multistep model 287–8
  gastric
    geography and race 264–5
    spread 292(f)
  hepatocellular 270–1
    geography 264(f)
  human papillomavirus 270
  in situ 255–6
  lung, small-cell 250(f), 289(f)
  metastases 18
  oesophagus 298(f)
  scrotum 265
  type *vs* site 262
cardiac enzymes 13, 216
  troponins 12, 13, 213, 216
  see also creatine kinase
cardiac failure *see* heart failure
cardiac output
  hypertension 204
  hypothermia 32
cardiac resuscitation, emboli 185
cardiac tamponade 218
cardiogenic shock 211, 212(f), 218
cardiovascular disease
  diabetes mellitus 195
  diet 198–9, 200–3
  hormone replacement therapy 193–4
  'lifestyle changes' 197–8

retina 190
risk reduction 198
see also atheroma; myocardial infarction
carotid arteries 231
  atherosclerosis 190
carriers, sickle cell disease 70
caseous necrosis 16–17, 118, 121(f)
caspases 22, 24
cataracts, diabetes mellitus 130–1
beta-catenin 282
causes, definition of 29
cavities, tuberculosis 120–1
CD4$^+$ T-lymphocytes 24, 153(t), 154
CD8$^+$ T-lymphocytes 153(t), 154
CD40 (B-cell surface receptor) 144
CD95 (death receptor) 24
CD antigens 153
cell cycle 282
  speed in tumours 291
cell-mediated hypersensitivity 49, 50(f)
cell-mediated immunity 143, 152–5
cell membranes *see* plasma membranes
cellular oedema 13
cellular oncogenes (c-*onc*) 275
central nervous system *see* brain
central vein occlusion, retina 169
cerebral aneurysms 207–8
cerebral emboli 185
cerebral infarcts 17(f), 228–37
cerolysin 35
Cervarix (vaccine) 270
cervix
  carcinoma 305–6
    human papillomavirus 270
    vaccination 161
  dysplasia 247, 248–9
  intraepithelial neoplasia (CIN) 247, 248(f)
  metaplasia 246
cetuximab 304
CFTR gene 59–60
chaperone-mediated autophagy 22, 23(t)
Charcot–Bouchard aneurysms 208, 237
chemical carcinogens 265–7
chemical mediators, inflammation 101–9
chemokines 103–4
chemotaxis 99
chemotherapy 25–6, 303
  on wound healing 134
Chernobyl accident, tumours 267
chimney sweeps, scrotal carcinoma 265
chloride, cystic fibrosis 60
cholera 7, 77–8
  toxin 37(f)

cholesterol 194
  metabolism 199
  reverse transport mechanism 199–200
  serum level reduction, coronary heart disease prevention 200
  see also familial hypercholesterolaemia
cholesterol ester transfer protein gene (CETP gene) 202, 203
chorionic villus sampling 65
chromatids 62(f)
chromatin, apoptosis 22
chromosomal abnormalities 57, 60, 61(f), 62(f), 65
  breakages 60
  deletions 62(f), 69
  maternal age 71–2
  tumours 273, 274(t)
  see also translocations
chronic granulomatous disease of childhood 101
chronic rejection, transplanted organs 158
chylomicron remnant particles 198
chylomicrons 198, 200(t)
  fat embolism 186
cilia
  Fallopian tubes 81
  respiratory tract 80
circle of Willis 231, 233(f)
circulatory disorders 165–8
cirrhosis, liver 135, 136(f), 137(f)
CJD (Creutzfeldt–Jakob disease) 43–4
classical pathway, complement system 108
claudication 165
clavulanic acid 87
clonal evolution, tumour cells 283(f)
clones, B cells 146
Clostridium botulinum 36
Clostridium difficile 80
Clostridium perfringens 35
Clostridium tetani 36
Clostridium welchii 18
cloudy swelling 13
clubbing, fingers 300
cluster designations *see* CD antigens
c-*myc* gene 279
  Burkitt's lymphoma 269
coagulation system 107, 108(f), 172–4
  wound healing 129
coagulative necrosis 15–16, 18
coarctation, atherosclerosis 194
codons 60, 61
coeliac disease 50–4
  IgA deficiency 147
cold
  frostbite 31, 32–3
  hypothermia 31–3

'cold diuresis' 32
collagen
  scarring 131
  vascular walls 174
  wound healing 130
collagenases, tumours 294
collateral vessels 169, 180
  heart 182(f)
colliquative necrosis 16, 18
colon
  adenomas 249
  splenic flexure, infarcts 229, 231(f)
  see also colorectal carcinoma
colony stimulating factors 104
colorectal carcinoma
  Dukes' staging 260(f)
  hereditary non-polyposis CRC 285
  multistep model 287–8
colour blindness 57
combination therapy, antibiotics 87
comminuted fractures 125(f), 126
comparative genomic hybridization 66, 289–90
complement, B-lymphocytes and 144–5
complement-fixing type III reactions 46
complement system 107–9
complete carcinogens 265
compound fractures 125(f), 126
  osteomyelitis 135
computed tomography
  coronary angiography 219
  strokes 232(f)
concentric atheromatous plaques 192
conducting system, heart 12–13
cone biopsy 305
congenital diseases 7
congestion, lung 111, 112(f)
conjugation, antibiotic resistance mechanism 84–5, 86(f)
connections, objects *vs* 6–7
consecutive clot 177, 178(f)
consolidation 5, 113
constant regions, immunoglobulins 148, 151
contact, infection 79
contact dermatitis 49
contact inhibition 294–5
continuous endothelium 94
contractures 135
copper deficiency 51(t)
coronary arteries
  atherosclerosis 190, 194, 214
  bypass surgery 219
  CT angiography 219
  occlusion on cardiac conducting system 13

coronary heart disease
  lipids and 198–200
  prevention 200–3
  risk reduction 198
  see also myocardial infarction
cor pulmonale 185
corticosteroids *see* steroid hormones
cortisol, hormone-secreting tumours on 250(f)
co-stimulatory cell surface molecules, B-cells 144
Cotswolds revision, Hodgkin's lymphoma staging 260(f)
cowpox 160
C-reactive protein 110–11
creatine kinase 9, 13
  MB isoenzyme 213
Creutzfeldt–Jakob disease 43–4
Crohn's disease 224
cross-linking, IgE 45
cross-reactions, autoimmune disease 155, 156
Cushing, Harvey 300
Cushing's syndrome 250(f), 299, 300
cyanosis 165
cyclin-dependent kinases (CDKs) 279, 282(f)
cyclins 279, 282(f)
cyclo-oxygenases 102, 104(f)
cystic fibrosis 59–60
cystic medial necrosis 208
cystitis 80
cysts, implantation dermoid 130
cytogenetics *see* genetics; molecular genetics
cytokines 103–4, 106(t), 111
  cancer treatment and 26
  granuloma formation 117
cytology
  breast lumps 252, 258(f)
  cervix 246
cytoskeleton, ischaemia 9
cytotoxic hypersensitivity, antibody-dependent 46, 47(f), 148, 154
cytotoxic T cells 143, 154
cytotoxins 34

Darwin, Charles 55
death receptor 24
debridement 124
decompression sickness 186
deep venous thrombosis *see* venous thrombosis
degranulation, mast cells 105
delayed–persistent inflammatory response 96
delayed type hypersensitivity 49, 50(f)
deletions 277
  chromosomal 62(f), 69
  RB gene 276(f)
Delta F508 mutation, cystic fibrosis 60

De Motu Cordis (Harvey) 167, 168
dendritic cells 141–2
  follicular (FDCs) 141–2, 145(f), 146
dental abscesses 115
dermatitis 49
dermoid cysts, implantation 130
'designer' babies 72–3
desmoplasia 251
dexamethasone test 250(f), 299
diabetes mellitus 189
  cardiovascular disease 195
  fatty change 15
  HLA haplotypes 63
  mumps 156
  retinopathy 130–1
  skin infections 83
  urinary tract infections 80
diapedesis (emigration), leucocytes 92, 99
diarrhoea, infectious 34–5, 38(t)
DIC (disseminated intravascular coagulation) 186–8
diet, cardiovascular disease 198–9, 200–3
differentiation, tumours 262
diffusion weighted imaging, MRI, strokes 232(f)
diploidy 66
directly observed therapy, short course (DOTS) 121
discontinuous endothelium 94
disease
  causes 7–28, 29–73
  defining 3–6
dispermy 60
dissection, aorta 208, 209
disseminated intravascular coagulation (DIC) 186–8
  fat embolism syndrome 186
diuresis, 'cold' 32
diuretic phase, shocked kidney 228
diversity regions, immunoglobulins 151
DNA 57, 66, 67(f)
  analysis 66–9
  antibiotic resistance transmission 84
  cancer treatment on 25–6
  'fingerprinting' 69
  genotoxic carcinogens and 266
  microarrays 290
  repair 284–5, 286(f)
    genes 275
  tumours and 263
DNA probes 67, 69
DNA viruses 39(t), 40(f)
  oncogenic 272
Doderlein's bacillus 80
dominant alleles 57
dominant oncogenes 273–4
double-barrelled aorta 209

double minutes (DM)   277
Down syndrome   71–2
  nuchal translucency thickness   64(f)
  triple test   64
drug-eluting stents   219
drug reactions, type II hypersensitivity   46
dry gangrene   18
ductal carcinoma   256, 258(f)
Dukes' staging, colorectal carcinoma   260(f)
dysplasia   247–9, 305
dyspnoea   184
dystrophic calcification   18, 19(f)
  tuberculosis   137

early genes, oncogenic DNA viruses   272
E-cadherin   282, 295
eccentric atheromatous plaques   192
ecchymoses   166
ECG, myocardial infarction   13
elastin   103(f)
elderly patients *see* age/ageing
electricity, wound healing   136
electrocardiography (ECG), myocardial infarction   13
electrocution   29–31
elongation factor 2, bacterial toxins affecting   36
embolism   165, 166, 180–6
  pulmonary   183–5
    shock   211, 213(f)
  strokes   230, 232(f)
  systemic   185–6
emigration (diapedesis), leucocytes   92, 99
empyema, tuberculosis   121
emulsion instability theory   186
encrustation theory (Rokitansky)   196–7
end arteries   231
endocarditis   175
  infective, embolism   185
  rheumatic fever   156
endogenous lipid pathway   198–200, 201(f)
endometrium, menstrual cycle   21–2
endothelins   205
endothelium   174–5, 202(f)
  adult respiratory distress syndrome   228
  angiogenesis   130
  damage in atherosclerosis   197
  hypothermia   32
  permeability in inflammation   94, 95(f)
endothelium-derived relaxing factor (nitric oxide)   105–7, 214
endotoxins, bacterial infections   33–4, 36(t)
Entamoeba histolytica   39(t)
enterococci, vancomycin-resistant   86
enterotoxins   34–5, 38(t)

environmental agents, tumours   265
enzymes
  bacterial toxins as   35–6
  cardiac   13, 216
    troponins   12, 13, 213, 216
    see also creatine kinase
  DNA analysis   66
  lysosomal   22, 102
eosinophilia, necrosis   15
eosinophils, inflammation   91(t)
epidemiology   77–8
  tuberculosis   117–18
epidermis, wound healing   129–30
epidermodysplasia verruciformis   269–70
epidermolytic toxin   35
epinephrine (adrenaline), for anaphylactic shock   46
epithelial–mesenchymal transition (EMT)   294
epithelioid cells   116, 117, 124
epithelium
  adult respiratory distress syndrome   228
  iron deficiency   224
  wound healing   130
epitopes   141
Epstein–Barr virus   145–6, 156, 268–9
Escherichia coli, heat stable enterotoxin   35
E-selectin   97, 98(t)
essential hypertension   205
evolution   55
exercise   198
  on high-density lipoprotein   202–3
  hypothermia   32
exogenous antigens   48–9
exogenous lipids   198, 199(f)
exons, immunoglobulin genes   151
exotoxins   81
  bacterial infections   34–8
    type III   35–6
expression arrays   290
extrinsic allergic alveolitis   48(f), 49
extrinsic causes of disease   29, 30(t)
exudates, inflammatory   89, 93, 94
eye
  defences   79
  trauma   155
  see also retina

Fab (variable end of immunoglobulin)   148
faeco-oral route of infection   79
fainting, hypothermia   32
Fallopian tubes, cilia   81
falx cerebri   234(f)
familial hypercholesterolaemia   57
familial polyposis coli   264, 282

familial tumour syndromes 284(t)
family history 69–70
  tumours 73, 263–4
farmer's lung 48(f)
Fas receptor (death receptor) 24
fat emboli 185–6
fat embolism syndrome 186
fat necrosis 17
fats *see* lipids
fatty acids 200–2
fatty change 13–15, 138
fatty streaks, arteries 190, 193
Fc receptors, NK cells 154
femoral head, avascular necrosis 70(f)
fenestrated endothelium 94
alpha-fetoprotein 64, 72
fetoscopy 64
fetus
  hydrops 58(f)
  passive immunity 147
fever 109–10
fibrillation 218
  atrial 236
fibrin 93–4, 129, 170–1, 173
fibrinoid necrosis 18
fibrinolysis, DIC 188
fibrinolytic system 107, 108(f)
fibrinopeptides 107
fibroblasts
  steroid hormones on 134
  wound healing 130
fibro-fatty lesions, atherosclerosis 190–1
fibroids, uterus 249
fibronectin 129
fibrous caps, atheromatous plaques 191
field effect, transitional carcinoma spread 292(f)
fine needle aspiration cytology, breast lumps 252
fingers, clubbing 300
fish oils 202
fluorescence *in situ* hybridization 65–6
  see also comparative genomic hybridization
foam cells, atherosclerosis 197
foamy macrophages 123
folate deficiency 51(t), 225
follicles, lymph nodes 142
  hyperplasia 143
follicular dendritic cells (FDCs) 141–2, 145(f), 146
food poisoning 34–5, 38(t)
foramen magnum 234(f)
foreign bodies, on wound healing 134
foreign-body giant cells 124
F plasmids 84
F prime plasmids 85

fractures 125, 126
  emboli 185
  healing 128, 131–3, 135
    abnormal 135
fragile X syndrome 59
frameshift mutations 60, 61
frogs, thyroxine 21
frostbite 31, 32–3
functional type III reactions 46
fungi 43
  tuberculous cavities 121
fusiform aneurysms 207(f), 210

gamma globulins 146
  see also immunoglobulin(s)
gangrene 17–18
Gardasil (vaccine) 270
gas gangrene 18
gastric carcinoma
  geography and race 264–5
  spread 292(f)
gastritis, alcohol 138
gastrointestinal tract
  defences against infection 80
  metaplasia 246
  splenic flexure infarcts 229, 231(f)
  tumours
    local effects 298–9
    see also colorectal carcinoma; gastric carcinoma
  watershed infarcts 229
  see also stomach
gefitinib 304
gender, atherosclerosis 193–4
gene therapy 272, 304
genetics 54–73
  atherosclerosis 194
  diagnostic tests 63–9
  immunoglobulins 151–2
  malignant tumours 263–4, 273–90
    see also targeted anticancer therapies
genotoxic carcinogens 266, 267
geographical factors, tumours 264–5
Ghon focus 118–19
giant cells 124
giant macrophages, multinucleate 124
Giardia 81
glandular fever 145–6
Gleevec (STI-571) 303–4
glomeruli, renal, Goodpasture's syndrome 46
glomerulonephritis 49, 101, 158
glucose, cholera and 37(f)
gluten, coeliac disease 51
glycylcyclines 87

Goodpasture' s syndrome   46
gp20 (HIV)   24
gp120 (HIV)   88
G proteins, bacterial toxins affecting   36
grading, tumours   256–8, 259(t)
graft-versus-host disease   159
gram-negative bacteria   34(t), 35(f)
gram-positive bacteria   34(t), 35(f)
granulation tissue
   in thrombus   177
   wound healing   130–1
granulocytes (polymorphs)   16, 90, 91(t),
   96–101
granulomatous inflammation   116–22, 124
   tuberculosis   118
Graves' disease   46, 157
Graves, Robert   158
greenstick fractures   125(f), 126
grey hepatization, lung   112(f), 113
growth disorders, benign   243–50
   atrophy   244–5
   dysplasia   246–9
   hyperplasia   243–4
   hypertrophy   243–4
   metaplasia   246–9
   neoplasia   249–50
growth factors   104
   atherosclerosis   197
   oncogene action   277–8, 279(f)
   wound healing   130, 136
   see also named growth factors e.g. insulin-like growth
         factor-1
growth fractions, tumours   291
growth inhibition, tumour suppressor genes   280–3
GTP binding proteins
   bacterial toxins affecting   36
   tumour growth   278–9

haematemesis   135
haematocrit, normal ranges   223(t)
haematomas   166
   fractures   131
haem groups   70, 71(f)
haemochromatosis   71
haemoglobin
   normal ranges   223(t)
   types   70, 71
haemoglobinopathies   69–71
haemolysins, thiol-activating   35
haemolysis   71
   disseminated intravascular coagulation   187
haemopericardium   218
Haemophilus influenzae type b vaccination   162(f)

haemorrhage   166
   intracranial   230, 232(f)
   tumours   298
haemorrhagic infarction   169
haemostasis   170–4
   wounds   129
Hageman factor   107, 129
haploidy   66
Harvey, William   167–8
Hayflick limit   285
healing see wound healing
health, disease vs   3
heart
   arrhythmias   12–13, 216–18
   collateral vessels   182(f)
   conducting system   12–13
   hypothermia   32, 33(t)
   pulmonary embolism on   185
   thrombosis   185
      myocardial infarction   175, 177
   see also coronary heart disease; myocardial infarction
heart block   13, 218
heart failure   218
   shock   211
heat loss   31
heat stable enterotoxin, E. coli   35
heavy chains, immunoglobulins   146
   diversity   151–2
heavy chain switch   146
Heisenberg, W., quoted   6–7
Helicobacter pylori   81, 225
helminths   43
helper T cells   143, 145(f), 153–4
   tuberculosis and AIDS   118
hepatitis, viral, as chronic   115
hepatitis B virus   38, 42(f), 270–1
hepatocellular carcinoma   270–1
   geography   264(f)
hepatocytes   91(t)
Her-2 oncogene   259
   action   278
   amplification   277
   antibody   303
hereditary non-polyposis colorectal carcinoma   285
heritability   63
herniation, brain   231, 234(f)
heterogeneity, tumours   291
Hib, vaccination   162(f)
high-density lipoprotein   194, 200(t)
   factors affecting levels   202–3
   obesity   198
Hiroshima, tumours   267
histamine   105

histiocytes *see* macrophages

histochemistry, myocardial infarction   216

histogenesis, tumour classification   262

HLA types *see* major histocompatibility complex system

Hodgkin's lymphoma
   Ann Arbor staging   260(f)
   Epstein–Barr virus   268(f), 269

Hodgkin, Thomas   269

homeostasis   3

homogeneously staining regions (HSRs) (chromatin
  bodies)   277

honeymoon cystitis   80

hormone replacement therapy
   cardiovascular disease and   193–4
   on high-density lipoprotein   202

hormones
   involution caused by   21
   reaction to stress   111
   see also named hormones e.g. oestrogens

hormone-secreting tumours   250(f), 299–300

hospital infections   83
   methicillin-resistant *S. aureus*   86

Howell-Jolly bodies   220, 225

human herpesvirus 8   271

human immunodeficiency virus (HIV)   38
   apoptosis   24
   drug resistance   87–8
   mode of infection   81
   tuberculosis and   118
   see also AIDS

human papilloma virus   269–70
   vaccination   161

human T-cell leukaemia virus-1 (HTLV-1)   271, 272

humoral immunity   143, 144–52

Hunter, John   89, 180

Huntington's disease, DNA analysis   67

hyaline arteriolosclerosis   206

hyaline membrane, ARDS   228, 229(f)

hybridization, DNA   67

hydrogen peroxide   101

hydropic degeneration   9, 13

hydrops, fetus   58(f)

hydroxyl ions   101

5-hydroxytryptamine   105

hyperacute rejection, transplanted organs   158

hyperaemia   166

hypercalcaemia, tumours and   300

hypercholesterolaemia, familial   57

hyperchromatism   255
   cervical dysplasia   247

hypercoagulable blood   174

hyperlipidaemia   194
   obesity   197–8
   secondary   200

hypermutation, antibodies   146, 148

hyperparathyroidism, calcification   18

hyperplasia   243–4, 245
   bone marrow   220
   lymph nodes   143
   neoplasia *vs*   249
   prostate   243, 244(f)

hyperplastic arteriolosclerosis   206

hypersensitivity   44–9, 50(f)
   antibody-dependent cytotoxic   46, 47(f), 148, 154
   coeliac disease   50–4
   immune complex mediated   48–9, 101
   tuberculosis   118–19

hypertension   203–7
   intracranial haemorrhage   230
   problems of definition   3
   renal   190, 205
   risk of cardiovascular events   194
   secondary   205–6

hypertrophic osteoarthropathy   300

hypertrophy   243–4, 245
   neoplasia *vs*   249
   right ventricle   185
   scars   135

hypervariable regions, immunoglobulins   148

hypochlorous acid   101

hypochromic anaemia   220, 221(t), 222(f)

hypoplastic bone marrow   220

hypotension, hypothermia   32

hypothalamic–pituitary–adrenal axis   111

hypothalamus, fever   109

hypothermia   31–3

hypovolaemic shock   211, 212(f)

hypoxia   6
   hypothermia   32

hysterectomy   306

ICAM-1 (adhesion molecule)   97–8

imatinib   303–4

imbibition hypothesis (Virchow)   196

immediate–persistent inflammatory response   95, 96(f)

immediate–transient inflammatory response   94, 96(f)

immobilization
   fractures   131
   wound healing   134

immune complex mediated hypersensitivity   48–9, 101

immune-mediated granuloma formation   116–17

immunity   139–62
   adaptive   81, 139, 143–55
   evasion   81–3
   innate   81, 139
   to tumours   296

immunization   159–62
   human papillomavirus   270

schedules (UK)   162(t)
  children   161(t)
  against tumours   296
immunoglobulin(s)   142, 144–9, 150(f)
  generation of diversity   151–2
immunoglobulin A (IgA)   147, 149(t), 151
immunoglobulin D (IgD)   148, 149(t)
immunoglobulin E (IgE)   148, 149(t), 151
  cross-linking   45
immunoglobulin G (IgG)   146, 147, 149(t), 150, 151
immunoglobulin gene superfamily   148, 150(f), 151
immunoglobulin M (IgM)   146, 147, 149(t), 150, 151
immunotherapy   303
implantation dermoid cysts   130
inactivating mutations   275, 280
inappropriate hormone production   299–300
incidence
  genetic diseases   57
    maternal age   72(f)
  tuberculosis   117–18
  tumours, by type   302(f)
incomplete carcinogens   265
Indian ink, endothelial permeability   94, 95(f)
infarction   166, 169
  central nervous system, healing   133
  cerebral   17(f), 228–37
  disseminated intravascular coagulation   187
  expansion (myocardial)   218
  kidney   15–16
  pulmonary   184–5
  spleen   17(f)
  tumours   299
  water-shed, brain   228–9, 231(f)
  see also myocardial infarction
infarction at a distance, myocardium   214
infections   79–88
  atherosclerosis risk from   195
  body defences   79–81
    evasion   81–3
  transmission   79, 81
  tuberculosis   117–21, 137
    antibiotic resistance   85–7, 121
  see also bacteria; viruses
infectious mononucleosis   145–6
infective endocarditis, embolism   185
inflammation
  acute   89–114
  chronic   90, 115–16
    role of macrophages   123
  granulomatous   116–22, 124
    tuberculosis   118
  lymphatic system   139–43
  systemic effects   109–14

wounds   129
  see also macrophages
influenza, susceptibility to infection   38
inheritance
  cancer   280, 281(f)
  Mendelian   55–7
  multifactorial   61–3
initiators, carcinogenesis   265
innate immunity   81, 139
insects, infection transmission   79, 81
insertional mutagenesis   272
in situ carcinoma   255–6
insulin-like growth factor-1, ageing   27
integrins   98
interferon(s)   26, 104, 106(t)
  immunotherapy   303
interferon-gamma, on atheromatous plaques   192
interleukins   26, 106(t)
  granuloma formation   117
  reaction to endotoxins   34
intermediate-density lipoprotein   200(t)
intestines see gastrointestinal tract
intracranial haemorrhage   230, 232(f)
intracranial tumours   297–8
intraepithelial neoplasia   247, 248(f)
intrinsic causes of disease   29, 30(t)
intrinsic factor   225
introns, between immunoglobulin genes   151
inversion, chromosomal   62(f)
involucrum   115
involution   245
  caused by hormones   21
iodine deficiency   51(t)
ionic channels, ischaemia   9
iron   223–4
  deficiency   51(t)
    anaemia   222(f), 223–4
  in inflammation   110
ischaemia   8–12
  kidney   15–16, 228
  myocardium   216

Japanese people, gastric carcinoma   264–5
jaundice
  anaemia   224
  haemoglobinopathies   71
Jenner, Edward   159
joining regions, immunoglobulins   151

kallikrein   107
Kaposi's sarcoma   271
Kaposi's sarcoma-associated virus   271
karyolysis   15
karyorrhexis   15

karyotypes 65
    tumours 273
keloids 135
keratinocytes, wound healing 129
KFERQ (amino acid sequence) 23(f)
kidney
    adult polycystic disease 59
    'cold diuresis' 32
    Goodpasture's syndrome 46
    hypertension 190, 205
    hypothermia 32, 33(t)
    ischaemia 15–16, 228
kinins 107
kit gene, mutations 276
Klinefelter's syndrome 57
Koch, Robert 117
Koch's postulates 117
koilocytosis, cervix 248(f)
koilonychia 224
Krukenberg tumour 292(f)
Kupffer cells 91(t)
kuru 43
kwashiorkor 49, 51(t)

labile cells, tissue regeneration 125, 127(f)
lactate dehydrogenase 13
lactoferrin 101
lacunar infarcts, brain 133
laesio functae 90
Lancefield group A *Streptococcus pyogenes* 140, 156
Langerhans cells 141(f)
Langhans giant cells 124
latent infections
    tuberculosis 119
    viral 39, 42(f)
law of segregation 57
lecithin-cholesterol acyltransferase 200
lectin binding pathway 109
leiomyoma, uterus 249
Leishmania 42(f)
leucocytes
    activation 99
    inflammation 92, 96–101
    polymorphonuclear 16, 90, 91(t), 96–101
    see also specific types e.g. macrophages
leucocytosis 220
leucoerythroblastic anaemia 220, 221(t)
leukaemia 220
    adult T-cell leukaemia/lymphoma 271
    chronic myeloid 273, 303
leukotrienes 102
Lewis adhesion molecules 97
LFA-1 (adhesion molecule) 97–8

lifestyle changes, cardiovascular disease 197–8
light chains, immunoglobulins 146–7
lines of Zahn 177, 178(f), 179(f)
lipid A 33–4
lipids
    metabolism 198–200, 201(f)
    strokes 232
    see also hyperlipidaemia
lipofuscin 27
lipo-oxygenase pathway 104(f)
lipopolysaccharide 33–4
lipotechoic acid 34
liquefactive necrosis 16, 18
Listeria monocytogenes 34
    toxin 35
liver
    cirrhosis 135, 136(f), 137(f)
    fatty change 13–15
    regeneration 125, 134, 244
    see also hepatocellular carcinoma
lobar pneumonia 4–6, 111–14
local vascular tone 204–5
loss-of-function mutations 275, 280
loss of heterozygosity 289
loss of polarity 255
low birth weight, atherosclerosis risk from 195
low-density lipoprotein 194, 200(t)
    metabolism 199
    obesity 197–8
    oxidation 197
    receptor deficiencies 57–9
low-density lipoprotein receptors, macrophages 123
L-selectin 98(t)
lung
    lobar pneumonia 4–6, 111–14
    see also entries beginning pulmonary…
lymph 140
lymphatic system 139–43
    tumour spread 292(f), 293
lymph nodes 140, 141(f), 142
    hyperplasia 143
    tumours and 293
lymphocytes 139–40, 143(f)
    atherosclerosis 197
    inflammation 91(t)
    see also B-lymphocytes; T-lymphocytes
lymphokine activated killer cells (LAK cells) 303
lymphomas 146
    adult T-cell leukaemia/lymphoma 271
    see also Burkitt's lymphoma; Hodgkin's
        lymphoma
lysogenic conversion 84
lysosomal enzymes 22, 102

lysosomes 101
   chemical mediators in 102
lysozyme 101

macro-autophagy 20, 22, 23(t)
macrocytic anaemia 220, 221(t), 222(f), 225
macrophages 91(t), 96, 122–4
   accessory cells 141
   alveolar 80, 113
   atherosclerosis 197
   steroid hormones on 134
   wound healing 129, 130
mad cow disease 43
magnetic resonance imaging, strokes 232(f)
major basic protein 101
major histocompatibility complex system (MHC system) 149–51
   ankylosing spondylitis 63
   coeliac disease 50–1, 54
   diabetes mellitus 63
   protection from NK cells 154–5
malaria, Burkitt's lymphoma and 269
malignant hypertension 204
malignant melanoma *see* melanoma
malignant neoplasms *see* leukaemia; tumours
malnutrition 49
   fatty change 14
mal-union, fractures 135
mammography, calcification 18
mannose binding pathway 109
Mantoux test 49, 50(f)
marasmus 49
Marfan, Antoine 209
Marfan's syndrome 208, 209(f)
margination, leucocytes 92, 96–9
markers, tumours 262
mast cells 105
   allergic reactions 44(f), 45–6
maternal age, chromosomal abnormalities 71–2
matrix metalloproteinases 192(f)
   stromelysin 3, on atheromatous plaques 192
mean corpuscular haemoglobin, normal ranges 223(t)
mean corpuscular volume, normal ranges 223(t)
megakaryocytes 91(t)
megaloblastic anaemia 221(t), 224–7
melanoma
   geography 264(f), 265
   lymphatic drainage 140
membrane attack complex 108
membrane phospholipid, platelets 172
Mendel, Gregor 55
Mendelian inheritance 55–7
menstrual cycle, endometrium 21–2

messenger RNA (mRNA) 66
metabolic syndrome 195
metamorphosis 21
metaplasia 246, 262, 305
metastases, tumours 18, 291–5
metastatic calcification 18
methicillin-resistant *Staphylococcus aureus* (MRSA) 86
methylation, on tumour suppressor gene action 277
MHC system *see* major histocompatibility complex system
microaneurysms, cerebral 208, 237
microangiopathic haemolytic anaemia 187
micro-autophagy 22, 23(t)
microcytic anaemia 220, 221(t), 222(f)
microglial cells 122
microsatellites 285, 289
microvasculature, inflammation 90, 92–6
miliary tuberculosis 119, 120(f), 121
mismatch repair genes (*MMR* genes) 275, 285
mitochondria
   apoptosis 23(f)
   ischaemia 9
mitosis counts, tumours 291
mitral valve, myocardial infarction 218
molecular family planning 72–3
molecular genetics, tumours 273–90
   see also targeted anticancer therapies
monoclonal antibodies, cancer treatment 303
monocytes 122
   inflammation 91(t)
monokines 103
monomers, IgG as 147
monosomy 60
Montagu, Lady Mary Wortley 159–60
mosaicism 65
mouth 80
MRSA (methicillin-resistant *Staphylococcus aureus*) 86
mucinous carcinoma, breast 258(f)
muco-ciliary clearance system 80, 81
mucosal contact, infection 79
Müllerian duct 21
multi-drug resistant tuberculosis 121
multifactorial disorders, genetic 61–3
multinucleate giant macrophages 124
multiple myeloma 146
multistep model of carcinogenesis 287–8
mumps, orchitis 155–6
mural thrombosis 218
muscles, wasting 245
mutations 31(f), 60, 61, 68–9
   activating 273
   B cells 148
   Burkitt's lymphoma 269
   cancer 263, 264, 267

mutations (*contuined*)
  CFTR gene 60
  frameshift 60, 61
  human immunodeficiency virus 88
  inactivating 275, 280
  kit gene 276
  in prions 44
  see also point mutations
myc genes 279
  N-*myc* gene amplification 277
Mycobacterium tuberculosis 117, 118
mycotic aneurysms 210
myeloma 146
myeloperoxidase 101, 102
myocardial infarction 8–13, 211–20
  gender 193
  pain 165, 211–12
  subendocardial 215–16, 229
  thrombosis 175, 177
  treatment 218–20

NADPH oxidase 101
naevi 249
Nagasaki, tumours 267
nails, koilonychia 224
beta-naphthylamine 265, 266
natural killer cells 152, 154–5
  type II hypersensitivity 46
natural selection 55
necrosis 15–19
  apoptosis *vs* 20
  avascular, femoral head 70(f)
  caseous 16–17, 118, 121(f)
  frostbite 33
  myocardial infarction 11(f)
nematodes 43
neoplasms
  benign 249, 250(f)
  see also carcinoma; tumours
nervous system
  apoptosis in development 21
  degeneration, autophagy 27(t)
  healing 133
  hypothermia 32, 33(t)
  see also brain
neural tube defects, alpha-fetoprotein 64
neuromas, traumatic 133
neurotoxins 34, 36, 38(t)
neutralization, antigens 148
neutropenia 220
neutrophils
  granules 102
  hypersegmentation 225

inflammation 91(t), 96
  wound healing 129
niacin deficiency 51(t)
nipple, Paget's disease 251
nitric oxide 105–7, 214
nitroblue tetrazolium, myocardial infarction 216
nitrogen dioxide 101
nitrogen emboli 186
N-*myc* gene, amplification 277
non-coding DNA 69
non-disjunction 60, 61(f)
  Down syndrome 72
non-steroidal anti-inflammatory drugs (NSAIDs) 102
non-union, fractures 135
normochromic anaemia 220, 221(t)
normocytic anaemia 220, 221(t)
Northern blotting 67
nose, defences 80
nuchal translucency thickness 64(f)
nuclear-cytoplasmic ratio 255
nuclear explosions 30(f), 267
nuclear oncoproteins 279
nutritional diseases 49–50, 51(t)
  wound healing and 134

obesity 49
  hyperlipidaemia 197–8
obstetrics, disseminated intravascular coagulation 187
occlusion, vascular 169–88
occupational causes, tumours 241
oedema 93
  pulmonary, ARDS 229(f)
oesophagus
  Barrett's metaplasia 246
  carcinoma 298(f)
  varices 135
oestrogen receptors, breast carcinoma 259
oestrogens, sexual development 21
oligonucleotides, DNA probes 67, 69
oliguria 228
omega 3 fatty acids 202
omega 6 fatty acids 202
oncogenes 272, 273–9
  growth factors 277–8
  mechanisms of tumourigenesis 276–9
  signal transduction proteins 278–9
oncogenic DNA viruses 272
oncogenic RNA viruses 271–2
oncoproteins, nuclear 279
ophthalmitis, sympathetic 155
opsonins 99, 142
opsonization 99
oral rehydration solutions 37(f)

orchitis, mumps   155–6
organ damage, perfusion deficiency   227–9
organization
    lobar pneumonia   113
    thrombus   177
orthopnoea   184
Osler, Sir William   235
    quoted   233–4
osmotic gradients, inflammation   92–3, 95(f), 140
osteomyelitis   115
    compound fractures   135
oval cells, liver   134
oxidative phosphorylation   9
oxidized lipoproteins   197
oxygen, hypothermia on uptake   32
oxygen free radicals   25, 101
    adult respiratory distress syndrome   228

p53
    inactivation by viruses   24
    protein   282–3
Paget's disease of the nipple   251
Paget, Sir James   252
Paget, Stephen, on tumour metastases   291–2
pain
    circulatory disorders   165
    myocardial infarction   165, 211–12
palliative cancer treatment   304
pancreatitis, fat necrosis   17
pancytopenia   220
pannus   115
papillary muscles, myocardial infarction   218
papillomas   269–70
papilloma viruses *see* human papilloma virus
paracetamol, on fever   110
paracortical hyperplasia, lymph nodes   143
paraneoplastic syndromes   300, 301
passive immunity   159, 161–2
    fetus   147
Paterson–Kelly syndrome   224
pathological fractures   126
pathology   3
pellagra   51(t)
penetrance   57
penicillin resistance   86
pentamers, IgM as   147
percutaneous coronary intervention (PCI)   219
perforation, gastrointestinal   298–9
perfringolysin   35
perfusion deficiency, organ damage   227–9
pericarditis   218
pericardium, leakage   218
perinatal autopsy, thymus   21

peripheral resistance, total   204–5
permanent cells, tissue regeneration   125, 127(f)
permeability, microvasculature   93, 94, 95(f)
pernicious anaemia   222(f), 225, 226(f)
persistent viral infections   39
petechiae   166
phages   84, 85(f)
phagocytosis   22, 90, 99–101, 122–3
phagolysosomes   101
phagosomes   101
Philadelphia chromosome   273
phospholipase C activity toxin   35
pituitary gland, effects of swelling   297
plague, mode of spread   79
plasma cells   144, 146
plasma membranes
    bacterial exotoxins affecting   35
    ischaemia   9
plasmids   84–5
plasmin   107, 174
plasminogen activators   174
    resolution of thrombosis   177
Plasmodium spp.   39(t)
platelet activating factor   104–5, 107(f)
platelet-derived growth factor   177
    atherosclerosis   197
platelets   170, 171–2
    activation   105
    aspirin on   172
    granules   171, 172
    haemostasis   129
    surface membrane receptors   172
    venous thrombosis   177
    see also antiplatelet agents
platyhelminths   43
pleomorphism
    cervical dysplasia   247
    malignant tumours   255
pleura, tuberculosis   121
Plummer–Vinson syndrome   224
Pneumocystis carinii   39(t)
pneumocytes, ARDS   228
pneumonia, lobar   4–6, 111–14
poikilocytosis   220, 225
point mutations   60, 61
    oncogenes   276, 278–9
    sickle cell disease   70
polarity, loss   255
polio vaccine   160
polio virus, cell damage   38
polyclonal B cell response   146
polycystic kidney disease, adult   59
polycythaemia   174, 220

polycythaemia rubra vera 174
polymerase chain reaction 69
polymorphonuclear leucocytes 16, 90, 91(t), 96–101
polypill 203
polyploidy 60, 66
polyunsaturated fatty acids 201, 202
portal hypertension 136(f)
positron emission tomography 294(f)
post-primary tuberculosis 119–21
Pott, Percival 265
precancerous adenomas 287–8
precipitation, antigens 148
predisposing factors 7
pregnancy
    anaemia 226–7
    breast hyperplasia 22
    ultrasound 63–4
    uterus 244
pressure sores 135(f)
primary complex, tuberculosis 119
prions 43–4
procollagen 130
progesterone receptors, breast carcinoma 259
programmed cell death 19–21, 23(f)
    in tumours 26
Prometheus 244
promoters, carcinogenesis 265
prostaglandins 102
prostate, benign hyperplasia 243, 244(f)
prostate-specific antigen 262
proteases, on atheromatous plaques 192
proteasomes 150
protein arrays (proteomics) 290
proto-oncogenes 272, 273, 275
protoporphyrins, metabolism in haemoglobinopathies 71
protozoa 39
P-selectin 97, 98(t)
pseudarthrosis 135
pseudomembranous colitis 80
pseudopodia 99–101
pulmonary embolism 183–5
    shock 211, 213(f)
pulmonary hypertension 185
pulmonary oedema, ARDS 229(f)
purine bases 66, 67(f)
Purkinje, Johannes 230
purpura 166
pus 93, 102
pyknosis 15
pyrexia 109–10
pyrimidine bases 66, 67(f)
pyrogens 6, 34, 38(t), 109–10

rabies virus 81
racial factors
    tuberculosis 118
    tumours 264–5
radiation 29, 30(f)
    carcinogenesis 267
radiotherapy 25, 301–3
    on wound healing 134
ras genes 276, 278–9
rats 79
RB1 gene 280, 282
reaction to injury theory, atherosclerosis 196–7
reactivation infection, tuberculosis 119, 120, 121(f)
recanalization 177–80
receptors
    growth factors 277–8, 279(f)
    leucocyte activation 99
    see also specific types
recessive alleles 57
recessive oncogenes (tumour suppressor genes) 275, 279–83
red blood cells 220–7
    haemoglobinopathies 71
    normal counts 223(t)
    phagocytosis 122
red hepatization, lung 112(f), 113
reduction, fractures 131
Reed–Sternberg cells 268(f)
regeneration
    liver 125, 134, 244
    wound healing 125–6, 127(f), 129–30
regional infarcts, myocardium 214, 215(f)
rejection, transplanted organs 158–9
remodelling 131
    fractures 132–3
renal failure, shock 228
renal glomeruli, Goodpasture's syndrome 46
renal tubular epithelium
    acute tubular necrosis 228
    hypothermia 32, 33(t)
renin, hypertension 205
repair 126, 131
    central nervous system 133
replacement phase, wound healing 130
replicative senescence 27, 287
reproductive system, development 21
resolution
    of thrombosis 177
    tissue repair 126
respiratory burst 101, 105
respiratory distress syndrome, adult (ARDS) 228, 229(f), 230(f)
respiratory tract
    defences 80, 81
    lobar pneumonia 4–6, 111–14

see also entries beginning pulmonary…
   restriction endonucleases 66, 67
restriction fragment length polymorphisms 67
restriction fragments 66–7
resuscitation, cardiac, emboli 185
reticulocytes 223
reticulo-endothelial system 122
retina
   cardiovascular disease 190
   central vein occlusion 169
   diabetes mellitus 130–1
retinoblastoma 264, 280, 281(f)
retroviruses 41(f)
   drug resistance 87–8
   tumourigenesis 271–2, 275
   see also human immunodeficiency virus
reverse transcriptase 87–8
reverse transport mechanism, cholesterol 199–200
reversible cell damage 9, 12, 13–15
rhesus incompatibility 46, 47(f)
rheumatic fever 156
rheumatoid arthritis 115–16
rhinovirus 81
rho proteins, bacterial toxins affecting 36
right ventricle, hypertrophy 185
ring formation, chromosomal 62(f)
risk (predisposing factors) 7
RNA 66, 67(f)
   translation 66, 68(f)
     tumourigenesis 277
RNA viruses 39(t), 40(f)
   oncogenic 271–2
Robertsonian translocation 62(f)
Rokitansky, K. von, encrustation theory 196–7
rupture
   aorta 209
   tumours 298–9

saccular aneurysms 207(f), 210
saddle embolus, pulmonary 183
Salmonella typhi 115
salt intake, hypertension 205
sarcoidosis 117(f), 121–2
sarcomas, spread 293
scarring 127–8, 131
   abnormal 135
   myocardium 8, 9, 10(f), 216
Schilling test 225
Schistosoma 43(f)
Schwann, Friedrich 133
scrapie 43
screening for cancer 288, 301
   cervical 246, 248–9
scrotal carcinoma, chimney sweeps 265

scurvy 51(t)
'seed and soil' theory 292
segregation, law of 57
selectins 97, 98
selenium deficiency 51(t)
Selnas method 72–3
senescence, replicative 27, 287
sensation, circulatory disorders on 165
septicaemia 143
septic shock 211
sequestered antigens 155
serotonin 105
serum sickness 48
sex pili 84
sex selection 72
sexual development 21
sexually transmitted diseases 79
shock 124, 211, 212(f), 218
   anaphylactic 45–6
   endotoxic 34
   organ damage 227–9
   pulmonary embolism 211, 213(f)
shock lung (ARDS) 228, 229(f), 230(f)
sickle cell disease 69–70
   DNA analysis 69
   haemoglobin 71(f)
signal transduction proteins, tumour growth 278–9
single-gene disorders 57, 60–1
singlet oxygen 101
sinusoidal macrophages 122–3
skin
   infections 81, 83
   tumours and ultraviolet light 267
   ulcers 134, 224
slow transforming viruses 271, 272
small-cell lung carcinoma 250(f), 289(f)
smallpox, immunization 159–60
smoking
   atherosclerosis 194
   bronchial metaplasia 246(f)
   on high-density lipoprotein 202–3
   lung cancer risk 247(f)
smooth muscle, atherosclerosis 197
snake venoms, work of Arthus 48
Snow, John 7, 77–8
sodium
   cholera 37(f)
   hypothermia 32
   transmembrane leakage 9
somatic cell hybrids 280
Southern blotting 67
space-occupying lesions, brain 231, 297–8
specific granules, neutrophils 102
sperm sorting 72

spherocytosis   122
spleen   125, 143
   infarction   17(f)
   sinusoidal macrophages   122–3
splenectomy   123, 125
splenic flexure of colon, infarcts   229, 231(f)
spongiform encephalopathies, transmissible   43–4
squamous cell carcinoma, human papillomavirus   270
stability, atheromatous plaques   192, 214, 232
stability genes   275
stable cells, tissue regeneration   125, 127(f)
staging, tumours   258–9, 260(f)
Staphylococcus aureus   35, 86, 115
stasis, thrombosis   175
statins   198
stem cells
   central nervous system repair   133
   liver regeneration   134
   tumours and   287, 304
steroid hormones
   involution caused by   21
   tumours producing   299
   on wound healing   134
STI-571 (Gleevec)   303–4
stimulatory hypersensitivity (type V)   46
stomach
   alcohol on   138
   carcinoma
      geography and race   264–5
      spread   292(f)
   Helicobacter pylori   81, 225
stop codons   60, 61
Streptococcus pneumoniae   111
   toxin   35
Streptococcus pyogenes
   Lancefield group A   140, 156
   toxin   35
streptokinase   177
stress, hormonal reaction to   111
stress fractures   126
strokes   229–37
stromelysin 3, on atheromatous plaques   192
ST segment elevation   213–14
subcellular infectious agents   43–4
subendocardial infarcts   215–16, 229
sublethal cell injury   9, 12, 13–15
sun exposure, tumours   267
superior vena cava compression   292(f)
superoxide   101
suppressor T cells   143, 154
suppurative inflammation   115, 116(f)
   see also abscesses; pus
surfactant deficiency, ARDS   228

sutures   124, 130
   strength   131
sweat test   59, 60
sympathetic ophthalmitis   155
syphilis, aneurysms   209–10
systemic embolism   185–6
systemic lupus erythematosus   157–8

tachycardia   6, 218
tamoxifen   303
tamponade, cardiac   218
targeted anticancer therapies   259, 303–4
tat gene, HTLV-1   271, 272
T-cell receptors   152–3
T cells *see* T-lymphocytes
tears   79
telomerases, tumours and   285–7
telomeres   27
   tumours and   285–7
temperate phages   84
tenascin   295
tensile strength, wound repair   131
tentorial herniation   231, 234(f)
testis *see* orchitis
testosterone, sexual development   21
tetanus toxin   36
tetracyclines   87
thalassaemias   70–1
therapeutic gene transfer   304
thiamine deficiency   51(t)
thiol-activating haemolysins   35
thoracic duct   140
thrombin   172
thrombocythaemia   220
thrombocytopenia   220
thromboembolism   181
   see also embolism
thrombolysis, for myocardial infarction   219
thrombophilia   174
thrombosis/thrombus   165, 166, 169–88
   atherosclerosis   197
   mural   218
   organization   177
   propagation   177
   strokes   230
thromboxane, ARDS   228
thymus, apoptosis   21
thyroxine, frogs   21
tissue factor   129
tissue-invasive toxins   34, 38(t)
tissue-type plasminogen activator   174
T-lymphocytes   143, 152–4
   CD4$^+$ 24, 153(t), 154

CD8$^+$ 153(t), 154
  inflammation   91(t), 140
  in lymph nodes   142
  MHC molecules on   150
  tolerance   156(f)
  type IV hypersensitivity   49
  wound healing   129
  see also helper T cells
TNM staging, tumours   258, 260(f)
tobacco see smoking
tolerance   155, 156(f)
toll-like receptors   99
tonsillar herniation   234(f)
tonsillitis   140
torsion   299
total peripheral resistance   204–5
Touton giant cells   124
Toxoplasma gondii   39(t)
transactivating genes
  hepatitis B virus   270
  HTLV-1   271
transactivating viruses   272
transcription
  DNA   66, 68(f)
  mRNA, tumourigenesis   277
transduction   144
  antibiotic resistance mechanism   84
  viral oncogenes   275
trans fatty acids   200–2
transfer RNA (tRNA)   66
transformation, antibiotic resistance mechanism   84
transforming growth factor-beta, tumour growth inhibition 282
transient ischaemic attacks (brain)   230, 231–2, 236
translation, RNA   66, 68(f)
  tumourigenesis   277
translocations, chromosomal   62(f), 72
  Burkitt's lymphoma   269, 276(f)
  chronic myeloid leukaemia   273
  oncogenes   276–7
transmissible spongiform encephalopathies   43–4
transmission of infections   79, 81
transmural infarcts, myocardium   214, 218
transplantation   158–9
  tissue matching   150
transposons   85, 86(f)
transudates   93
trastuzumab   259, 303
trauma see fractures; wound healing
traumatic neuromas   133
Trichomonas   39(t)
triglycerides   198
triple test, Down syndrome   64

triple vessel atheroma   215(f)
triple X syndrome   59
triploidy   60
trisomy   60
tropocollagen   130
troponins   12, 13, 213, 216
Trucut biopsy, breast lumps   252
tuberculin test   49, 50(f)
tuberculosis   117–21, 137
  antibiotic resistance   85–7, 121
  caseous necrosis   16–17, 118, 121(f)
  primary   118–19
  secondary   119–21
tubular epithelium, kidney
  acute tubular necrosis   228
  hypothermia   32, 33(t)
tumour necrosis factor   24, 26, 106(t), 123, 301
  cancer treatment with   303
  granuloma maintenance   117
  reaction to endotoxins   34
tumour necrosis factor receptor   25(f)
tumours
  benign   249, 250(f)
  causes   263–72
  classification   259–62
  clinical features   251–8
  coeliac disease   54
  emboli from   186
  family history   73, 263–4
  growth rates   291
  heterogeneity   291
  historical aspects   241
  hormone-secreting   250(f), 299–300
  immunity   296
  incidence by type   302(f)
  local effects   297–9
  local excision   301
  malignancy
    clinical signs   251, 257(f)
    macroscopical features   252–5, 257(f)
    microscopical features   255, 257(f)
  molecular genetics   273–90
    see also targeted anticancer therapies
  prognostic factors   255–9
  spread   18, 291–5
  systemic effects   299–301
  treatment   301–4
    apoptosis   24–5, 26
    see also chemotherapy; radiotherapy
  viruses causing   42(f)
  see also carcinoma
tumour-specific antigens   296
tumour suppressor genes   275, 279–83

turbulence
   atherosclerosis   191
   thrombosis   175
Turner's syndrome   57, 58(f), 59
two hit hypothesis (Knudson)   280, 281(f)
tyrosine kinases, tumour growth   278

Ukraine, tumours   267
ulcers
   malignant   298
   skin   134, 224
ultrasound
   pregnancy   63–4
   venous thrombosis   179(f)
ultraviolet light, tumours   267
union, fractures   132
unstable atheromatous plaques   192, 214, 232
urinary tract, defences against infection   80
urokinase-like plasminogen activator   174
uterus
   leiomyoma   249
   pregnancy   244

vaccination *see* immunization
vacuolar degeneration   9, 13
vacuolar myopathies, autophagy   27(t)
vagina, defences against infection   80
valvular disease
   calcification   19(f)
   myocardial infarction   218
vancomycin-resistant enterococci   86
variable regions, immunoglobulins   148, 151
variant Creutzfeldt–Jakob disease   43–4
varices, oesophagus   135
vascular endothelial growth factor, antibody   304
vascular endothelium *see* endothelium
vascular occlusion   169–88
vascular supply
   bronchi   184–5
   wound healing   134
vasculitis, systemic lupus erythematosus   158
vasoactive amines   105
vasoconstriction, wounds   129
vasoconstrictors   205–6
vasodilatation
   inflammation   90
   wounds   129
vasospasm, coronary   214
veins, tumour spread   293
venous embolism   185
   see also pulmonary embolism
venous thrombosis   169, 176–7, 178(f), 179(f), 180
   see also pulmonary embolism

ventricular arrhythmias   218
ventricular septal defects   218
verotoxins   36
vertebral arteries   231
very low-density lipoproteins   194, 200(t)
vinca alkaloids   26
vinyl chloride   265
Virchow, Rudolf   169–70
   imbibition hypothesis   196
   on tumours   241
Virchow's triad   170, 174–7
virulent phages   84, 85(f)
viruses
   gene therapy   304
   infections
      apoptosis   24
      classification of organisms   39(t)
      diabetes mellitus   63
      direct cell damage   38–9, 40–2(f)
      hepatitis   115
         see also hepatitis B virus
      suppressor T-lymphocytes   154
   mode of infection   81
   oncogenes (v-*onc*)   271–2, 275
   resistance to antiviral agents   87–8
   tumours from   267–72
      antigens   296
   see also specific viruses
visual fields, pituitary tumours   297
vitamin D, calcification   18
vitamin deficiencies   51(t)
   B_{12} 225
   on wound healing   134
von Willebrand factor   129
   atherosclerosis   197

Warthin–Finkeldey cells   124
warts   269–70
wasting, muscles   245
water-shed infarction, brain   228–9, 231(f)
water supplies, cholera and   77–8
Western blotting   67
wet gangrene   18
Willis, Thomas   208
Wolffian duct   21
women, atherosclerosis   193–4
worms   43
wound contraction   127–8
wound healing   124–31
   failure
      local factors   134–5
      systemic factors   134
   by primary intention   126–7, 128–9